Clinical Medical Ethics:
Cases in Practice

Clinical Medical Ethics: Cases in Practice

Terry M. Perlin, Ph.D.
Professor of Interdisciplinary Studies
and Fellow, Scripps Gerontology Center,
Miami University, Oxford;
Consultant in Medical Ethics,
University of Cincinnati College
of Medicine, Cincinnati, Ohio

LITTLE, BROWN AND COMPANY
BOSTON/TORONTO/LONDON

Library of Congress Cataloging-in-Publication Data

Perlin, Terry M., 1942–
    Clinical medical ethics: cases in practice / Terry M. Perlin.
        p.   cm.
    Includes index.
    ISBN 0-316-69959-4
    1. Medical ethics—Case studies.   I. Title.
    [DNLM: 1. Ethics. Medical.   W 50 P451c]
    R724.P425   1992
    174'.2—dc20
    DNLM/DLC
    for Library of Congress   92-12544
                                                                     CIP

Printed in the United States of America

RRD-VA

2677

WA 255   e ✓

To Roberta, Jenny, and Daniel
with love and gratitude for all
you have taught and given.

Contents

Preface

Twice on clinical ethics rounds in acute care hospitals I have heard patients make the same request of a physician: "Can't you just give me something so that I can die?" On the first occasion, the patient was 70 years old and was slowly dying from a painful head and neck cancer that had rendered him immobile. The second patient was a young man in his early 30s, in the final stages of AIDS; he was having difficulty breathing. The two doctors—one a woman, one a man—gave virtually the same response. "It's impossible; it's against the law. We'll try to keep you comfortable." Afterward, the physicians spoke, earnestly and with some anxiety, about the difficulties of facing such requests. "How," they asked, "do we know what the right thing to do is?"

No book can answer that probing question with certainty. *Clinical Medical Ethics*, however, is a start in the direction of wondering, thinking, worrying, and reflecting about ethical dilemmas and conflicts of values faced in a variety of health care settings. By raising central issues and by giving the reader an opportunity to work through an assortment of difficult cases, this book provides a foundation for reaching sound, fair, and useful judgments about difficult choice determinations. Many of the cases are set in the emergency department, the operating room, the intensive care unit, or the medical-surgical floor of acute-care hospitals. Others are set in the out-patient clinic, the long-term care or nursing care facility, at home, and in the physician's office.

Details of the cases in this book have been changed in order to preserve the confidentiality of patients, families, friends, and caregivers. Nearly every case, however, is *real*. That is, the medical situations and ethical problems have emerged from actual clinical experiences. Some have come from reports, case conference discussions, and grand rounds presentations. Others have emerged from informal discussions with physicians, nurses, psychologists, social workers, and allied health care professionals. Many more have come from my observations and ethics consultation activity. A few cases have been paraphrased from reports in the clinical literature. (These are acknowledged and cited in the text.) Cases have been selected because they are representative. Few, if any, are sensational or flamboyant. This book provides a recognizable set of materials, of cases in practice.

No single volume can say everything about clinical medical ethics. Multi-volume works are devoted to quite specific and limited questions (e.g., heart transplantation ethics). But we must begin somewhere. This book's goals and assumptions can be stated explicitly:

1. This book is designed for medical students and residents, physicians, and other health care workers, including nurses, social workers, administrators, and attorneys. It is nearly jargon-free and can be read by a general audience.
2. The book is introductory in the sense that it assumes no extensive background in philosophy or moral theory. It is also intermediate, in the sense that it presumes that readers have had or are beginning to have authentic experiences in patient care, and thus have faced the kinds of dilemmas described.
3. Every effort was made to be clear. The book is written in accessible language. The terms ethical and moral are used interchangeably. The goal is to avoid excessive philosophizing and to open difficult topics for sustained analysis and discussion. More issues are raised than resolved. Not unlike medical practice itself, much uncertainty remains when the day is done.
4. Many views are heard in this book. The duties, roles, and responsibilities of the physician are emphasized, but the voices of patients, families, nurses, social workers, consultants, administrators, lawyers, and policy makers, are also in evidence. In each chapter, in the Voices section the perspectives and clinical experiences of specific health care providers are stated in the first person.

5. This is not a cookbook or a set of guaranteed approaches to ethical issues in clinical medicine. No such work could be written. We live in a society in which values are often in conflict and in which authority is more likely to be challenged than blindly followed. Thus, this book raises issues, demands clear thinking, invites reflection, and asks us all to do the best we can. No more, but no less, than this is required.

Clinical Medical Ethics: Cases in Practice begins (after an introductory chapter) with a substantive discussion of essential approaches and concepts in medical ethics. Subsequent chapters focus on the clinical settings in which real, difficult-choice cases are encountered on a routine basis. This topical focus begins with issues found at the beginning of life: during pregnancy and childbirth and in the neonatal period. It proceeds with chapters on ethics in family practice/primary care, in pediatric and adolescent medicine, in medicine and surgery, in psychiatry and psychotherapy, and on ethical dilemmas found at the end-of-life for adult patients. It concludes with chapters on the professional responsibilities of doctors and on the allocation of scarce health care resources.

Each chapter is structured around the presentation of five essential cases, clinical dilemmas that demonstrate basic ethical problems, concepts, or challenges found in real-life settings. By scrutinizing actual clinical cases, the book gives a context to such problems. These essential cases are presented, analyzed, and discussed. The concept or dilemma found in each case is both specific and general. For example, the problem of securing agreement from a teenager to treat is quite concrete; but the issues of competence and consent are found among many age groups, in many contexts. Such cases are applicable in a variety of health care institutions and practices. No single chapter attempts to exhaust the ethical dilemmas faced in a specific medical field or area. Taken together, the essential cases studied throughout the book provide an overview of the major concepts and problems in clinical medical ethics.

After the five essential cases, a more detailed examination of a related clinical problem, a complex and difficult case, is evaluated. An approach to understanding and analysis of cases unique to this book is called the PRACTICE model. The PRACTICE model is the basis for more detailed case analysis. It provides a systematic method of examining clinical, psychosocial, and ethical dimensions of cases in a comprehensive fashion.

At the end of each chapter are two special sections:

In Voices a member of the health care team speaks about her or his perspective on clinical medical ethics, based on collaborative activities in providing health care. These voices present real-world commentary and show how, in most situations, the doctor-patient relationship can best be understood in its real-life setting. This context is team-based and collaborative. Learning to hear these voices is an important part of one's education in clinical medical ethics.

Think Pieces present a challenging problem or conceptual dilemma that goes beyond cases and individual decision-making to reflection and analysis. These think pieces invite the reader to consider matters of social policy, of the relationship of medicine to other professions, and of ways of determining values and duties in one's personal as well as professional life.

In addition, each chapter includes Cases for Discussion and Recommended Reading. Toward the end of each chapter are two cases that are related thematically to chapter material. The cases are followed by a series of questions meant to begin a discussion of central issues. Each case can be scrutinized in detail by applying the PRACTICE model of analysis. Recommended Reading is a short list of relevant books at the end of each chapter. The standard texts or studies noted contain further bibliographic references on the subject. Readers are also referred to *Medline* and *Bioethicsline* computer data bases for references to the journal literature.

T.M.P.

Acknowledgments

This book is full of cases. I have relied on many others in assembling and in retelling the stories embodied in these clinical summaries. The medical and psychosocial data, the interpersonal texture, and sometimes the confusion and complication in these cases have been provided to me by specialists and generalists, believers and skeptics, doctors and other health care personnel, patients, families, students, lawyers, administrators, and many friends. I am grateful for the trust they have shown and for the immense amount they have taught me.

Research and seminar experiences were funded by both the National Science Foundation and the National Endowment for the Humanities. The opportunity to study with the late Mulford Q. Sibley, University of Minnesota; Tom L. Beauchamp, Kennedy Institute of Ethics, Georgetown University; and James Childress, University of Virginia, was unforgettable. The idea for developing and writing *Clinical Medical Ethics* was suggested by John Hutton, M.D., Dean of the College of Medicine, University of Cincinnati.

My principal guides in this project have been three doctors— Robert V. Brody, Colin Macpherson, and Barbara Morris—and three attorneys—William Fischer, Gary Harris, and Rosiene Weaver. Their humanity and sensitivity have provided needed encouragement; their concern for justice as well as for the lives of clinical patients have made them indispensable role models.

The cases and perspectives found in this book emerged from conversations with practitioners and patients and their families. Working with dedicated professionals as they agonized over difficult choices both upset and inspired me on various occasions. The honesty and integrity of those who have helped me so much have my lasting admiration.

Among the physicians who have been both my native informants and teachers are: Carrie Angus, Sharon Attaway, Clarke Baxter, Joseph Bateman, David Bienenfeld, Robert Bower, Deborah Borchers, Marcelle Cedars, Judith Daniels, Cindi DeLaat, Peter Dignan, Mark Dine, Edward Donovan, Betty Lou Eilers, Craig Eisentrout, Fred Elkus, Michael Farrell, Andrew Filak, Josef Fischer, John Flege, Herbert Flessa, Tim Freeman, Marjorie Gass, Saad Ghosn, Paulette Gillig, Jack Gluckman, Stephen Goldberg, R. Jeffrey Goldsmith, Charles Hattemer, Jeff Heck, Theodor Herwig, J. Randolph Hillard, Paula Hillard, Loren Hiratzka, Kay Jabin, Jay Kammer, Jerold Kay, Rena Kay, Uma Kotagal, Peter Kotcher, John LaPuma, Edward Larson, Douglas Lehrer, Robert Lerner, Warren Liang, Audrey Ludwig, Robin Luke, George Lundberg, Herbert Magenheim, Simon Magowan, E. Gordon Margolin, Charles Margolis, Christine McHenry, Bud Muehler, Al Muhlman, Martin Myers, Kenneth Newmark, Donald Nofziger, Jennifer O'Flaherty, Sonya Oppenheimer, Anna Ornstein, Deb Pillow, William Polanka, Elizabeth Rabkin, Robert Rebar, T.J. Redington, Robert Rothenberg, Robert Ruan, Denise Saker, Edward Saeks, Raymond Sawaya, William Schubert, Richard Selzer, Mark Siegler, Deborah Silverman, Marcia Slomowitz, John Stone, Walter Stone, Bruce Swarny, Ole Theinhaus, Stanley Troup, Richard Vilter, Nita Walker, Greg Warshaw, Michael Webb, Scott Wilkinson, and Phil Zeitler.

Members of many health care teams, including nurses, social workers, psychologists, therapists, support personnel, and clergy, and educators in several institutions, have taken the time to make suggestions, offer help, and sometimes comfort. They include: Mila Ann Aroskar, Robert Atchley, Sheila Atchley, Larry Bahr, Debbie Beckman, Edward Beiser, Linda Blackstone, Muriel Blaisdell, Ellin Bloch, Ellen Bloomfield, Jean Braucher, Barbara Burnett, Ellen Burns, Hirsch Cohen, Stephen Cohen, Phil Cottell, Dax Cowart, Richard Daniels, Jan DeCosmo, Christopher DeSerna, Cynthia DeSerna, Mark Dinkelacker, Karen Donnelly, Kathleen Driscoll, Janet Earhardt, Curtis Ellison, Elaine Englehardt, Roger Fischer, Beth Frederick, Victor Fredericksen, Alan Fuchs, Carol Fuchs, Ellen Galbraith, Earl Gilreath, Leon Goldman, Elizabeth Gothelf, Lesha Greengus, Lisa Groger, Jackie Gruer, Ann Hager, Linda Harpster, Mary Heider, Carol Helle, Anne Henderson, Linda Hill, Anne Hunsacker, Tim Jabin, Andrea Jacoby, Margaret Jendrek, Patricia Beattie Jung, Marshall B.

Kapp, Robert Katz, Cynthia Kelley, Bert Klein, Barry Kogan, Jack Kues, Tom Long, Anne Lovell, George Luthringer, Marjorie Marks, Pam Mayberry, Sue McCloskey, Laurence McCullough, Paul Miller, Rick Momeyer, Sue Momeyer, Nancy Morwessel, Tom Mozeley, Peggy Muncie, Tom Murray, Linda Nathan, Sue Nicodemus, Lois LaCivita Nixon, Nancy Ogg, Howard Ottenheimer, Paul Pearson, Roberta Perlin, Beth Polanka, Jane Readnower, Robert Reece, Gina Reid, Clarissa Rentz, M. Kathy Robbins, Tara Rosnell, Jean Rothenberg, Diane Ruether, Debbie Rumpler, Ida Schick, William Scrivener, David Schwallie, Meryl Seidner, Mildred Seltzer, Richard Sexton, Sandro Spinsanti, Doug Spitler, Terre Stout, Connie Tabb, David Tabb, Kevin Tabb, Betty Tedesco, Joseph Tomain, Ruth Torok, Judith Van Ginkel, Norma Wagoner, Virginia Warren, Barry Weinstein, Robert Weir, Cass Williamson, Sam Williamson, Donna Woodman, Diane M. Wright, and Anne Zimmerman.

I have not mentioned the names of the hundreds of patients who spoke with me, often while they were in hospital beds; nor have I listed their family members, many of whom I saw in moments of anxiety or grief. The preservation of privacy must prevail. To all of them I express heartfelt gratitude. In addition, numerous medical students and residents, law students, and undergraduate and graduate students talked with me in ways both academic and personal. Members of institutional ethics committees and nursing ethics forums have allowed me to collaborate on their important projects as a teacher and consultant.

The institutional settings for the reading, observation, and discussion that led to the writing of this book have been the School of Interdisciplinary Studies and Scripps Gerontology Center, Miami University (Ohio); University of Cincinnati College of Medicine; University of Cincinnati College of Law; University of Virginia; Georgetown University; Academy of Medicine of Cincinnati; Children's Hospital Medical Center (Cincinnati); The Jewish Hospital of Cincinnati; Drake Center, Inc. (Cincinnati); Bethesda Hospital (Cincinnati); Court Psychiatric Clinic of Cincinnati and Hamilton County; University of Cincinnati Hospital Psychiatry Emergency Service; San Francisco General Hospital; The Shanti Project (Berkeley and San Francisco, California); the Hospices of Middletown and Cincinnati, Ohio and Louisville, Kentucky. The Florida Endowment for the Humanities invited me to be a scholar-in-residence during 1989. Over the course of several months I had a chance to meet people of all ages and backgrounds in seven Florida cities as they debated priorities in allocating resources for health care. As a member of the advisory board of the Urban Health Project in Cincinnati I have been able to track young medical students as they first encounter the problems of patients with only limited access to the health care system.

Assistance in preparation of this book came from the patient Lois Simmons, Bernie McMacken, Virginia Moore, and Daniel Perlin. My editor at Little, Brown and Company, Laurie Anello, brought comfort, cheer, and wit to a project that has made us friends.

The entire manuscript was read and criticized by Dr. Barbara Morris. Her comments were clear, balanced, and fair; her wisdom is incorporated into the book itself. I hope that her compassionate concern for patients is evident in the text as well.

Clinical Medical Ethics:
Cases in Practice

▪1▪
Getting Down to Cases: An Introduction to Clinical Medical Ethics

The possibilities for medical advances are almost beyond imagination! We can now replace broken, diseased, or worn-out kidneys, livers, hearts, even bone marrow. Will brains be transplantable in a few decades? Only a few years ago, babies born a month or so early died; today premature infants (tiny babies with genetic disorders or grave complications) leave the womb at 28 weeks, survive, and go home. There was hope 10 years ago for increasing sophistication in diagnosing fetal disease through noninvasive techniques. We can now see into the womb and are beginning to perform surgery on the unborn. Life for those who are dying can be extended, not quite forever but for long periods, due to technologically supplied respiration, hydration, and nutrition and the use of new medications.

Such innovations did not develop in a vacuum. They are the culmination of years of basic and clinical research, and they cost a great deal, not only in dollars. Such new treatments raise fundamental questions about what human life is, or ought to be. They force all of us to ask: What are the costs society is willing to expend to create life, nurture it, and sustain it? Every medical decision presupposes a doctor-patient relationship. In an era of highly specialized medicine, especially in large cities and in immense hospitals, the nature of that relationship is problematic. In addition to a primary care physician who provides the gatekeeping role of getting the patient into the system, an ill patient may see a variety of specialists, medical residents and students, highly trained nurses, and other health care personnel (psychologists, social workers, respiratory, occupational, or rehabilitation therapists) in the course of a single hospital stay. Roles, and rules, are changing all the time. Advances in medical technology have heightened societal expectations of physicians and their support staffs. For physicians it is increasingly hard to navigate the waters of health care. Knowing what to do is difficult enough. Doing not only the medically but the morally right thing is more difficult still.

Some problems in medical ethics, however, at the surface seem more easily resolved than others.

■ THE CASE OF MRS. H. ■

An 87-year-old woman, Mrs. H., had spent the last 4 years in a nursing home, and was admitted to the hospital for tests. She had reported difficulty breathing and was weak and run down. She had been diagnosed as having breast cancer 6 months earlier and had a mastectomy that had never healed completely. In fact, her anterior chest wall was one large wound. Generalized spread of the cancer (metastasis) was discovered on her return to the hospital. Mrs. H. was alert and oriented, but she was blind. She specifically asked her caregivers at the hospital and, earlier, at the nursing home not to revive her if she should suffer a cardiac arrest. She also said, "I do not want any more treatment for the cancer. I know that the situation is hopeless." Mrs. H. was a widow and had no immediate family or friends available. The nursing staff asked the attending physician about "code status" for Mrs. H. Should she be designated in her chart as "do not resuscitate" (DNR)? The nurses told the doctor that this seemed the clear preference of the patient.

The attending physician refused to write a DNR order in Mrs. H's chart. In fact, he ordered chemotherapy for the patient without her knowledge and apparently against her wishes. There was seemingly no person outside the medical staff who visited this patient. Arrangements were being made to prepare Mrs. H. for chemotherapy.

Few clinical situations *seem* as clear-cut and obvious as that of Mrs. H. First, she was dying and her death was imminent. Second, she was mentally aware of her surroundings and her clinical status. She had the *capacity* to make choices about her medical care. Third, Mrs. H. had expressed her views about her care or, to put it more specifically, about nontreatment. Finally, there was an authentic difference of opinion about treatment options. The nurses advocated for Mrs. H. The doctor acted in clear opposition to those views.

The case of Mrs. H. is a relatively rare one. Few patients of advanced age with terminal cancer—either in long-term care or acute-care facilities—have on-the-record statements about treatment or nontreatment. It is also unusual to see such a clear-cut illustration of the physician-nurse conflict. Right and wrong appear terribly obvious in this vignette. Are they?

THE PRACTICE MODEL

If we scratch the surface of any serious medical case, we find forces and factors that demand scrutiny. Many of them are not strictly medical or clinical but rather are ethical issues or questions. Strategies for identifying and ultimately resolving ethical dilemmas in medicine involve a serious and determined effort. Understanding theories and principles is indispensable. Trying to estimate the consequences of one choice over another is challenging. Sorting out personal and professional values is very important. Looking at like cases and (often) at the law pertaining to such situations can be most useful. But the first requirement, the essential prerequisite, is getting a detailed and concrete sense of the literal situation. To practice clinical medical ethics we must take a systematic and careful approach to a difficult ethical problem. The **PRACTICE** model is a method of analyzing, discussing, and, ultimately, helping to resolve serious ethical dilemmas in clinical medicine.

Traditionally, there are two fundamental questions that must be addressed in situations demanding ethical analysis: Who decides? and What is the right decision? Neither question is easily answered. Determining the appropriate decision-maker would appear to be easily decided in most clinical settings. The patient, we are told, makes the necessary choices. This is a useful, but limited, response. In hard-choice situations (e.g., Do I accept the recommendation for chemotherapy for the cancer that is likely to kill me even with treatment?) few patients are alone or have the experience (not to mention the wisdom) to act autonomously. Family members have views; patients are often, quite rationally, depressed; physicians have biases for or against treatment; and the cost of care is another factor. Who decides on treatment is an even more difficult question to answer when patients are either incompetent or indecisive. Infants, by definition, lack the capacity to make medical-care decisions. But so do older persons in the final stages of Alzheimer's disease (senile dementia). Our long-term care facilities are filled with patients for whom difficult and controversial decisions must be made. Court-appointed guardians are sometimes designated as decision-makers. But who is to guard the guardian?

Even if we were, somehow, to determine exactly who was to make a specific decision, it is notoriously hard to know just what the right choice is. In matters of life and death all sorts of value conflicts emerge. Religious and secular views and their contradictions make such choices controversial. The challenge of doing clinical medical ethics is never-ending, not because (as we often hear) "there are no right answers," but because right answers are hard to find. The **PRACTICE** model is not meant to be a panacea. It is provided as a means of getting closer to the resolution of essential ethical issues.

P Patient (medical and psychological facts)
R Relationships
A Advocacy (rights and duties)
C Conflicts
T Treatment or nontreatment options
I Interests (of the various parties)
C Consequences (short- and long-term)
E Ethical principles at stake

Let's look at the case of Mrs. H. from the perspective of each element of the **PRACTICE** model.

Patient

We know that Mrs. H. is very sick and that her cancer has spread throughout her body and that she is unlikely to live for a long time. We make this conclusion based not on her age — to do so would be age-ist — but as a result of the objective tests regarding her condition that appear in the medical record. Patients with advanced breast cancer and significant metastases have a very limited life expectancy, even with surgical, radiologic, or chemotherapeutic intervention. That does not mean that some treatments for Mrs. H. would be completely futile. Alleviating her suffering—relieving the pain from bone metastases, for example—will always be an option. But Mrs. H. will never be cured.

We also realize that the patient is blind but can hear and speak and, thus, can communicate her views to her caregivers and others. What we *do* know in any medical ethics case must be supplemented by an acknowledgement of what we *do not* know. Here, we are uncertain about the status of her heart and lungs (though we do recognize she is having difficulty breathing) and cannot accurately predict a cardiopulmonary incident that might impair her or lead to her death. We would want to read her medical record very thoroughly. We would also certainly want to talk with Mrs. H. in an honest fashion about her choices.

We are also in the dark about Mrs. H.'s psychological status. We can assume that she is in pain. But treatment for that pain (narcotics, for example) might impair her cognitive capacity and have an impact on her mood as well. The nurses seem to think that Mrs. H. can express her preferences in a reasonable fashion. If she were to receive analgesic or sedating medications—morphine might be the drug of choice—her capacity to ask questions and make decisions could be substantially or totally impaired.

Relationships

Mrs. H. is a widow without available friends or family; since her admission to the hospital she has been without visitors. Her relationships for the past 4 years have been with staff and residents in the nursing home. We know little about the content of those relationships, but if we wished we could find out more. She also has connections with her present caregivers: The nurses in the hospital have come to know her; the attending physician knows the condition of his patient, but only directly during the present hospital stay. Is there a private physician who has known Mrs. H. for some years? Finding a family attorney who has spoken with Mrs. H. in the past, discovering just who has been responsible for her financial matters while she was a nursing home client could provide access to her prior sense of herself and her interests. While some unknowns will always remain, a search for a thorough, psychosocial history of this patient is clearly in order.

Can anyone determine future interests in this case? Without a family, does Mrs. H. wish to bequeath her estate to a charity? Will many days in the hospital deplete her funds and diminish future-oriented relationships? Mrs. H. is still coherent and can be approached for answers to these qeustions. But who will take the responsibility to act on her behalf?

Advocacy

In most hard cases, the patient is in possession of the authority to make decisions or to refuse treatment. The fundamental right of autonomy and the corollary duty to respect the decision of persons with decision-making capacity is inherent in contemporary health care law and ethics. But autonomy is rarely an absolute. For patients deemed incompetent (by legal authorities, mainly courts), autonomy can no longer be exercised. A substitute decision-maker must be appointed. But Mrs. H. has no court-appointed guardian. She has a legal right to make decisions for herself. But realistically, for very ill patients or moderately demented persons or even for patients who are so sick that they cannot make informed judgments readily, respecting autonomy is a goal for which we aim, not a certainty.

Mrs. H. cannot move about on her own, cannot demand information and cannot read her own chart. She is dependent on the care of her nurses and the authority of her doctor. Who will speak for Mrs. H. in this situation? Who will act in her presumed best interest? All health care professionals are advocates in some sense. Nurses, especially, are trained to hear and to speak for those who are silent or silenced. Physicians are pledged to do their best for patients and, above all, not to harm them. Who will empathize with Mrs. H. and argue for her interests?

One resource—given that there appears to be no family member available to serve as Mrs. H.'s advocate—might be found in the nursing home in which she previously resided. Nursing or other staff may have a medical or clinical interest in helping with the care of Mrs. H. If Mrs. H. resided in a state that provided either for a living will or a durable power of attorney for health care process, while competent she could have designated a surrogate decision-maker to speak in her voice were she to be incapable of choosing to accept or to refuse treatment. This person could legitimately advocate for Mrs. H.

Conflicts

There are several apparent conflicts in this case. Clearly, the wishes of Mrs. H.—to cease treatment for cancer and to refuse resuscitation should she suffer a cardiac arrest—are contested by her physician. The nurses and doctor are also in disagreement. We know nothing of the views of other, prior caregivers; their involvement might lead to even more dispute. The hospital hierarchy is not yet involved in this debate. But if the physician's orders are contested, many other people may become part of this case: nursing supervisors, the chair of the medical department, risk managers and other hospital personnel, even the courts.

There are conflicts of a wider nature that go beyond the specifics of Mrs. H.'s care that should also be noted. Is there a right to die? Must physicians who disagree with a patient's wishes respect such desires? Medical decisions are made collaboratively most of the time. The doctor-patient relationship presumes conversation and discussion. But physician orders are what put into effect clinical procedures. The prerogatives of nurses when physician orders are questioned are real, if limited. What party or parties might be called into the case? Other doctors, the nursing supervisor, and even the institution's ethics committee might have an interest in the case. But setting such a process in motion requires someone aside from the treating physician. A nurse, resident, or perhaps a medical student might raise the issue. Mrs. H. does not seem to have the knowledge of what is coming or the physical capacity to shift the prospective course of action.

Treatment or Nontreatment Options

On the surface, this seems to be an either/or situation. Either we treat the cancer or cease such therapy and allow the patient to die. But a wider perspective entails other possibilities. Can cancer treatment ever be considered not curative, but palliative (i.e., designed to relieve symptoms and to make the patient more comfortable)? If a DNR order is written into Mrs. H.'s chart, what does this mean with regard to treating her for infections, for labored breathing, or for other possibly treatable organ failures or illnesses that occur along the way? Does DNR mean do not treat?

If cancer treatment does *not* proceed, there are options to consider for the patient's care too. Should she return to the nursing home?

Would she prefer hospitalization in order to better manage pain? Which hospital unit is best for Mrs. H., the intensive care unit or a general medical-surgical floor? Could she be admitted to an inpatient hospice unit, a place that provides terminal care? If the patient retains consciousness, she will need forms of treatment that skilled and gifted professionals can provide: pain relief, psychological support, religious counseling, and a death with other persons present, if desired.

Interests

Mrs. H. seems to have an interest in nontreatment. Does that mean that her best interest is her painless death? Some might argue that if she becomes unconscious, Mrs. H.'s interests dissolve. Others might claim that due respect for her earlier views and for her present *dignity* oblige us to exercise her refusal of treatment. Finding someone who speaks for silent patients is a challenge often encountered in medical-ethical dilemmas. Do we work on the assumption that a prior expression is always the best guide to future treatment decisions? How can such interests be codified, even guaranteed?

The physician seems to have an interest in continuing to treat his patient. Assuming that his reasons are benign (i.e., he wants to give her the best care he can; he wishes to extend her life for as long as possible), can we assign him authority in acting on behalf of Mrs. H.? The physician also has a professional interest in having his orders followed. Medicine is *not* totally hierarchical, but physicians do rely upon nurses to carry out their treatment decisions. Precedent-setting is a worry in this case.

The hospital nurses seem to have an interest in contesting the physician's orders. Are their motives purely those of patient advocates? Or could there be a hidden agenda, even a political one, here? What about other staff who may not share the nurses' opinions. Finally, the hospital has a legal and ethical interest in providing quality health care that respects patient wishes and maintains staff morale. Such an interest may become central as the case of Mrs. H. unfolds.

Consequences

Making determinations in health care based on the possible consequences is both useful and (at times) pointless. This is because we always seek the best results, but medical (and moral) uncertainty renders prediction difficult. Trying to project both short-term and long-term consequences is always wise in dealing with hard-choice dilemmas. In the case of Mrs. H., we can state with relative certainty that if she receives no further cancer treatment she will die soon, but it is also possible that chemotherapy could accelerate her dying. If she gets treatment against her expressed wishes, then her loss of autonomy is also a consequence: It might cause her to become angry, depressed, or even to seek legal counsel. The consequences of this last possibility are also unpredictable.

Another short-term concern centers around the nurse-physician debate. If the nurses' viewpoint is sustained, their dual sense of successful advocacy and of the establishment of a credible nursing viewpoint within the hospital is encouraged. If they ultimately agree, perhaps reluctantly, with the physician's order, their self-perception changes significantly. Here the shift from short-term to long-term consequences is apparent.

The results are hard to predict in this case. If we set a precedent we can hope that sustaining Mrs. H.'s wishes will lead to greater respect for patient preferences, or physicians who want to exercise treatment choices for reluctant patients will have to find more creative (perhaps even manipulative) ways of doing so. If the doctor rescinds his chemotherapy order and writes a DNR order in the patient's chart (even reluctantly), his morale may suffer and, more generally, a physician's sense of being under siege from many forces—nurses, bureaucrats, insurance companies, the government—may be reinforced.

Ethical Principles

There are fundamental norms in health care called essential ethical principles (Fig. 1-1). They are rarely absolutes and they often come into conflict, but they are a foundation for analyzing any hard case. In a preliminary way, we can mention a few such principles that seem applicable to Mrs. H.'s case.

First, there is the principle of *autonomy*, the affirmation that competent adult patients have the guaranteed right to make determinations about essential personal matters (e.g., the nature of the health care they receive). Mrs. H.'s autonomy takes expression in her refusal of treatment. It is abridged if she is forced to accept the cancer care she has stated she does not want. But as we shall see, not all patients can exercise their autonomy with equal dexterity.

AUTONOMY: Deliberate choice-making; self-legislation; rooted in the right to privacy and the notion of individual freedom; fundamental to the idea of informed consent

VERACITY: Truth-telling; the basis of promise-keeping and other fiduciary relationships; the premise of an open health-care professional–patient relationship

BENEFICENCE: Doing good; promoting the well-being of others, especially those to whom care is offered; essential to the professional obligation to help others in need

NONMALEFICENCE: Avoiding harm to others; the obligation to protect persons from danger, pain, and suffering; rooted in the Hippocratic oath and other ancient medical traditions

JUSTICE: Being fair; respecting human equality; concern for the allocation of scarce resources on an equitable basis; necessary for the implementation of social policy

---

Fig. 1-1. Five fundamental principles of medical ethics.

Second, the principle of *veracity*, or truth-telling, is manifest in this case. Here, as always, we would like to know more. What, precisely, has the doctor told his patient? Has he used euphemisms to disguise the care he is recommending? Is he being completely open and honest? With regard to the role of the nurses in this case: Are they obliged to affirm the principle of veracity by reporting the doctor and speaking the truth to those not directly involved in the case? How far does the commitment to truth-telling extend? Should whistle-blowers go to the media in pursuit of an essential principle?

The principle of *beneficence*, rooted in the health care professional's obligation to promote the well-being of patients, is at stake in Mrs. H.'s case. There are clearly divergent views of what that well-being means. The physician seems to think that continuing treatment leading to extended life is a primary good; the patient and nurses regard a death without great suffering as a fundamental good.

The three principles sketched here are clearly related: In order to benefit the patient, her views must be known. She must hear the truth in order to exercise her autonomous choice-making capacity. The physician's desire to promote patient benefit cannot proceed in isolation: He must hear the other parties and make determinations that can be morally validated.

VALUES IN CONFLICT

Doctors and patients, lawyers and hospital administrators, religious and secular advocates, not to mention medical students and residents, have concerns and conflicts about what's right and what's wrong in the area of medical care. Newspaper headlines and television panel shows are filled with discussions and debates about such dramatic matters as "should we transplant organs from babies born without any chance of surviving on their own?" Reasonable and passionate persons legitimately differ about the morality of undertaking such activities. The presumption of all who join in the effort of debating and discussing the difficult problems encountered in health care is quite simple: How can we serve those who are ill or dying in a manner that is based on fairness, justice, and compassion?

No health-care problems are merely medical: All involve values. The discussion of contemporary dilemmas in medical ethics is a beginning, a chance to sort out our priorities and values in situations that must inevitably be faced. It is now possible to keep very ill patients biologically alive by means of remarkable technological equipment such as the ventilator (respirator) for an indefinite period of time. Persons whose hearts stop beating or whose breathing has ceased may be revived. Those who are unable to feed themselves can be artificially hydrated and nourished. Organ transplantation is a burgeoning field. None of this was possible 30 years ago.

This new technology was never meant to make decisions. Using it requires us to make choices. Our increasing capacity to extend life raises difficult questions. How do we determine what is appropriate treatment for a patient dying of incurable cancer? How do we discover the desires of those who (because of Alzheimer's disease, for example) can no longer communicate? The questions are only beginning.

In this epoch of conflict over values and public-policy decisions, a new approach to problem solving has emerged. *Clinical medical ethics*, a field that combines efforts at finding the optimal approach to patient care with a serious concern for the feelings and viewpoints of patients, families, and providers, has been at the forefront of an attempt to confront value conflicts and provide reasoned ways of charting difficult problems and solving moral dilemmas. Nearly all schools of medicine have incorporated courses that introduce students to ethical issues in medicine. Hospitals and nursing homes have established institutional ethics committees and have hired ethics consultants to help with seemingly intractable problems. Commissions at the federal and state levels have explored such questions as the right to die or the use of DNR orders in medical emergencies. Efforts at grassroot discussions about the allocation of scarce health care resources have engaged a wider community in such endeavors. And everyday practice reminds physicians and physicians-in-training that ignoring values conflicts in medicine will not make them go away.

The need to confront matters of life and death—especially decisions made at a time of crisis—occur regularly for doctors, not only in their professional lives. Physicians are also the children of aging parents, are sometimes parents themselves, and lead lives in which they too fall ill, and comfort friends and relatives in their grief. Ultimately we all die. To recognize that health-care problems are more than scientific challenges, that they involve ethical and often legal perspectives, is a part of this new approach to medical education and continuing education. How we regard our rights, our duties, our obligations to others necessarily has an impact on our decisions, sometimes in ways we do not quite comprehend. The discussion of our contemporary dilemmas is a *beginning*, a chance to sort out our priorities in situations that must be faced. It is not an abstract debate. It is a subject in which real life and death decisions must be made in actual clinical cases.

■ FIVE ESSENTIAL CASES ■

Case 1-1

All dilemmas in medical ethics involve doctor-patient relationships. Acting in the best interest of a patient, though desirable, can also be problematic.

Dr. R. has been the primary care physician for Mr. L. for 10 years. The patient is 56 years old, an executive at a local company, and a chain smoker. Dr. R. has been warning Mr. L. about the dangers of smoking and has tried to help him quit. Mr. L. has tried twice to do so—once via a behavior modification group approach—but has failed. After a routine examination, Dr. R., wanting to help her patient but seeing no easy way to make the necessary impact, sends Mr. L. a letter that tells him that "preliminary tests show what seem to be early signs of emphysema. You should stop smoking immediately." In reality, all of Mr. L.'s test results are normal. On receiving the letter, Mr. L. is shocked by the news and ceases smoking by going cold turkey. In subsequent visits (for the following 3 years), the patient expresses his gratitude to Dr. R. for improving the quality of his life. He tells the physician that "I guess I had a real scare, but I think it worked for me."

The doctor-patient relationship is the basis of quality health care. We can be certain that the physician in this case made this bold effort to manipulate her patient into giving up smoking for beneficent reasons: She knew that smoking is the leading preventable killer (via cancer and heart disease) of older American males, and she knew that Mr. L.'s earlier efforts had been in vain. Had she sent such a letter after knowing a patient for 2 months, we might be very dubious. The nature of the doctor-patient relationship between Dr. R. and Mr. L. has now changed, however, because the physician but not the patient is aware of a clear informational imbalance. Still, Mr. L. is very happy with the results: He has stopped smoking and his physician has become a heroine to him.

A variety of questions emerges regarding the relationship of physician and patient. Doing what's best for the patient seems to have moved the physician to lie, or at least to shade the truth. In determining the rights and wrongs in this situation, there are clear principles at stake: For example, truth-telling seems compromised. But if good results are the focus of our attention, the story does seem to have a happy ending. One challenge is to try to imagine alternative scenarios: Are there ways of dealing with a recalcitrant smoker not noted in this case? Dr. R. did not write her letter without a lot of earlier intervention. Could others have done more?

It may also be useful to place yourself (subjectively) in a hard-choice case. If you were a partner of Dr. R. and she told you about this case, how might you respond? Would your instincts lead you to applaud the consequences? Or might you have some reservations about the precedent set by duplicitous statements in the name of . patient welfare?

<u>Case 1-2</u>

Ethical issues in medicine often involve legal questions. Physicians are sometimes caught in the middle in conflicts involving the law.

Dr. S., a board-certified psychiatrist, treated Mrs. T. on an out-patient basis for schizophrenia for 2 years. Prior to that, Mrs. T., who is now 26 years old and married, had been voluntarily hospitalized twice, after experiencing auditory hallucinations. During the past 2 years, the patient had been maintained on a psychotropic drug (haloperidol) and had received supportive psychotherapy from Dr. S. In one of their therapy sessions, Mrs. T. mentioned that the stress of caring for her 4-year-old son Gregory was very burdensome and noted that she would "really feel free if she could only get rid of that kid."

One morning, a month later, Mrs. T. drowned Gregory in the bathtub. She told the police that she was sorry, but that he was just "too much trouble to take care of." She was arrested for first-degree murder. Her court-appointed lawyer immediately told the authorities that Mrs. T. was seeing a psychiatrist and that she had a prior history of major mental illness.

■ ■ ■

The legal system weighs on health care decision-making in various ways. (Expressions of outrage about malpractice litigation and consequent insurance costs are ubiquitous in the medical journals.) Doctors are often called on by lawyers and courts to give testimony, to serve as expert witnesses, and to provide care for those caught up in the criminal justice system. The doctor-lawyer relationship, in the abstract at least, has not been a happy one. In this case, Dr. S. may be involved in the prosecution of Mrs. T. He may also be the subject of a lawsuit, perhaps by Gregory's grieving father, Mr. T. Should Dr. S. have taken greater care to protect Gregory after hearing Mrs. T.'s statement about wanting to "get rid of that kid?" The standards to which we hold psychiatrists are often determined not only by peer behavior and review but also by what judges and legislators decide.

This case asks us to consider the role of doctor-patient confidentiality (a legal protection in most states). In hindsight, we may wish that Dr. S. had abridged the confidentiality implicit in his therapy with Mrs. T. He might have taken his patient's threat more seriously and, had he acted upon it, Gregory might still be alive. Retrospective condemnation is perhaps too easy. Still, a grieving father might consider Dr. S.'s failure to warn an act of malpractice. Only a court (or, perhaps, an insurance company) could settle that legal issue.

When law and medicine interact, it is not unusual for larger questions to emerge. General questions about human behavior and moral responsibility are asked. Beyond the specific role of the physician in the case of Mrs. T., do we see her behavior as *bad* and thus requiring legal, criminal sanction or *mad* and thus mandating treatment by mental health professionals? Doctors, psychiatrists especially, are influential in determining the kind of "punishment" a person with a history of mental disease and treatment deserves. Dr. S. may find a conflict of roles: In the courtroom is he an advocate for Mrs. T., or does he take the viewpoint of the state in trying to achieve justice?

Case 1-3
Most medical ethics cases involve families and other health care providers, not just the named patient.

Mrs. B. was growing increasingly confused. Aged 86, a widow with three adult children, Mrs. B. was experiencing memory loss and wandered around the neighborhood. When she was taken to the emergency room, she was referred to an interdisciplinary geriatric assessment center where she was diagnosed as having Alzheimer's disease, an irreversible senile dementia. The physician who made the diagnosis, Dr. A., did not tell Mrs. B. immediately, but he conferred with her three children. Two of the family members said, "Don't tell Momma. She will get depressed and won't understand anyway. We will take good care of her at home, as long as possible. Then we can afford to put her in a nursing home." The third sibling was unsure of how to proceed. The nurse practitioner, part of the geriatric team, was in the conference room when this statement was made. She believed as a matter of principle that Alzheimer's patients in this stage of the disease have a right to know what the future is likely to bring. Dr. A. thought that the family was right and that it would be cruel to burden Mrs. B. with this information.

Division of opinion within family groups and within health care practice groups is not unusual. Medicine is a human profession: Reasonable people differ, sometimes vociferously, about hard choices. It is rare for a patient to lead a totally solitary life: Most have families or friends involved in a case; others are protected by social service agencies or court-appointed guardians. Often a patient has several physicians who have provided care. (We might ask, at the outset of this case, Was there a physician responsible for Mrs. B. before she was seen at the geriatric assessment center?)

It is in the rich interplay of interests and perspectives that we see varying viewpoints about patients in need of care. Mrs. B.'s family is itself unsure what course of action to take, just on the issue of telling the patient. A patient who is at present confused but not severely demented does not lose her "rights." But in affirming her autonomy, some people believe we are harming her. Should an important principle override a family's concern about their mother? Is veracity indispensable? If a climate of trust does not exist in medical settings, chaos could reign. But truth can take many forms: kind, clear, brutal, or "half." Dr. A.'s initial response is to consult with the family. He, at least for the moment, bypasses the patient. Is this duplicity?

The case will go on, no matter what Mrs. B. discovers. At some unpredictable but certain point in the future, she will become totally incapable of making decisions (for example, about the nature of home health care, about institutionalization, about planning for the end of life). By that time it will be much too late for the patient to have made her wishes known, either formally via an advance directive (such as a living will or durable-power-of-attorney for health care document) or informally. Some person or persons will have to become the surrogate decision maker(s) for this patient. Families, often in conflict about the right thing to do in putting together a treatment plan, can divide acrimoniously or be helped into forming a useful and caring whole. Physicians, witnessing family anxiety and ambivalence, often believe that they must remain neutral, though involved in a nonjudgmental and supportive manner. Detachment itself can become a moral position.

Within the health care team—here, between doctor and nurse practitioner—differences of opinion provide an opportunity for detailed discussion. How patient, family, and providers proceed will be only partly a function of Mrs. B.'s disease. Determinations will also reflect long-held religious and secular values, economic issues, and the intricacies of familial relationships. Hardly anything in the realm of clinical medical ethics happens in isolation. Understanding the context of decision-making is required.

Case 1-4

Physicians are responsible not only to patients and families but to their profession and to society at large.

Dr. W. is a prominent cardiothoracic surgeon with 19 years of postresidency experience and is highly regarded for his work doing coronary artery bypass graft (CABG) surgeries. A cardiologist has referred Mr. C., a 49-year-old patient, to Dr. W. The cardiologist's report states that Mr. C. is in great pain from angina. An angiogram reveals three-vessel disease (an indication for surgery) and that the patient is HIV positive. Dr. W. calls the cardiologist; she says that Mr. C. has agreed to the HIV screening test.

This is Dr. W.'s first experience (to his knowledge) of being asked to do surgery on a patient who is HIV positive. His professional organization and his state licensing board tell him that his obligation is to treat patients in a nondiscriminatory manner, but Dr. W. is still worried. He tells his surgical colleagues, privately, "I have a lot of anxiety about doing this one. I know about precautions, but they are never total guarantees. The real thing is I want to live to see my grandchildren. Why should I have to operate on this guy?"

Public health issues create demands on physicians. The extent of the AIDS epidemic could not have been foreseen by Dr. W. when he entered medical school. His ambivalence about accepting Mr. C. as a patient is not irrational. Cardiothoracic surgery often involves needle sticks and cuts from bone shards. AIDS is a deadly disease, and HIV infection is communicated by bodily fluid exchange, but Dr. W.'s colleagues are likely to remind him that a former surgeon general once called physicians who refused to treat HIV positive or AIDS patients unprofessional and irrational. National and state medical societies have issued policy statements mandating care of such persons. If several peers discover Dr. W.'s reluctance to accept this patient, his hospital privileges may be in jeopardy. Refusing to care for Mr. C. has implications for other cardiothoracic surgeons, for surgeons in general, and for the public's perception of physicians.

Doctors and other professionals enjoy unique privileges. High status and prestige, substantial incomes, and, perhaps especially, the ability to regulate peers are marks of the medical profession. In a complex world, expectations of medicine are rising. Physicians play multiple roles: Primary care doctors act as "gatekeepers," providing entry for patients into the world of the medical center; specialists act as admired consultants providing high-technology assessments and interventions; administrators govern large institutions while trying to keep costs from rising. The medical profession is larger and more complex than ever. Dr. W.'s determination about whether or not to accept the referral from the cardiologist is not simply a matter of the patient's condition or the physician's fears. The physician represents the profession as a whole. A single, discrete patient-care decision may be intricately tied to public health law and practice and to matters of social policy as well.

Case 1-5

Making ethical decisions in medicine involves both reason and emotion. Analytic skill and intuitive awareness are essential in reaching sound judgment to resolve clinical ethical dilemmas.

David N. is 16 years old and has had leukemia for 3 years. He comes from a small rural community and has been in foster care all his life. The county social service agency is his legal guardian and makes health-care decisions for him. David has been in and out of the Hospital for Children for many years and the staff on the hematology-oncology floor has come to regard him with a lot of affection. The attending physician and many nurses call him Davy, bring him small gifts, and celebrate his birthdays with him. All efforts at achieving a remission of his cancer have been without success. David is now experiencing difficulty in breathing, and a decision has to be made about placing him on a ventilator. Without such support he is likely to die very soon. With the ventilator, he may live for many months, in the hospital, and (perhaps) in some pain. He has no relatives available; prior foster parents do not visit.

The unit staff has talked with David about the decision regarding ventilation. He says that he cannot decide. He is a minor and someone must speak on his behalf, presumably in his best interest. The social services agency has a policy regarding such a decision: David must be intubated and placed on the ventilator. Extending his life is the fundamental goal. The agency operates not only as guardian for many children like David, but also in a political climate in which accusations about child neglect are viewed negatively. The attending physician, two pediatric residents, and several nurses think that David would be better off if "nature could take its course." They have seen many other children die lingering deaths from this kind of leukemia. They express an honest affection for this patient—one nurse states, "He's like one of my own kids!"—and they feel that the agency's policy is wrong. They also know that it is unlikely to be changed and that a probate court would sustain the agency's decision.

■ ■ ■

A purely rational approach to this case would recognize that children cannot, by law, make their own health-care decisions and cannot give either informed consent or make informed refusals. Usually parents fulfill the roles of decision-makers. For some minors, an agency or court-appointed surrogate must act on behalf of the child. This is the way the system operates, and in general it works well. Reasonable medical personnel also know that they must work with such agencies frequently and that a collaborative attitude is valuable.

The doctors and nurses involved in David's care also feel that their patient is closer to them than the average child under their care. They see David daily, they have watched him grow weaker, and they accept that eventually he will die. As professionals they speak very little of these things, but they are quite reluctant to perform the procedures and provide the life-sustaining interventions that the social service agency requires of them. They are also the only hospital in the area that can do this work.

Is it possible to achieve an equilibrium between a rule-based, pragmatic approach to this case and an empathic, perhaps agonizing, and emotional response to David's situation? Ethics in medicine is never simple. It is never totally objective either. Understanding the intuitive, affective dimension of care-giving is indispensable to further work on this case. Providing a legitimate forum for discussing not only the rights and wrongs in David's case but also the anxieties, fears, and psychological projections that inform our worries about the patient is an important part of case analysis in medical ethics.

Professionals have their own values, beliefs, and standards. Nurses and doctors must live with their decisions and must respond not only to the scrutiny of peers but to their own consciences. Clarifying such personal values entails the open admission that many of our rational statements are influenced by gut feelings and by emotional states. Medical ethics discussions are opportunities for an honest confrontation with such emotional bases, and, in fact, may provide a chance to view other professionals as caring individuals.

■ CASES FOR DISCUSSION ■

Each of the five cases we have reviewed would be an apt subject for a thorough analysis via the **PRACTICE** model. We hope that you will do so. The following cases are presented without commentary. Only a few suggestive questions are included. These cases have emerged from the clinical practice of medical students, residents, private physicians, and hospital staff. Ask yourself: What other concerns would I have, if I were involved in this case? How would I attempt to gain the views of all appropriate parties? How might I attempt to resolve the dilemmas seen here?

Case A

Miss J., a 30-year-old woman, is a member of the Jehovah's Witness sect and, as a matter of religious conviction, refuses any blood transfusions. She is admitted to the hospital with gastrointestinal (GI) bleeding, which is diagnosed noninvasively and requires surgery for repair. The patient has lost a great deal of blood, and her red blood count is dangerously low. She is informed about the potentially fatal consequences of her refusal. The staff are shocked. Aside from the treatable internal bleeding, Miss J. is in good health and has led a vital and community-involved life. She has no children, nor is she married, but her parents express great love and affection for her. Courts have held, almost uniformly, that competent adults cannot be forced to receive blood in similar circumstances.

Questions

1. What other facts about Miss J. would be useful to you right now?
2. What values are in conflict in this case?
3. If Miss J. dies today, as a member of the treatment team what (if any) is your responsibility?
4. Would the case have a different outcome (for you), if Miss J. had a 3-year-old child?

Case B

Mr. W., age 23, is an admitted male prostitute and IV drug user. He is taken to the emergency room (ER) one evening after a street fight. When a nurse attempts to draw blood from the patient for a drug screen, he injures himself with a needle. The patient refuses to consent to an HIV test, even though the staff explains that it is important both for the nurse who was stuck and for the patient's well-being. A recent state law gives the hospital the authority to order the test, but the patient, who is not badly hurt, says that he is going to leave the ER now, against medical advice.

Questions

1. What rights and duties are in conflict in this case?
2. What questions of a legal nature do you have here?
3. How might a policy approach to this case head off the present difficulty?
4. Short of physical coercion, what strategies that might lead Mr. W. to accept the HIV test now are ethically appropriate?

■ THINK PIECE: CLINICAL ETHICS ■

In a much-publicized trial, retired engineer Roswell Gilbert received a sentence of life imprisonment in a Florida court for having shot his wife. Mrs. Gilbert, aged 73, was suffering from dementia (Alzheimer's disease) and osteoporosis. Her husband shot her several times in their apartment in Winter Garden, Florida. The Gilbert story was transformed into a made-for-television movie. Mr. Gilbert was released from prison after serving several years.

A less well-known case, in a different Florida county, involved Mr. and Mrs. Hans Florian. They had been married for 33 years when he shot her to death. Her brain had deteriorated significantly due to Alzheimer's disease and, after she could no longer feed or bathe herself (and her vocabulary had shrunk to two words in her native German, pain and fire), she was placed in a nursing home. Mr. Florian stated that he killed her because he was 17 years older than his wife and did not want to die first and leave her alone. He could have been found guilty of first degree murder, but the Florida grand jury refused to indict Mr. Florian.

In Michigan, Dr. Jack Kevorkian designed and built a self-described suicide machine and talked about it several times on a nationally televised show. Several women facing a future of intractable pain or psychological suffering, including one recently diagnosed as having Alzheimer's disease, asked the physician to assist them in dying. Dr. Kevorkian, a pathologist, hooked these people up to his suicide machine. Each woman clearly retained decisional capacity; each voluntarily pushed the buttons that set the suicide device into action. Three fluids then flowed into their vein. The last fluid contained a potassium chloride solution that caused a fatal arrhythmia. Dr. Kevorkian was charged with murder by legal authorities. No matter what the outcome for this particular physician, the issues he raised about the appropriateness of physician-assisted suicide will not go away.

Alzheimer's disease remains an illness of unknown cause and without effective treatment. Possible causes are genetic predisposition, a slow virus, an environmental toxin, immunologic changes, and perhaps the abnormal accumulation of proteins. Drug therapies are limited to treatment of behavioral problems. Alzheimer's patients exhibit frequent agitation but also display anxiety, depression, apathy, delusions, have sleep problems, and wander. Caregivers for Alzheimer's patients are often overworked, fatigued, and frustrated. Home health care and long-term care options are available but are rarely reimbursed by insurance plans or government coverage. Support groups for family members are widely available. The best present estimate is that there are about 4 million persons now in some stage of Alzheimer's disease in the United States. It is the fifth leading cause of death among older persons.

What are the medical and ethical differences, if any, among these three cases? Can we make useful distinctions among them? Clearly, in the case of Dr. Kevorkian we have a physician involved (assisting?)

in the suicide of patients. In the Gilbert and Florian cases, a male spouse kills his wife. Uniting the cases is the diagnosis of Alzheimer's disease, a deteriorating brain disorder that takes many years to lead to the death of the patient.

A 1988 Roper public opinion poll asked whether a physician should be lawfully able to end the life of a terminally ill patient at the patient's request: 58% of respondents said yes; 27% said no; 10% were undecided. In the Netherlands it is estimated that between 5000 and 10,000 patients are assisted in death by doctors each year, by measures that include the injection of a lethal dose of a short-acting barbiturate followed by a paralyzing agent. The American Medical Association, at the policy level, has rejected physician-assisted authority as an ethical practice.

Judicial authorities in Florida reached different results in the Gilbert and Florian cases. But even supposing that both men *had* been found guilty, does that make their acts *unethical*? Mr. Gilbert was quoted as saying that he did not believe he committed a murder and that the laws must be changed. What is the essential difference between helping someone die by connecting her to a suicide machine so that she can push the button and shooting her? What, for that matter, is the difference among injecting a suffering patient with a bit more pain-killing narcotic than is required, hastening the death of a terminally ill person, and using a pistol or shotgun? We can make analytic evaluations of such acts—based on motives, relationships, goals, and practices—but are they distinctions without a difference?

■ VOICES: PHYSICIAN AND MEDICAL SCHOOL PROFESSOR ■

I've been a doctor for about 45 years in several countries. Most of my practice has been in large American cities. I've been affiliated with several medical schools and with many hospitals and countless colleagues. I have taught medical students and residents for three decades. Ethics in medicine—simply the awareness that problems exist—has evolved slowly but surely. During the time in which I've been practicing, we've gone from zero to a rather modest peak. There surely are plenty of people today who give lip service to ethical practice. Forty years ago there were many more such practitioners. Now, at last, there is an environment in which there can be a meaningful expansion of the scrutiny of medical practice from the ethical point of view. Most of this change has come from forces outside medicine. Patient activists and advocates, outsiders who have an interest in our field, have asked hard questions. The revelation of Nazi medical experiments during World War II shocked many doctors, as has the revelation of torture around the world, sometimes committed by physicians. These revelations have pushed medicine into coming to grips with its humanistic essence.

Things are better today, but I'm still not happy. The law is a source of anxiety and this indirectly influences ethical behavior in medicine. But this is a case of people doing the right thing for the wrong reason. More positively, doctors are beginning to realize that the quality of their daily lives will be improved by talking about ethics issues with their patients and with colleagues. Another incentive for raising consciousness has been the activities of minorities, women, nurses, and other health care professionals. The criticism from nurses, for example, has been going on for a long time. But at last doctors are beginning to listen.

I'm not sure you can teach virtue, but you can try. Number one, you've got to start with people who are willing to look at issues of what's right and what's wrong. Second, you need some group, preferably one with prestige, and a leader who has the respect of colleagues, who will lead to a broader understanding. Third, and most important, you've got to find a forum for doctors to practice ethically and to be rewarded for doing it.

There surely are problems galore today. No one seems in charge of health care in the United States. It's a mess. We've got real disagreements about fundamentals: For example, should there be a national health plan in order to take care of the medically indigent? Should HMOs or PPOs get our support? Should private practice be preserved? Now, I am a pluralist. But if you care about the availability and the equity of giving medical care, you can't just accept the present mix of medical delivery systems. Doctors have to be citizens and exercise their political, as well as medical and ethical, responsibilities. Our long tradition of individual, entrepreneurial medicine is passé. Even the independent practitioner suffers from many restrictions today. I can't imagine a system that will be perfect. But I can tell you that at the moment we don't have a system at all.

Another lingering problem is that biases continue to pervade medical practice. The lack of care for the disenfranchised, the homeless, and those who lack access to the health care system due to un- or underemployment is a disgrace. That number seems to be growing, and this is based on impoverishment. Because the poor lack political clout, there's not much chance for getting attention. I sometimes wonder if there's a built-in age bias in our care delivery system. Older people are often poor and lack social contacts; people over 70 tend to be less combative and more deferential to their physicians. So they are often treated unfairly.

I have come to think that male and female doctors and medical students are different, and this shows in the values by which they live. The female medical students are more caring, more sensitive, more concerned about the humanitarian elements of medicine. They are less interested in the technical parts of medicine; men are more turned on by machinery. Women just seem more sensitive, though there are clearly many men who have such attributes. Women probably make better primary care doctors. But if you want someone to take your brain out and clean it and put it back neatly, men tend to be more interested in such things. Maybe 20 years from now these characteristics will be distributed better. Even among the men we have greater diversity than we did 30 years ago. We don't have the premed jocks, who know nothing but undergraduate science.

I don't know if doctors should be held to a standard of moral accountability higher than that of the general public. We should not hold doctors to a higher standard because we believe they are better people. We should be demanding of physicians because we want them to be better and know that they are trying to be better. Personal benefits should become second-level priorities for physicians.

I'd say to younger practitioners and medical students who want to practice medicine ethically: If you project 30 years ahead, I can guarantee that what you say to your friends and perhaps your children is this—the things you *got from* medicine are not as important as the things you have *given* to it.

RECOMMENDED READING

Beauchamp, T.L., and Childress, J.F. *Principles of Biomedical Ethics* (3rd ed). New York: Oxford University Press, 1989.

Childress, J.F. *Who Should Decide? Paternalism in Health Care.* New York: Oxford University Press, 1982.

Englehardt, H.T. *The Foundations of Bioethics.* New York: Oxford University Press, 1986.

Jonsen, A., and Toulmin, S. *The Abuse of Casuistry.* Berkeley: University of California Press, 1988.

Kass, L. *Toward a More Natural Science: Biology and Human Affairs.* New York: Free Press, 1985.

Katz, J. *The Silent World of Doctor and Patient*. New York: Free Press, 1984.

May, W.F. *The Patient's Ordeal*. Bloomington: Indiana University Press, 1991.

Veatch, R.M. *A Theory of Medical Ethics*. New York: Basic Books, 1981.

■2■

Responsibility in Clinical Medical Ethics: Basic Concepts

Practicing clinical medical ethics ought to be hard work. The task does not involve learning an orthodox way of seeing medical problems and dealing with them virtuously. There is no ethics cookbook. Such a text exists only in utopia. Clinical problems are too complicated, too individual, to be solved by guaranteed formulas. Rather, the perspective of clinical ethics suggests ways of seeing medical problems as rooted in human choices and, thus, human fallibilities. The goal is to be a responsible practitioner. What does it mean to enjoin an ordinary person (or a practicing professional) to be responsible?

First and most obviously, being responsible *usually* means obeying the law and following agreed on policies and procedures. (The doctor who fails to document an intervention, whether a successful or a faulty one, is behaving irresponsibly.) The term *usually* is italicized only to emphasize that merely following the strict letter of the law may not be enough and that on occasion lawful mandates or standardized policies may be ethically dubious. (South African physicians, until very recently, were prohibited by law from serving black or coloured [mixed-race] patients in certain hospitals. Those doctors who violated that law did so in conscience, for moral reasons.) In general, however, the law is followed by responsible practitioners.

Second, there is a cognitive aspect. Put in positive terms, a responsible person sees things in the world that irresponsible people either ignore or fail to apprehend. Some persons can walk by homeless people as if they were invisible. They feel little or nothing and have no sense of commonality with those persons hovering in doorways; those with a positive cognitive sense of responsibility both see and feel concern for those living on the street. They at least care about the pain in the lives of others. Viewed negatively, a responsible person does *not* seek immediate gratification but considers the needs of others. A surgeon does not leave the operating room because he or she is hungry and wants a midmorning snack.

Third, a responsible person has a commitment to some measure of human choice and freedom. She rejects the argument that everything about the world—or about the medical profession—is a given, set in concrete, and incapable of change. Relying on cliches such as, "Well, it's impossible to do anything about medically indigent patients. The poor will always be with us," means that we either have no duty to help change dangerous situations or will not exercise our wills in such a direction. Responsible persons reject predestination and expend energy imagining futures, considering alternatives, and pondering possible consequences.

Fourth, responsibility entails reflection. Stopping, pondering, questioning, even criticizing business as usual are modes of moral reflection. Not just doing, but *thinking* about what we are doing, means talking with others about rights, obligations, and duties. Using a moral vocabulary—being judgmental when appropriate—means holding others morally responsible. For physicians in training, those at the bottom of the totem pole, this is no small task, and for those long in practice, who value their colleagues' sentiments and favors, it is also not easy to use a moral vocabulary, which includes terms of praise and condemnation, readily. No one claims that responsibility is a light burden to carry. Happily, groups such as institutional ethics committees exist to provide a forum for discussing ethical dilemmas and a group milieu for resolving such issues.

Since ancient times, in the Hippocratic Oath (see Appendix A) and reaffirmed by professional societies and physician behavior, the central responsibility in medicine has been a devotion to the patient. This requires an attitude toward the patient of respect and concern. It also mandates a thoroughness in diagnosis, prognosis, and treatment that goes well beyond scientific understanding. The whole patient is the subject of the doctor's inquiry and care, and no matter what model of patient-professional relationship one advocates— whether it is the doctor as partner, friend, collaborator, mentor, or "priest"—the arbitrary exclusion of any central aspect of the patient's life is irresponsible. As a result, professional responsibility entails a concern for patient values. Not only what's wrong but also what's important morally and humanly for the patient become prime questions. This means that a patient's (or family's) religious as well as secular views are appropriate territory for exploration and understanding. Though clinical medical ethics may be analytically distinguished from religious ethics, in practice the division often appears to be an artificial one. Patients and practitioners have ideas and ideals, about matters of illness and wellness and about life and death, that blend theological, philosophical, and scientific knowledge, insights and intuitions. To recognize that the patient is a person—an embodiment of the rich textures of human problems and possibilities—is a commitment to the highest kind of medical responsibility.

Two very specific perspectives have helped to frame discussion (and debate) about what is right and what is wrong in clinical medical ethics. These frameworks, the *utilitarian* and the *deontological*, differ from one another in concept and in mode of analysis (Fig. 2-1). Utilitarians project toward the future and attempt to find solutions to hard-choice dilemmas that, by balancing benefits and burdens, lead to the greatest sum of good over harm. A cost-benefit analysis (often found in assessing a new surgery's potential improvement over older techniques) is clearly utilitarian. "Getting the best results" is a catch phrase that embodies such a *consequentialist* viewpoint.

The deontological perspective emphasizes maxims, rules, and principles that inform decision-making. Doing one's duty (the Greek

---

Two basic approaches to decision-making in clinical ethics:

1. **UTILITARIANISM:** The attempt to maximize good consequences over bad ones by pursuing the long-term best interest of all parties. Utilitarians try to increase good over harm by focusing on projected results of an action or decision. For utilitarians, a thing is right if it serves the goal of increasing the balance of good (or pleasure or right) over harm (or evil or wrong).

2. **DEONTOLOGY:** The act *itself*—its essential features—determines its moral worth. Without regard for consequences alone, deontologists emphasize the principles, rules, maxims, and duties that must be followed. A moral value is based not on results but rather on the essence of a fundamental principle.

Fig. 2-1. Utilitarian and deontological perspectives

term *deon* means duty) is an obligation without specific regard for consequences. Deontologists may differ in their affirmation of specific principles and duties. But most contemporary medical ethicists agree that five fundamental principles are at stake—and sometimes in conflict—in clinical judgments involving values (see Fig. 1-1). These two frameworks are simply different ways of ordering and seeing; they are not "keys to the kingdom." Each may serve as a useful check. Asking the blunt question, "How is this case likely to come out?" invites a utilitarian calculation. Inquiring about concrete principles, "Will a basic duty be violated if I affirm this decision?" may reaffirm for the practitioner a commitment to an important obligation. Taken together, utilitarian and deontological perspectives provide a useful, human, and reflective context for making judgments in clinical medical ethics.

■ FIVE ESSENTIAL CASES ■

Case 2-1

Conflicts in clinical medical ethics often result from clashes of principles. Not only "what's right" may be at stake, but "who decides" can be at issue. When living or dying are central concerns, the pressure to "get the best results" is routinely present as well.

William B. was 70 years old when he was admitted to the hospital, a religious facility with strong policies, based on Christian principles, about critical care. Prior to admission Mr. B. had been suffering for about 6 years from many illnesses, including emphysema, arteriosclerosis, chronic respiratory failure, and an abdominal aneurysm. His wife reported that he was often depressed, due mainly to his conviction that he was dying. In the hospital a routine chest x ray revealed a lung tumor. The lung collapsed upon biopsy, due to advanced emphysema, and could not be readily reinflated. Mr. B. had a tracheotomy and was placed on a ventilator. Efforts to wean the patient from the breathing machine were unsuccessful.

Mr. B. remained conscious and was able to communicate with his physicians and family, initially by writing on a pad. On several occasions, however, Mr. B. tried to disconnect the ventilator. He was placed in soft restraints. Mrs. B., his wife of many years, asked the hospital and the treatment team to remove the ventilator. In response to questions by many persons, Mr. B. indicated that, of course, he wanted to live. But he stated that he did not wish to live in the "intolerable conditions forced upon me ... being continuously connected to this machine which sustains my every life and breath." He said that he did understand that disconnection from the ventilator might lead to his death.

The hospital and the physicians caring for Mr. B. refused this request. They declared that according to their ethical precepts it was morally wrong to "disconnect life-support systems from patients whom they viewed as having the potential for cognitive sapient life." The administration also refused to allow Mrs. B. to take her husband home or to another facility. To permit this, the hospital felt, would be to aid in the commiting of suicide.

(Based on Bartling v. Superior Court [Glendale Adventist Medical Center] 209 Cal. Rptr. 220 (Cal. App. 2 Dist. 1984))

Life or death is the "stake" in this case. All parties seem to agree that Mr. B. is very ill and is likely to die, no matter what the level of intervention, relatively soon. (Definitions of *terminal illness* vary considerably; hospices routinely accept patients likely to die within 6 months; in nursing homes a dying patient is often seen as one who will not live more than a few days.) Neither the hospital, this patient's physicians, nor his family expect him to recover from his many ailments or to be restored to a previous level of function. But agreement about Mr. B.'s condition has led to a seemingly implacable conflict. The patient and his spouse base their demand that he be removed from the ventilator on a claim of autonomy, a most fundamental principle of medical ethics (see Fig. 1-1). The hospital and its staff, however, in refusing to collaborate with the B. family and, even more forcefully, in attempting to mandate the maintenance of the respirator, center their ethical position on the principles of beneficence (hoping to help Mr. B.) and nonmaleficence (arguing that to let this patient die in this manner would be to cause him harm). In addition, the hospital feels that there is a religious value, the Christian principle to preserve life and the corollary sanction against assisting in suicide, that forces them, in conscience, to resist the patient and his family's wishes.

Just who should be making the decision in this case is seemingly problematic. As a general rule, patient management is self-management (Fig. 2-2). But such freedom to choose, or to reject, treatment is never total. No patient can demand a new heart and expect to get it. Similarly, physicians, nurses, institutions, and society as a whole (often manifested through legislation or court action) are implicated in some difficult cases. The hospital is denying Mr. B.'s autonomy for what it believes is a good reason—that his death would be a moral wrong. In doing so, it is tacitly stating that the doctors and the institution are the appropriate and exclusive decision-makers in this case. Mr. and Mrs. B. affirm patient self-determination as the paramount interest. Mr. B. is an adult; he appears to understand the consequences of his refusal of treatment; and he has advanced serious reasons for rejecting the ventilator.

If we place ourselves in the situation of the treating physician in this case, the dilemma is sharpened. The doctor is pledged to resist disease, to help patients who are sick or suffering, and to preserve health if possible. Mr. B.'s doctor, if she follows her patient's stated wish, will have to remove ventilatory support and, if she is a loyal caregiver, watch as Mr. B. gasps for air, thrashes about, and in effect drowns. This withdrawal of the ventilator, a quite routine medical technology, is never easy. Symbolically and literally, such a taking away of this life-sustaining equipment creates great psychological burdens for caregivers. (Another example: Many end-stage kidney disease patients decide to go off dialysis. All die within a few weeks. Such decisions are very often difficult for nephrologists and their team members to accept.)

But if this same doctor, joining with her institution's administration, tells Mr. B. in effect that he must stay tethered permanently

---

1. A clear concise statement of the patient's condition, disease, disorder, or problem must be presented.
2. The nature and purpose of the proposed treatment (or course of therapy, or drug regimen) must be stated, in language specific and clear enough to be commonly understood.
3. The risks and consequences of the proposed treatment must be described.
4. Any feasible alternative to treatment must be stated to the patient.
5. The patient must be told his or her prognosis if the proposed treatment is not given.

Fig. 2-2. Elements of informed consent

to the ventilator, the physician (though perhaps acting in accordance with a basic principle) has responded in a way that can only be called *paternalistic*, saying by her actions that "I know better than you do what is in your best interest." The motive for such an argument may be rooted in the principle of beneficence. A decision about the case of Mr. B. moves us to prioritize our principles. Reasonable persons, and sometimes courts of law, will differ about such prioritization.

Case 2-2

Patients can make treatment choices and reject treatment recommendations if they retain decisional capacity (a clinical term, often referred to as "competence" in the legal system) (Fig. 2-3).

Mr. O. is a 59-year-old married man with three adult children. A merchant for more than 30 years, Mr. O. was admitted to the hospital last year for surgical resection of a primary carcinoma of the colon. It was believed that the entire cancer had been removed. But 2 months ago, the patient was readmitted due to a persistent cough and abdominal distention. A complete workup showed extensive metastatic disease; prognosis was a range of 3 months to 1½ years, depending on the level of treatment. The oncologist believed that radiation and chemotherapy could extend Mr. O.'s life considerably and that side effects could be managed effectively. Mr. O. agreed to the recommended treatment plan and checked into C. Hospital on a weekday morning.

That afternoon, Mr. O. told his primary care physician, Dr. N., that he was not interested in radiation or chemotherapy. On inquiry the patient said, "Let's face it, my life is over." Dr. N. observed the patient to be anxious and upset. Mr. O. showed signs, often seen in very ill persons, of

---

1. Speak with the patient *more than once* to determine if he or she understands the medical facts of the case and the clinical situation.
2. Determine the patient's appreciation of the options of both treatment and nontreatment and his or her understanding of the consequences of the various choices.
3. Examine the patient's reasoning process in this situation and clarify how it is set into the context of his or her values and goals.

Fig. 2-3. Determining decisional capacity: a checklist

cognitive "fuzziness." He seemed to be generally "with it," but in response to questions he seemed distracted and vague in his answers. A preliminary screening for depression showed that Mr. O. was indeed despondent. His affect is sad, and he says that he does not want to suffer a great deal of pain and does not wish to become a burden to his wife and children. He has disclosed to the physician that he has made a will and provided for the sale of his business and other property. Dr. N. asks Mr. O. if he will agree, just once, to meet with a consultant-psychiatrist. The patient agrees. The psychiatrist reports to Dr. N. that Mr. O. is "a seemingly rational and engaging person. He is not suffering from any major psychiatric disorder, although he is clearly upset and saddened by his limited future prospects. I think that this patient is depressed, though not psychotically. His refusal of any further cancer treatment seems to me part of his desire to see his life end as soon as possible. I would not rule out the possibility of this patient's taking his own life in order to forestall pain and suffering."

Legal and medical experts as well as patient advocates agree: Competent persons have a clear right to accept or refuse medical treatment proposed by their physicians. *Competence* is a legal term, not a psychiatric judgment. Only a court or legal authority can declare a person incompetent. The medical term that parallels competence is *decisional capacity*. Patients who seem to lack such capacity—and it is usually the physician or the consulting psychiatrist who renders an assessment of that capacity—may eventually be declared incompetent. In such cases choices are frequently made for them, often in opposition to their declared desires. Mr. O.'s decisional capacity is a crucial element in this case. If he has lost it, he may be confined, lose his liberty, and be forced to accept cancer treatment against his will (see Fig. 2-3).

The physical condition of the patient may present problems not only of decisional capacity but also of *assessment*. Persons with moderate mental retardation, for example, may be unable to understand complicated explanations and their seemingly incomprehensible responses may be a product of faulty question formation. Substance abuse (drug and alcohol ingestion) may be temporary impediments in assessing decisional capacity, as may the side effects of prescribed medications. Sometimes, simply waiting for recovery is enough. Mental illness is often assumed to be an automatic disqualifier. But symptoms of thought and mood disorders can overlap, and further investigation by specialists may be required. Not all demented patients are alike and even persons with Alzheimer's disease may, in the earlier stages, have sufficient memory to deal with medical decision-making.

In a very general way, competence (and decisional capacity) flow from the ability to make reasoned choices. The patient must, of course, be given sufficient and clear information in order to evidence such choices. No patient need have medical expertise: a cogent explanation that a lay person can comprehend is sufficient. But *knowing* what is happening is only the general foundation of decisional capacity. In addition, the patient must understand his or her own medical problems at present and be able to deal with information in a useful and rational manner. Finally, patients need, at a minimum, some way of communicating choices to caregivers. The stroke patient in "locked-in" condition, while perhaps knowing the details of diagnosis and prognosis, remains totally without the means to state a choice. He thus lacks decisional capacity until communication can be restored.

Mentally ill persons can be competent. Someone suffering from schizophrenia may at times be nondelusional and, if asked to consent to surgery, be fully capable of understanding and deciding rationally. Conversely, incompetence is often the result of mental incapacitation or illness. The comatose patient clearly lacks decisional capacity, as does the person in an alcoholic stupor. But most cases in which decisional capacity must be determined are not so clear-cut. (By legal definition, minors in most circumstances are deemed incompetent; people of all ages with extensive mental retardation who are under the supervision of court-appointed guardians are also incompetent.) Courts have been reluctant to stipulate precise definitions for competence. Still, competence is presumed for adults. Just as one is assumed, by law, to be innocent until proven guilty, so a person is said to be competent until the opposite can be satisfactorily demonstrated.

In medical settings, it is rare for a patient who agrees with a physician's recommendation for treatment to be evaluated for decisional capacity. The tacit assumption is that if the patient follows the physician's advice, he or she must be rational because an approved choice is being made. But when patients say "no" or question the basis for a doctor's proposed course of care, especially if there is even a minimal reason to suspect that the patient's cognitive or affective status has changed of late, the next step is usually to investigate decisional capacity. When Dr. N. asked Mr. O. to see the psychiatrist, this is precisely what occurred.

The consultant tells Dr. N. that his patient is *not* suffering from a serious mental disorder. The psychiatrist suggests that Mr. O. is rational. But this single term surely demands exploration. Does it mean that Mr. O. knows that without cancer treatment his life will be shortened? Or does it simply show that the patient, knowing his terminal status, has made a reasonable plan for disposing of his property? Because this patient is terminally ill, his rejection of recommended care will not be seen as unusual. But is it the product of thoughtful consideration or a reaction rooted in fear and desperation? Any assessment of decisional capacity, in order to be thorough (if not completely secure), needs to be based on an examination of the patient's actual, living context.

We need to know many complicated things in order to pursue that context: Mr. O.'s relationship with his family; his medical and mental health history; his sense of himself as he has experienced the recurrence of cancer. Because the psychiatrist has noted the possibility of suicidal thoughts in this patient, another realm of investigation seems warranted. Is Mr. O. serious about killing himself? Does he have a plan? Will he tell others in advance and perhaps ask for assistance? While the possibilities are fascinating, they do not touch on the issue of Mr. O.'s competence. Even some psychiatrists, well-trained in characterizing whether a patient is suicidal as the result of mental illness, might think that this patient's desire to take his own life is a rational choice!

There is no definitive test of reasonableness. We commonly tolerate the refusal of treatment when a religious belief is cited, even though our own vision of hell (or heaven) would never countenance the rejection, say, of blood products in a life-threatening situation. If one patient says that being a Jehovah's Witness is the basis for treatment refusal and another bases the same rejection on grounds of "personal preference," we are hard pressed to give reasons that affirm the former while rejecting the latter.

In Mr. O.'s case, we must look at much more than the patient's mental status or medical condition. His refusal of treatment may upset many people, family as well as health care professionals. A determination of his decisional capacity will be crucial in making future patient care plans. If Mr. O. is deemed incapable of exercising choice, his treatment refusal will not be respected and a surrogate decision-maker will be appointed to act on his behalf. His freedom to choose will cease and another person will have to consent to his medical care.

Case 2-3

A competent adult has the right to make an informed decision. The process of achieving *informed consent* is basic to the doctor-patient relationship (Fig. 2-4).

In the emergency room of City Hospital (a large, university-affiliated teaching institution), Dr. L. is the physician on duty. Late in the evening he is called to see a patient who has come into the ER, apparently on his own. The patient, D.V., presents with a slashed Achilles tendon. He refuses to say just how he was injured but states that the wound was not self-inflicted. Dr. L. calls in a surgeon who examines the injury and states that if the tendon is sutured within 24–36 hours, the patient will recover completely. If it is not treated, D.V. will have a chronic limp.

Dr. L. tells these facts to D.V. and attempts to admit him and prepare him for surgery. He refuses to be treated. He replies, "The doctors are going to try to kill me. They give you hypodermic needles and I know they contain poison."

During the history and physical examination, D.V. told Dr. L. that he is receiving psychiatric treatment—he did not mention the reason—and stated that he was taking no medication at present. D.V. says that he lives alone and can care for himself. Hearing his treatment refusal, Dr. L.

Check the patient for:
1. Primary thought disturbance
2. Hallucinations or delusions
3. Disturbing or aggressive behavior
4. Difficulties in communication
5. Affective disorders
6. Disturbances of memory, orientation, and cognition
7. Severe mental retardation
8. Suicidal or homicidal ideation

Fig. 2-4. Psychopathology and informed consent

calls in a psychiatrist for a consultation. She feels that if D.V. were given antipsychotic medication, which has a clear tranquilizing effect, he would become more reasonable and would consent to treatment. The psychiatrist also states that, at present, she does not find D.V. dangerous to others or to himself (i.e., he is neither homicidal or suicidal). This patient is clearly confused, the psychiatrist says, but he does know that surgery is medically recommended and understands the consequences of saying "no" to the treatment. She does not find him to be so psychopathologically impaired as to be incapable of making an informed decision about the tendon.

D.V. continues to refuse the surgery, repeats his statement about the syringe and tells Dr. L., "I can go to another hospital where they won't try to kill me." He says that he is going to leave the ER, against medical advice (AMA).

Immediate questions emerge from the story of Mr. D.V. Does this patient have the right to refuse to be treated in the emergency room? Do the doctors have an obligation to treat this patient, even if he resists care? What weight must we give to his (apparent) irrationality in telling the doctors that he fears they will "kill me?" Should we respect D.V.'s refusal of treatment, or should we in some way compel him to remain in the ER? More generally, though the consulting psychiatrist states that D.V. has the decisional capacity to consent to treatment and thus the capacity to refuse treatment, is this the end of the story?

Rooted in the ethical principle of autonomy is the ideal of informed consent. The rule of thumb, in virtually every jurisdiction is that: *a competent adult has the right to make an informed decision*. Legally, a physician or health care professional who fails to gain the informed agreement to treat runs the risk of being charged with battery, the tort of unlawful touching, even if no real injury has resulted.

In order to go ahead with the surgery, a physician must gain the informed consent of D.V. (see Figure 2-2). This does not mean filling out a form or signing an agreement. Gaining informed consent entails a process of information giving and doctor-patient exchange and includes the possibility of informed refusal of recommended treatment. Patients about to undergo surgical procedures usually have some time to contemplate the possible risks and benefits of treatment. In the ER setting there is little time for contemplation. Still, the need to engage in the informed consent process with D.V. remains important.

The doctrine of informed consent has historic roots in the ideal of individual freedom and in the right to privacy, which, though not specifically noted in the U.S. Constitution, has been upheld by courts, at least since the early twentieth century, to be a fundamental and enforceable liberty. From both utilitarian and deontological (see Fig. 2-1) perspectives, the benefits of informed consent seem apparent. The promotion of individual autonomy, self-governance, is obvious. When patients choose their treatments and understand the implications of such choices, a better and clearer doctor-patient relationship may develop. Physicians are encouraged to be honest and to avoid even the appearance of duplicity.

Informed consent recognizes the expertise of the health care professional but roots it in openness and honesty. Informed consent contests paternalism: It suggests that, though patients and doctors are obviously persons of differing skills (and problems), the professional encounter depends on mutual trust and respect. Finally, informed consent encourages rational decision-making, not acquiescence or angry rejection. Having patients participate in decisions about care, many physicians would state, is good for all parties concerned. The differential education and experience of patient and doctor, of course, make full disclosure a challenge. If the anesthesiologist tells the potential surgery patient that the chance of cardiac rhythm disturbance is 1 in 100 and that the risk of myocardial infarction is 1 in 2000, it is hard to know what, subjectively, the patient takes such information to mean. Still, the goal of informed consent is an admirable one—providing adequate information so that the autonomous patient can make an intelligent choice.

There are several widely recognized exceptions to the necessity to gain informed consent. The *emergency exception* states that in serious and emergent life-threatening situations (e.g., a patient with head trauma as the result of a motorcycle accident) the treating physician or staff need not obtain informed consent. The notion of *implied consent* suggests that with many minor, commonly encountered procedures with little or no risk, such as taking a blood pressure, the very lifting of the patient's arm in response to the offering of the blood pressure cuff provides a tacit agreement.

Finally, the exception of *therapeutic* privilege allows the forgoing of the informed consent process if it will entail risk of great harm to the patient. This exception can surely lead to all sorts of paternalistic justifications; it is rarely advocated for this reason (Fig. 2-5).

If we think of informed consent not as a goal (I got the form signed) but rather as a process—one with unique human prospects and problems—we will glimpse the complexities of actual medical decision-making. Certainly, from the physician's perspective, informed consent is an information-giving procedure. From the patient's viewpoint, it is an opportunity to learn, to contemplate, and to decide. But by focusing exclusively on the goal, we may miss some of the nuances. Doctors, as we have noted, know from experience and from attention to recent studies the risks and benefits of proposed interventions, both statistically and anecdotally. While physicians are rarely manipulative in an overt manner, how doctors communicate data, with what emphasis, and in what tone of voice, not to mention in what words, will have a manifest influence upon most patients. Patients who are ill, fearful, or naturally deferential to authority will often (in a seemingly willing fashion) agree to almost

---

Informed consent to medical, surgical, and pharmacologic treatments is required for all competent patients or their surrogates, but may be bypassed in certain situations:

WAIVER. The patient insists that he or she does not want to know the details of treatment. [Such a statement should be regarded as an invitation to further dialogue.]

EMERGENCY. In a life-or-death situation, caregivers may assume that the patient would want intervention to save life. [An emergency must be a serious and imminent threat; when the crisis has passed, the requirement of informed consent is restored.]

IMPLIED AGREEMENT. Commonly encountered procedures with little or minimal risk to the patient can be performed without specific consent (e.g., routine blood work). [Any doubts about implied consent should be resolved by consulting with the patient.]

THERAPEUTIC PRIVILEGE. If informing the patient will cause him or her serious and identifiable harm, the informed consent need not proceed. [Opportunities for paternalistic abuse of this exception may result from the physician's fear of provoking anxiety or depression in the patient; this is not deemed an adequate cause for abridging the consent process.]

Fig. 2-5. Exceptions to the doctrine of informed consent

anything offered by a physician. But does such agreement attest to an autonomously given consent?

What happens when patients will not agree to treatment, when instead of giving consent they offer refusal? The doctrine of informed consent is a two-way street. If patients were asked to agree and always did so, the encounter would be a perfunctory, merely mechanical, act. Informed consent implies the ability to give informed refusal. If all patients had to accept medical wisdom, informed consent would be a meaningless process. We believe that *informed consent implies the right to exercise informed refusal.* Patients who do state their unwillingness to accept the best medical advice are often regarded as management problems, noncompliant, or even difficult or hateful patients. Many are! But treatment refusal, like treatment acceptance, is a complicated notion, deserving of in-depth exploration.

Let's look at the case of Mr. D.V. He seems to have entered the ER voluntarily; there is no evidence that he was brought there by friends, relatives, or civil authorities. He is in pretty bad shape, although his slashed tendon is not likely to lead to death or to serious long-term disability. His response to the offer of surgery, which is not guaranteed but is most likely to correct his problem, is negative, but its basis remains unclear. He seems irrational and his prior history of psychiatric care might lead us to believe that he had a history of mental illness. The consulting psychiatrist has checked out the mental status of Mr. D.V. (Fig. 2-4). She tells us that there is no plausible way in which he can be held against his will; he does not meet the minimal criteria for involuntary civil commitment. Not only is he refusing to give his informed consent, he is heading out the door. Mr. D.V. seems to be expressing his autonomy. We are assuming that he understands the explanation given to him about the proposed surgery and the likely outcome if he accepts or refuses it. At this point he is doing so by simply saying "No!"

Is this treatment refusal in the patient's best interest? Probably not, medically speaking. A relatively simple operation, which would involve the usual risks, including being administered anesthesia, could fix him up and he would be on his way in a few days. But he will not be reasoned with. Most people would not behave in this manner. Should we allow him to leave the ER? Or, to put it in the language of ethical principles, should we allow autonomy to trump beneficence? From the utilitarian viewpoint, can we accept the bad result of a decision to refuse surgery?

For the treatment team, the case of Mr. D.V. suggests a very basic ethical conflict. Validating the patient's treatment refusal affirms his autonomy. But he limps away from the hospital clearly in need of some kind of medical treatment. The physician's duty to care for the ill or injured is a similarly strong obligation. But if we hold Mr. D.V. against his will, or inject him with a tranquilizer to gain his acquiescence, we have repudiated his right to make health care choices independently.

Case 2-4

The promise to maintain a *confidential* relationship between patient and clinician is a serious one, but there may be occasions in which the obligation must be rethought for reasons of public policy or concern for others.

Mr. F. is a 55-year-old truck driver with 30 years on the road. He is a union member and spends as many as 3 weeks away from home when doing a long-distance haul. Every 5 years his employer (and the union contract) require a physical examination. Seeing one's family physician is acceptable under this policy. Last month Mr. F. was examined by Dr. M. who, after a series of careful tests (including EKG) and a thorough history, suspected ventricular tachycardia, a condition that can result in fainting spells and loss of consciousness. Mr. F. told the physician that he had never passed out. Dr. M. referred the patient to a cardiologist for further studies.

The specialist examined Mr. F., had him wear a Holter monitor, which records cardiac and other functions continuously for a 24-hour period, and confirmed the diagnosis. She recommended medical treatment and careful follow-up. Mr. F. told Dr. M. that he would "take my medicine religiously." Dr. M., wanting to make sure that the drugs were working to correct the patient's condition, told Mr. F. that "we need to do a few more Holter monitor assessments over the next month or so. In the meantime, I want you to stop driving the truck." The patient became upset. He told Dr. M. that if he asked to stop driving, his employer and his family would know immediately that something was wrong.

Dr. M. said, "We have to know if this drug is working." He also asked Mr. F. to consider the potential danger to others on the road. Mr. F. said, "I can handle it. I only have 2 years until retirement, and I don't want to lose my pension. Don't worry, I'll be careful." Dr. M. is aware of the relevant state law that mandates a report to the Department of Health if the patient "has ever experienced a lapse of consciousness or is likely to do so while driving." If this report is filed, the motor vehicle department will be notified and may revoke the patient's driver's license.

Dr. M. suggests that Mr. F. talk things over with his wife, but the patient says, quite adamantly, "No way! All this is between you and me, doc. I can deal with this. I just want to work for a couple more years so we can retire to Florida."

The request from Mr. F. to his physician to "keep things quiet" is fundamental to the doctor-patient relationship. The Hippocratic Oath, which originated in the fourth century B.C., pledges the doctor to "keep to myself" information about treatment (and beyond) regarded as personal and confidential (see Appendix A). Subsequent codes pledge physicians never to betray a promise to keep matters secret. A respect for privacy is indispensable if autonomy is to be cherished. The consequences of violating confidentiality are, in individual cases and for society per se, awful to contemplate. If a doctor shares information about a patient with impunity, whether it be about diagnosis, prognosis, and treatment or about the financial, familial, or sexual aspects of a case, then the intimacy necessary for functional health care will be impeded. Patients will pull their punches and tell doctors only selectively about their true concerns and worries.

Oddly enough, doctors rarely discuss confidentiality with their patients. When a waiver is requested (e.g., to provide information to third-party payers), this is routinely done by signing a form and is administered by office staff. The nature of such common abridgements of confidentiality is rarely explored: How much detail can an insurance company demand in return for its promise to reimburse physician or patient? Only at crisis time, and we may be approaching such a moment in the case of Mr. F., will the subject emerge.

In general, confidentiality is taken as a given. Usually breaking confidentiality is discussed only if legal duties or public policies are at stake (e.g., requirements to report gunshot wounds or sexually transmissible diseases). Curiously, among health care workers, the problem of confidentiality has another face. An embarrassing volcano of private information inundates the daily lives of doctors, nurses, and other providers. Observers note that elevator conversation and hallway chitchat about patients, procedures, and problems are omnipresent. In the big city teaching hospital, a patient may be seen by 20 caregivers, and may be read about by countless clerks, transcribers, and administrators in a single day; each has the chance to read the chart and, later, to gossip about the case. The computerization of medical records has made this phenomenon even more apparent.

When Mr. F. asks his family doctor to keep his condition secret, he presents challenges commonly faced by the physician in the realm of confidentiality. The demand for confidentiality may sometimes conflict with the physician's sense of what the patient may really need: The depressed person who asks the doctor to keep a suicide threat quiet usually does not have that wish respected. But is Mr. F.'s request comparable? Doctors also have an obligation to be concerned about the public's welfare (See Appendix B). That is the basis of the duty to notify public health authorities regarding communicable diseases. More recently a duty to warn specific third parties about imminent danger (e.g., the threat of murder or bodily injury) has been established by some courts and legislatures. But is Mr. F.'s situation really analogous to that of the mental patient who threatens to kill his girlfriend?

Dr. M. must feel conflict. He wants what is best for his patient and, naturally, wants to maintain the relationship with Mr. F. that he has developed over the years. If he tells the employer or the department of health about Mr. F.'s condition, there is a better-than-average chance that Mr. F. will be forced out of his job. Taking a moderate stance, arguing that "maybe you can work in the office for the next few years," may prove fruitful. But Mr. F. is likely to state, quite legitimately, that "those jobs pay half of what I get as a truck driver. And my pension is based on what I earn in my last 2 years of employment." Assuming patient rejection of this bargaining request, what should Dr. M. do?

We might pose the problem in terms of authority. Exactly who possesses the information about Mr. F.'s condition? Is it exclusively the property of the patient, or does Dr. M. have joint ownership? If the worst case scenario happens—if Mr. F. continues to drive, passes out, and injures or kills another driver—would Dr. M. be obliged to testify about the preexisting medical condition of his patient? Probably not. The evidentiary privilege rules that guarantee that a patient's confidential information be protected in legal proceedings would apply. Here the patient's right to retain information trumps the physician's obligation to reveal it. But Dr. M. would not want this case ever to come to court. His dilemma remains in the area of effective patient care. How does he balance his concern for Mr. F. with his worries about the potential consequences of agreeing to remain quiet? Should the physician cajole or coerce Mr. F? Should he threaten to tell Mrs. F? Should he offer some form of counseling? No matter what middle course we seek, the confidentiality dilemma remains: In the never-absolute realm of privacy, who governs the flow of information?

Case 2-5

The obligation to tell the truth, rooted in the principle of veracity, is *assumed* in clinical practice, but actually doing so may become difficult.

B.J., a 45-year-old female, comes into the ER with complaints of shakiness and auditory hallucinations. Routine examination and swift laboratory evaluation suggest alcohol withdrawal. She tells the physicians on duty, "I am feeling fine; I just need some time to get my act together. Don't make me take no pills or stuff."

Against her will, the patient is given ativan, thiamine, multivitamins, and magnesium sulfate 1 gm ivpb over 30 minutes—the standard regimen. B.J. is placed in a quiet area in the ER and further care is contemplated by the team. Her sister, who has been sitting at the patient's bedside during this time, comes running toward the physicians shouting, "She's not breathing!" Full resuscitation is undertaken; after 20 minutes of CPR, the patient regains a blood pressure and pulse and is admitted to the medical intensive care unit (MICU) in coma. Lack of oxygen to the brain for that long a period indicates that recovery of consciousness is unlikely.

An extensive workup is undertaken to establish the cause of the presumed respiratory arrest. The patient's initial magnesium level was 1.20 mg/dl (normal). After the CPR, during which she did not receive magnesium, the level was reported to be 9.4 mg/dl (toxic level). Multiple repeat measurements taken over the next several hours confirm markedly elevated magnesium. It is likely that this is the result of an iatrogenic origin (that is, it was caused by something in the health care environment, most probably the result of human error in this case).

B.J.'s family wants to know what happened. They approach an ER physician who tells them (without consulting with the MICU team), "We don't know why this occurred. It may have been a problem with her heart." The patient's husband does state that he remembers a doctor telling B.J. some years ago that she had a heart murmur and that she should watch her blood pressure.

■ ■ ■

Telling the truth clearly depends on knowing the truth. In B.J.'s case an unusual occurrence that as yet is inexplicable has resulted in severe damage to the patient. A response to the inquiry about causes depends on two factors: (1) knowing, or wanting to know, what happened; and (2) wanting to communicate that "truth" or even suspicion to B.J.'s family. It would be very easy to finesse this problem; the patient's husband seems deferential and quite willing to hear a vague explanation based on a previously existing medical condition. B.J. will perhaps never recover consciousness and will never ask questions. The standard reason offered for telling the truth (that is, a mark of respect for the patient's autonomy) does not quite figure in this case. B.J. is quite likely "out of it" permanently. Applying the principle of veracity to the patient's family becomes the central issue.

Truth-telling has an inconsistent pattern in contemporary health care. American physicians, as reflected in the *Principles of Ethics of the American Medical Association*, (see Appendix B) seem not to be obligated to follow the principle of veracity. Corollary duties, such as providing information necessary to give informed consent, presume the telling of the truth. If a patient is enrolled in an experimental protocol, for example, it is a clear violation of trust (and of law in many cases) to withhold a careful assessment of risks and benefits. Beyond institutional strictures, physicians want to tell the truth. An alliance between doctor and patient may fail if the atmosphere is a deceptive one. Still, the duty to tell the truth remains a contested notion for at least two reasons. First, definitions of truth and lying are notoriously complex; is a tiny lie a true dishonesty? Second, physicians sometimes justify deception on utilitarian grounds. Giving a placebo is the prime example: "A sugar pill certainly won't hurt this guy; it's likely to make him feel much better in fact!" Deception, in other words, can be characterized as benign or even beneficent.

Lying could also benefit the caregiver. In the not-so-distant past, efforts were made at covering up surgical mistakes. Injury or even death might be explained away by the phrase "there were severe complications." If no one outside the operating room staff revealed the facts, that could be the end of the story. More recently, with hospital, government, and third-party payer scrutiny, the likelihood of such duplicity has been reduced. Morbidity and mortality conferences routinely probe the reasons for unpredicted patient deterioration or death. An unexplained death within a hospital is often the occasion for an autopsy. Still, the physicians in the case of B.J. could avoid further investigation quite easily.

Complicating this case is the fact that several physicians are participants. The ER team knows what happened; the ER doctor has been approached by the family. In the MICU another team, led by a physician and including several medical residents, is concerned about B.J.'s status. If the ER physician puts the family off, they may pursue the matter "upstairs." Nurses and physicians do not always communicate about what families may or may not know. The chances of an unmanageable conversation taking place are great here.

There is also a high probability that the institution's risk management department will be called in. That group (whose job is to deal with potential lawsuits and to ensure compliance with standards of health care) is often revered for its protection of vulnerable physicians and others from legal threats. Would the risk management team advise silence, a limited response, openness, or simply further investigation? There are many ways to lie: evasion, the doling out of important information, and stating facts in obscure language come to mind. The iatrogenic factor in this case may never be discovered. (We assume that no intentional cause exists.)

B.J.'s situation presents a set of questions that inform much of clinical medical ethics. To what standards of ethical responsibility do we hold physicians? When doubts about the reality of a clinical situation remain, how much of this uncertainty must be communicated to other interested parties? What is the balance of fidelity owed to patients per se and to their families? Should doctors, working in a field in which perfection is often demanded but is rarely achieved, always tell as much of the truth as they know?

■ PRACTICE MODEL CASE ■

Mr. Howard is a 77-year-old man with metastatic squamous cell carcinoma of the lung. Surgical intervention was ruled out early on. He has previously refused any other treatment for his disease, agreeing only to regular examinations. Recently, his primary care physician Dr. M., noting that the patient has become increasingly anorectic and cachectic, has told Mr. Howard that he is getting worse. At an office conference attended by the patient and his adult son, Dr. M. initiates a discussion of resuscitation status and ventilatory support if, and when, Mr. Howard gets sicker and must be hospitalized. Dr. M. is quite factual, pointing out that Mr. Howard's disease is not treatable and noting that he has other co-morbid problems, including end-stage heart disease and pulmonary fibrosis. The doctor encourages a family meeting and provides the patient with a blank living will form. Mr. Howard, who still lives at home, independently, schedules an appointment for the following week.

Mr. Howard and his son meet with the two other family members (children of the patient). On returning to Dr. M.'s office, Mr. Howard makes the following statement, "We've talked it over. I don't want to die. I'm not filling out one of those death forms. I want you to do everything. If I stop breathing you should revive me. Use all the machinery you've got." Dr. M. is quite disconcerted by this reponse. He asks Mr. Howard's permission to speak with the son privately. Mr. Howard agrees and moves to the waiting room. On inquiry, the son tells Dr. M. "We tried to reason with him. Neither my sister or brother or I want to see him put through this misery. We're ready to let go, but dad isn't!"

Nine days later the patient is admitted to the hospital with a significant deterioration. He is having great trouble breathing and requires pain medication. He is not consistently responsive to questions from the health care team. He is getting worse every day. Without resuscitation (in the event of an arrest) or intubation, Mr. Howard is likely to die very soon. His family remains clear that they would prefer only a limited care plan for their father.

Patient

Mr. Howard is now a hospitalized patient and is very ill. Many medical choices must be made for this patient (e.g., should he be sent to the intensive care unit?). The clinical situation, no matter how "managed," is unlikely to result in longevity for Mr. Howard. His lung cancer, inoperable and spreading, is a virulent disease that (statistically) will result in death quite soon. Mr. Howard's pulmonary situation is influenced by multiple factors: the primary tumor, fibrosis in the lungs, and his heart disease, which will lead to fluid accumulation. Modes of treatment that will decelerate this disease process are available. Mr. Howard has said, prior to this hospitalization, that he wants maximal treatment. Unlike many patients who give advance directives, either formally via document or informally via conversation, Mr. Howard has told Dr. M. that he wants to be resuscitated and intubated.

Is this patient dying? The clinical "measurement" of death may be relatively secure. The irreversible cessation of breathing and circulation or the termination of whole brain activity or both are the most commonly accepted definitions. But dying is a less tangible notion; its essence is harder to grasp. Clinicians often speak of death being imminent (see Appendix D), but imminence is itself widely debated as a concept: Does it mean tomorrow, the next day, or within a few months? Of one thing we can be certain: Mr. Howard will not survive long without some form of intervention.

The fact that this patient is receiving pain medication is also medically significant. Metastatic lung cancer can cause great suffering, especially if it has spread to the bones, a frequent occurrence. But the type and dosage of pain medication need to be chosen carefully. Morphine and its derivatives can numb Mr. Howard's pain; they can also shorten his life, for respiratory suppression is among their side effects. Finally, from the clinical perspective Mr. Howard (if dramatic kinds of treatment are to be offered) will be placed in the hands of a variety of specialists (i.e., intensivists, pulmonologists, cardiologists, oncologists) who are strangers to this case. Although the patient may not be able to communicate with these physicians, life and death decisions will be made by them.

Relationships

Who is Mr. Howard? The barebones sketch provided in most case summaries provides important facts (for example, he has lung cancer that has spread beyond the primary site), but (as in all such brief reports) says very little about the patient himself. What has his life been like? He is a widower: How did he experience the death of his spouse? While age may be a factor in this case—cancer risk rises with longevity—it may be of interest not just clinically but symbolically. Mr. Howard's children have tried to reason with their father, to get him to accept his dying and to persuade him to accept limited, or palliative, care. How does his life-long connection to these offspring figure in this family's constellation? Who has traditionally governed? Who has been taking responsibility for Mr. Howard during his recent months of illness?

The autonomy model of patient decision-making is well established in both law and practice. Going by the book we can affirm Mr. Howard's prior statement by saying that aggressive treatment was his desire. At present, however, we cannot confirm with the patient this earlier claim on the health care providers. Should we now, while Mr. Howard is so sick that he cannot speak, defer to the family's wishes? Does autonomy disappear with pulmonary deterioration?

The role of families in medical decision-making is central. But either/or choices (i.e., obey Mr. Howard's earlier "commands" or bypass his prior wishes in favor of a present determination by his children) tend to ignore the complexities of real, systemic family realities. When Mr. Howard's children failed to secure his agreement to a limited treatment plan, the schism seemed evident. A deeper and sustained exploration of that difference might have elicited an understanding of family values. From the beginning an effort at collaborative decision-making by the patient in his family might have transpired. Is it now too late for such a strategy to be tried?

Advocacy

Mr. Howard's present condition, one in which his decisional capacity is probably permanently impaired, could make him the object rather than the subject of clinical concern. Asking the question, "Who will speak for the patient?" presumes the loss of competence and the inability to give informed consent on Mr. Howard's part. While many can assert their views about what his best interests might be, who (if anyone) will speak authentically for those interests?

When family members are in conflict about the care of a dependent patient who lacks decisional capacity, a legal alternative is to petition a probate court for guardianship. The conditions of this legally sanctioned surrogate decision-making process are scrutinized by the court. Sometimes a family member will be named guardian. Often, when families are arguing, another person, say a lawyer or a health care administrator, is appointed. This person is by definition a patient advocate, but in Mr. Howard's case such a scenario is unlikely because the siblings seem in agreement that aggressive treatment cease.

In the absence of a court-appointed decision-maker, who will serve to advance Mr. Howard's now silent desires? Dr. M. certainly knows that his patient has stated quite cogently that he wants continuing treatment. Is it the physician's obligation to speak for the patient in these circumstances? We may surmise that Dr. M. was less than enthusiastic about resuscitating and intubating Mr. Howard. Must Dr. M. now pursue this plan reluctantly? A beneficence argument could go either way. It would surely promote (or at least give symbolic respect for) Mr. Howard's earlier declaration if Dr. M. works to honor the request for intervention. On the other hand, a relatively painless though earlier death might also be said to benefit the patient. He will be spared the physical burden of resuscitation and the somatic suffering of terminal lung cancer if he is simply allowed to die. Advocating what's best for Mr. Howard will be no easy task.

Given the complexity of the relationships (see above) aspect of this case, perhaps a family conference, which might air both the overt and covert issues in Mr. Howard's situation, would help to clarify the essential motives and values surrounding these hard choices. At the very least, the health care team could begin to get a sense of who was speaking for the patient's interests and who was promoting the needs of those who will survive Mr. Howard's death.

Conflicts

From the health-care team perspective, an important question emerges at once: Must physicians provide services that will surely prove futile? Does the fact that Mr. Howard asked for certain forms of care mandate giving it? Physician judgment is partly scientific, partly psychosocial. No patient can demand any intervention and expect to get it; legal and moral obligations are rarely absolute. For example, the end-stage kidney patient who yells for a transplanted organ "now" will still have to wait a turn for access to this scarce commodity. Physicians, particularly primary care doctors in their gatekeeper roles, are involved in cost containment and allocation (or rationing) determinations every day. Can Mr. Howard demand 20 more days in the ICU (at great financial cost) just because he wants everything done? Money aside, Dr. M. must ask himself if resuscitating and intubating this patient is medically or ethically responsible.

There is also a conflict between Mr. Howard and his children. Their earlier dispute was never resolved. Most hospitals, in the absence of an advance directive, look to the family for advice and consent. A type of pyramidal hierarchy is a common decision-making model. Top priority for surrogate decision-maker usually goes first to spouse, then to parent(s), adult children, siblings, and others. In Mr. Howard's case, the children will be consulted and uniformly ask for palliative measures. Should they do so readily? Or should be mandated to consult Mr. Howard's prior "self?" Do earlier views vanish with the loss of communicative ability or consciousness? At the very least, can the family members talk about this concept?

Finally, there is a possible issue among the health care providers. Even if Mr. Howard has full code status, his medical condition statistically makes it very unlikely that he will ever leave the hospital alive. Nurses, residents, and medical students will surely respect written orders in his chart, but were Mr. Howard to arrest, the aggressiveness and the duration of efforts at resuscitation are not quite predictable. He would surely not get the effort that, say, a child who had drowned might receive. But should his history and condition disqualify him from a concerted effort at resuscitation? Informally, one still hears about "slow codes," in which the bedside emergency is approached in a more lethargic manner than usual. Anticipating such dubious and illegal solutions to this conflict may be called for here.

Treatment or Nontreatment Options

Mr. Howard, under very different circumstances, could be a typical hospice patient. He is dying; his cancer has a terminal trajectory, though the precise timing and the nature of his death remain unknown. In addition, the patient has children who could provide home health care as he is dying; hospices usually require a primary caregiver who will take responsibility in the home. He is old enough to qualify for Medicare reimbursement for such palliative care. Hospices require, as a condition of enrollment, that code status be DNR; ventilators are also not an option. Giving adequate pain medication is a hospice strength, and, here again, Mr. Howard will need such an individually designed drug regimen.

But nontreatment (or, more positively, palliative care) has been rejected by the patient. Now in the hospital, unless his family moves him to a hospice setting, he will get some kind of conventional medical intervention. Eventually, a quality assurance or third-party payer official will ask a very concrete question: "What good is the treatment we are providing doing for Mr. Howard?" If the answer is "little" or "nothing," then the pressure will be on to transfer the patient, either home or to a long-term care facility. Outside the hospital, a limited treatment plan may be required, but within that plan will be a statement about what must happen if the patient gets notably worse. Will Mr. Howard be one of the countless patients to be sent to a nursing home only to return very soon by the revolving door of the ER or the admissions office?

If treatment within the hospital is chosen for this patient, there is clearly a range of possibilities (see **PATIENT**). While persons in Mr. Howard's condition are found in the ICU, their presence is rarer in this era of economic awareness. Mr. Howard will probably be admitted to a general medical-surgical service. His physicians, in the absence of a thorough reexamination of the ethical issues in this case, may elect to attempt resuscitation and other kinds of treatment. Eventually, Mr. Howard will die. How and when that occurs can be an object of negotiation, planning, or simply "letting nature take its course."

Interests

Legally it will be very hard to assert Mr. Howard's earlier desires in a definitive manner because he would not complete a living will. Perhaps if it had been explained to him that an advance directive can be used not only as a means of *limiting treatment* but also as a way of *requesting treatment*, he might have filled out and signed such a document. Access to his interests is deducible. His statement to Dr. M. should count for a great deal. Earlier declarations (to family members, to clergy, or in writing via letters, diaries, or journals) should be sought. But in most such cases, the patient's "statements" are general, vague, or nonexistent. Mr. Howard has at least said something.

Does this patient's desire to remain alive via medical technology advance his interests? If we define such interests as including the limitation of pain, perhaps we should say "No!" But if the interests also entail a continuing concern for personal integrity—a sense that decency includes trying to keep promises or respect prior declarations—then another scenario would develop. Even without cognitive awareness, Mr. Howard's interests may survive and impose on us an obligation to at least consider his wishes.

What about family interests? Some might argue that the children of Mr. Howard have a claim. Should they lose their patrimony through futile expenditures? Should they have to watch the suffering of their father during his last months, tethered to a variety of complicated machines? Should families in general have their interests weighed in balancing benefits versus burdens of continuing care? The danger does exist that a family's needs will betray a patient's interests. Is that a peril in this specific case?

Consequences

It's life or death for Mr. Howard. And more than that. There is also a matter of precedent, ethical if not legal. What are the policy implications if futile treatments are granted to patients in situations like Mr. Howard's? If we go in the opposite direction, and grant the family its choice, we are saying in effect that formerly competent patients who leave no written documentation of their treatment wishes will be at the mercy of families who disagree with their prior oral expressions. Both choices have far-reaching consequences.

The virtual certainty of the death of a patient does not end consequentialist worries. For example how we provide pain medication will have an impact on the number of days, and the quality of those days, Mr. Howard will survive. Conscious patients can sometimes administer their own drugs for pain. Mr. Howard is hooked up to an IV drip or a central line. A great deal of morphine will put him into deep and presumably painless sleep. If he dies very soon, have we set a precedent worth emulating? Or are we, in making death "easier," cheapening life itself?

Focusing on ends or results naturally leads us to think about the family. They will survive Mr. Howard's dying. And though we must not place their interests above that of the patient, we need not neglect them either. They will have to grieve for their father whose last days have been spent in a most frightening milieu — the hospital. Their feelings and their sense of satisfaction with the quality of care given Mr. Howard are very important. If Mr. Howard's treatment plan is a limited one, the fact that he got good and respectful care (including excellent hygienic attention and pain control) will be appreciated by the family, but if Mr. Howard is shunted off to a corner and neglected or given only minimal attention, the family will bear a scar of resentment toward the health profession that will surely remain for a long time.

Ethical Principles

One way of probing patient autonomy is to ask two concise questions. If Mr. Howard were (miraculously) alert, conscious of his condition, and could speak to us, what might we ask him? More importantly, what would he choose for himself? While there is no certain way of discerning an answer to these hypothetical questions, just asking them forces us to focus on this patient's individuality. Did his earlier conviction emerge from a well-considered sense of his past and future? How did it fit into the value scheme that Mr. Howard routinely consulted as he made his life choices? More concretely, what did Mr. Howard's desire to stay alive represent? Was it a response to the fear of death? Was it produced by apprehensiveness about being abandoned? Did Mr. Howard's determination reflect earlier family conflicts? In saying he did not want to die, was Mr. Howard commiting himself to the use of possibly futile technological strategies? Understanding autonomy requires the probing of contexts.

There is certainly a justice issue present. Is it fair to give Mr. Howard the intensive care he desired? The resources he has demanded are not exotic—he does not request a left ventricular assist device while awaiting potential heart transplant—but they are limited. Not only is ICU space at a premium, the literal time of intensivists is a cost not often calculated. But if we deny intensive care to Mr. Howard, we are faced with a corollary justice question: Is this patient being offered only palliation because he is old, very ill, and near death? Do we want to make it public policy that, after a certain age, patients no longer have a claim upon the public weal regarding health care?

If Dr. M. thinks that it would harm Mr. Howard to provide CPR, (that is, if he thinks that physical and chemical resuscitation have minimal efficacy and run grave risks) is it a violation of the principle of nonmaleficence to agree with the patient's earlier directive? Sorting out this question is subtle. It is easy to slip to self-affirming conclusions through rationalization. By saying that the principle of preventing harm means that I should allow Mr. Howard to die as easily as possible, Dr. M. could be smuggling into the calculation a quiet kind of paternalism. He could be saying that the physician knows best what the patient truly wants and needs.

■ CASES FOR DISCUSSION ■

Case A

Mr. H., a 32-year-old male was admitted via the emergency department to the coronary care unit (CCU) with extreme chest pain. After 24 hours, myocardial infarction was ruled out and his hospital course was unremarkable. Further testing in the CCU was ordered. Late the next night, Mr. H. had the nurse page the intern on call; he said that he had an important matter to discuss with her. The intern, Dr. N., came in almost immediately. The patient told her, insisting upon confidentiality, the reason he thinks he was so upset and required hospitalization. He says that in the early morning of the day prior to his hospitalization, he intentionally struck another person with his car. This man was the member of a motorcycle gang who had been threatening Mr. H.'s daughter. Mr. H. says that when he found out that this man had died a short time afterward (in the surgical intensive care unit) of the same hospital, he began to experience chest pains. The intern asks if anyone else is aware of this incident. Mr. H. says, "No, not the police, not my wife, no one. And you promised not to tell!"

Questions
1. What are the intern's legal obligations in this matter? How would you find out the answer to this question?
2. What ethical principles and practices inform the argument not to tell anyone about this incident?
3. What ethical principles and practices inform the argument to reveal the details of Mr. H.'s experience?
4. Suppose that Mr. H. tells the intern that he intends to harm other members of the motorcycle gang? What should be done then?

Case B

Mr. D. is a 72-year-old man, married for 50 years, who was admitted to the hospital with a history of shortness of breath and marked exercise intolerance. An angiogram showed coronary artery disease, aortic valve disease, and depressed ventricular function. Mr. D. also had a long history of hypertension and diabetes along with chronic obstructive lung disease. In the year prior to his admission, he had had two episodes that seemed to indicate small strokes; they cleared without residual neurologic effect.

The consulting surgeon discussed with Mr. D. his risk factors, which were multiple, and the significant operative risk. Mr. D., his wife, and the doctor agreed that an operation should take place. Accordingly, Mr. D. underwent replacement of his aortic valve and coronary artery bypass graft (CABG) surgery. A few days after surgery Mr. D. awoke, was able to follow commands, and gave no evidence of neurologic deficit. His pulmonary function was poor, however, and he remained intubated for 5 more days. In the step-down unit, Mr. D. appeared to be confused and often sleepy. He was taken back to the intensive care unit (ICU) for aggressive pulmonary treatment.

The next day Mr. D., while sitting in a chair, became unresponsive with severe respiratory distress. He was reintubated and placed on a ventilator. His right side was flacid; his left side could be moved spontaneously and responded to painful stimuli. He could neither communicate nor move on command. Mr. D. remained ventilator dependent and required a tracheostomy. Nutrition was supplied at first by hyperalimentation and later by tube feeding. Mr. D. spent 3 months in the ICU in this condition. The physicians approached his wife and asked her opinion about resuscitation, should Mr. D. arrest, and about continuing his intensive care.

Questions

1. Who should be making decisions about Mr. D.'s care?
2. What are some ethical bases for deciding to withhold or withdraw life-sustaining respiratory and nutritional support?
3. When should determinations about care for a patient unlikely to recover essential function be made?
4. On what grounds could we argue that Mr. D. should stay in the ICU until he dies?

■ THINK PIECE: CONCEPTS ■

An elemental assumption in medical education is that the practice of the science/art of healing can be taught. We can take this to mean that the structure and function of the body can be demonstrated and investigated; that the origin and progress of diseases and disorders can be studied, charted, understood, and often reversed; and that professionals can be educated to do the noble work of preventing and curing illness. Let us take this as a central value assumption and not challenge it.

What are the parallel assumptions about practicing medicine ethically? Few would claim that there is a standard or verifiable method of behaving ethically, in any profession. Codes and covenants have surely been available since ancient times, but their languages are often so general as to be vague (see Appendixes A and B). Medicine, the rational pursuit of the art of healing, has a long commitment to ethical behavior, but even the briefest of historic glances shows how perspectives have changed. It was commonly deemed better to withhold the diagnosis of cancer from patients only 30 years ago. The medical and ethical premise underlying this deceptive practice was a beneficent one: It might harm the patient ("We'll rob her of any hope.") to deliver a statement about a possibly terminal condition. Today, nearly all physicians routinely communicate such diagnoses, adhering to the legal and ethical mandates of informed consent and to the principle of veracity.

Admitting that value perspectives change should not lead to surrender in the attempt to help physicians behave ethically. Even if we cannot achieve the horizon, we can still struggle to get closer. The larger question, however, remains problematic. *Do we know how to educate physicians (or anyone else) so that they will act ethically?* Though courses and texts abound, few would claim that teaching ethics is a science. On the contrary, in a society in which value conflict seems to be the norm (controversies about abortion or about the right to die are illustrative), achieving predictability, no less than certainty, is always a frustrating goal. There are many suggestions about how to "make" physicians ethical. Emphasizing good role models is one. Selecting students who demonstrate sensitivity to human needs is another. Providing experiences in classrooms and on the wards in which careful moral reasoning is emphasized has also been recommended. Simply telling medical students and residents a fundamental truth, that central events in the life cycle such as pregnancy, birth, and death, are not only medical moments, is a start. Stressing the necessity of health care providers' viewing patient choices as more than technical, as most often psychological and value-laden would seem to be a beginning. Shifting the responsibility for patient care (often claimed to be a burden) from the physician per se to a shared partnership in which common interests are discussed and debated is an obvious goal.

Will such a strategy help to create physicians who act ethically? It is hard to say right now. We can be quite sure, however, that medicine, always more than a science, will not suffer by complementing its emphasis upon acute observation, careful methodology, rational analysis, and verifiability with attention to the subjective, choice-making experience of doctors and patients. And if we can figure out how to focus attention on the doctor-patient collaboration, we can perhaps discover ways of teaching physicians how to gain that needed appreciation for the impacts of their decisions, to see that to live is to choose.

■ VOICES: RISK MANAGER (HOSPITAL ATTORNEY) ■

I'm a pretty rare type of lawyer: Doctors trust me. Part of my job is defending doctors who get in trouble or who are being sued for malpractice. I see a lot of anxiety out there. I hear the worst stories. Most doctors I know are fine people who are doing their best. Sometimes mistakes are made. My job is to deal with problems before and, unfortunately, after they occur. Attorneys who represent suing patients are seen by doctors in a very negative light. Physicians tend to look at malpractice lawyers, at plaintiff's lawyers, as unethical and too zealous. Doctors see lawsuits as attacks on their competence and on their profession. They see lawyers as wanting to recoup money and not understanding anything but the patient's side. They (the lawyers) are overzealous because they don't take the time to fully review the case. They just go for the jugular.

Those doctors I know who have been sued have been changed by the experience. The resident who is 6 weeks out of medical school is sometimes devastated. When residents get sued they often respond with anger, or sometimes depression. If the resident has actually acted negligently, his or her behavior is likely to be modified right away. For example, if the malpractice case involved a failure to document, the resident usually becomes an extremely faithful documenter. I can never tell, incidentally, if these responses come from the resident's becoming a better doctor or emerge from fear of another lawsuit. Older doctors are less likely to change their behavior and look upon a suit as a one-time situation. Let's remember that getting sued doesn't mean you have made a mistake. Most malpractice suits are not meritorious.

I often wonder whether or not patients who sue doctors get a lot of satisfaction from such an action. Patients sometimes have to wait years and spend a lot on such lawsuits. For some patients the original goal gets lost. Others hang in there and seek vindication. When patients lose a case, they always blame their attorney or criticize the system. When they are victorious, they sometimes say that they have changed the physician's behavior and feel like pioneers.

I spend a lot of time working on credentialing and I see a number of incompetent physicians. These doctors we have to take out of the system. We cannot tolerate physicians who can't do the job; they should be removed, immediately, from patient care activities. Hospitals are responsible for doctors who perform incompetently. Many court cases show this. Unethical physicians do exist. If a doctor is unethical, he is likely to harm patients. If a doctor conveniently lies to patients, a possible charge of incompetence exists. If physicians cover up for themselves or others it is unethical, and I regard such doctors as incompetent and would take measures either to change their behavior or toss them out of the system. Medicine is more than just diagnosing or treating sick people. It includes being ethical.

I wish that physicians would pay more attention to confidentiality. There are too many breaches of privacy. Repeated violations should be grounds for summary suspension. That's a kind of middle ground punishment, between immediate termination and just pressing the problem on the head of the department or service, especially if the violation were negligent rather than intentional. But I take confidentiality to be very, very important, and state statutes and policies also mandate it. I would say to a doctor who was violating confidentiality all the time, "You have breached the policy; it will not be tolerated. You are going to be suspended until such time as you can appreciate the gravity of what you're doing. A responsible physician cannot be cavalier about confidentiality. It creates a liability for the hospital and for you. Most important, privacy counts for a lot in this institution. Anyone who violates that is not practicing competently."

Whistle-blowers (people who see what they think of as unethical actions in the hospital) often call me or visit my office. I depend, in some ways, on such persons. The nurse in the operating room who tells me, "Doctor X didn't get an informed consent," is someone I really need. However, I have to be careful. The status and the motives of the reporter matters. If the call comes because of a concern for patient care, fine.

But if it comes from an ongoing battle with this particular doctor, then I am suspicious. The institution has to have a policy to protect whistle-blowers.

My best advice, as a risk manager, for physicians and for doctors-in-training, is pretty obvious. Above all, you need to learn how to communicate clearly and truthfully with patients and with families. If you don't, you get into trouble. Medicine seems inherently paternalistic. Doctors often think, "I'll tell them the good news and I'll hold on to the rest." I think that doctors have to give the bad news when they know it. And if doctors do not know what is happening, they have to learn how to say, "I just don't know." You have to sit down and talk with the patient and family when you can't predict results.

It's important for physicians to document. A problem may not come up for 2 years. If you've charted accurately and thoroughly you can defend your care. Also, in general you need to follow-up on your patients. Patients don't drop off the end of the earth when you're not there on a Sunday. You need to keep in touch, for medical, ethical, and legal reasons. It satisfies the patient because the personal approach, which has declined since the '50s and '60s, is what medicine should be all about. Doctors should at least give the impression that they care.

As a risk manager, it is encouraging to see the growth of ethics committees and, more generally, to see doctors talking at last about situations that have moral and ethical ramifications. Just asking me, as a lawyer, "Is there a state statute that covers this problem," will never be enough. Nowadays, within medical departments and nationally, doctors are pursuing ethical issues and anticipating problems and crises. I am glad that doctors have gotten into the boat, have secured the oars, are leaving the bank, and getting ready to cross the river. Physicians do face ethical dilemmas, and I believe that the law alone cannot solve their problems. Getting these issues out in the open is a positive first step. The more they can hear from nonphysicians and from patients, the better off we will all be.

RECOMMENDED READING

Beauchamp, T. and Walter, L., eds. *Contemporary Issues in Bioethics*, 3rd edition. Belmont, CA: Wadworth, 1989.

Buchanan, A. and Brock, D. *Deciding for Others: The Ethics of Surrogate Decisionmaking*. New York: Cambridge University Press, 1989.

Burt, R. *Taking Care of Strangers: The Rule of Law in Doctor-Patient Relations.* New York: Free Press, 1979.

Faden, R. and Beauchamp, T. *A History and Theory of Informed Consent.* New York: Oxford University Press, 1986.

Gorovitz, S., et al. *Moral Problems in Medicine,* 2nd edition. Englewood Cliffs, NJ: Prentice-Hall, 1983.

Reich, W., editor, *Encyclopedia of Bioethics,* Volume 1–4. New York: Free Press, 1978.

■3■

Ethics at the Beginning of Life: Birth/Perinatology

Birth and death are elemental subject areas in clinical medical ethics, both qualitatively and quantitatively. Certainly the ongoing debate about the meaning and quality of our existence is centered around these moments in the life cycle. Concerns about pregnancy, abortion, birth, and infant survival (and the corollary concerns about the end of life, usually at advanced age) involve millions of persons each year. Few of us evade for long the significant life moments of birth and death, if not our own, then those of our friends, family, or other intimates. Around the beginning of life, in the realm of perinatology, value assumptions weigh heavily in decision making.

Today the law, or perceptions of what courts, legislators, and sometimes even prosecutors will do, influences decisions in obstetrics and gynecology as well as in perinatal and neonatal medicine. Patient expectations regarding medical professionals run high; the quest for the perfect baby is no utopian dream. Obstetricians have glorious new tools available, including ultrasonography, amniocentesis and chorionic villi sampling, continuous fetal heart rate monitoring, and fetal blood analysis via the umbilical cord. Keeping up with new developments presents a challenge to the obstetrician who delivers ten babies per week. So much can go wrong! Patients are better educated than ever, and, according to some physicians, also more demanding than ever. Doctors are no longer treated as oracles.

Sociologic changes have reinforced this revolution of rising expectations. Families are often limited to one or two children; each child is, thus, very special to parents. The rising desire for home birth (part of the demythologization of physicians' traditional roles) also at times presents an increased risk of medical emergencies. The feminist movement, including the important grass roots push for self-care and for women's autonomy, has also created anxiety for many conventional practitioners. Finally, issues involving birth inevitably precipitate controversy because they deal with sexual behavior and with mores (e.g., teenage pregnancy) that reflect societal uncertainties.

The medical model for pregnancy in late twentieth century North America instructs the physician to see the fetus and the mother-to-be as two separate patients. Intuitively, we may acknowledge the existence of separate entities, but the existence of the fetus and the pregnant woman are entirely intertwined. There are reports of brain dead women (one for 9 weeks, another for 107 days) being maintained on artificial life-support systems to allow for the growth and development of an infant born alive. Most pregnancies proceed smoothly, but when conflicts emerge the interests of the two parties may come into ethical conflict. Social norms promote the view that parenthood is a virtually indispensable part of an individual's life: Most people think that someday they will have children, that it is quite natural, and that it is necessary for personal and interpersonal fulfillment.

Such perspectives are taken for granted and work most of the time. For women who wish to resist medical advice about problem pregnancies or for couples who experience difficulty in achieving pregnancy and who must rely on new reproductive technologies, significant problems may emerge. The wonders of medical technology provide solutions for old problems and, often, create new ones. For example, the ability to see the fetus with ultrasound and new methods of prenatal diagnosis and treatment create pressures on potential parents, physicians, and the state to regulate conduct during pregnancy. The creative modes of bringing about the birth of a child via artificial insemination, in vitro fertilization, or with the aid of surrogate mothers entail dilemmas of choice and responsibility.

Though no subject has polarized Americans more than abortion, the wider areas of reproductive rights and, especially, of women's interests in making determinations about medical and moral matters have had a deep impact on health practice and policy as never before. A corollary social concern for newborns, especially those born with abnormalities that are sometimes life-threatening, has raised the issue of personal and social justice in the field of perinatology and particularly in neonatal intensive care.

Issues in medical ethics that center on the beginning of life have changed during the last decade. The 1960s and 1970s debate concerned abortion. Of course, substantial and often savage arguments persist about the moral validity of terminating a pregnancy. In the years since *Roe v. Wade* the practice has become widely established. Today, as the abortion controversy continues to fester, participants have interest in the outcome of another debate about the treatment, or nontreatment, of imperiled newborns. Very premature (less than 28 weeks' gestation) and very tiny (less than 1000 g in weight) newborns survive, almost routinely, in neonatal intensive care units (NICUs). Whether they live or die has become a societal, not only a medical or parental, issue.

With the use of respirators, feeding mechanisms, biochemical support, and sensitive monitoring devices, it is possible to sustain the growth of such newborns. Many leave the hospital. Others die in a matter of days or weeks. Still others are permanently and irreversibly disabled. Some are left dependent on the technology that saved them—permanently attached to a respirator or an intravenous line or tube for feeding. Some grow up and are just fine. Data change almost daily, but statistical analyses, though informative, do not settle discussions about who lives and who dies. Knowing for example, that 20 percent of 500-g babies born prior to 26 weeks' gestation survive says nothing about "our child" or "this patient." Medical uncertainty about any specific newborns makes it difficult to predict the future course of such babies' lives. Imprecision about prognosis creates anxiety.

Another complication is a government mandate (the so-called Baby Doe regulations) that requires reports concerning infants from whom medical treatment is withheld (see Fig. 3-1). Such legislation may intrude on the decisions of pediatricians and families. The search for objective measurements and rules is a frustrating one. Should all infants be treated, without regard to their individual quality of life? Should every form of intervention (e.g., neonatal kidney dialysis) be attempted in every case? Once a treatment modality has been started for the premature infant, may it ever be withdrawn? Is doing so a form of euthanasia? How is treatment itself to be defined—does it include medications, pain relief (which may sometimes suppress breathing itself), and any and all types of surgery? As in other clinical realms, the determination of precisely who is to decide is crucial. Legal and medical precedents suggest that parents have the right to make such determinations. But can a

---

In 1985, after a series of court cases and legislative struggles, government and physician groups agreed to implement rules that would govern the care and treatment of newborns with severe and profound birth defects. Passed by the U.S. Congress as amendments to the *Child Abuse and Neglect Prevention and Treatment Act*, the law mandates state child protective service agencies to scrutinize cases in which "medically indicated treatment" for infants may be withheld. Failure to provide such treatment that, in the treating doctor's professional judgment, will be effective or will overcome all life-threatening conditions is prohibited by the regulations. Particular attention is paid to providing "appropriate nutrition, hydration, or medication."

There are exceptions, however. Treatment may be withheld if the infant meets one of the following criteria:

- The infant is chronically and irreversibly comatose.
- The provision of treatment would merely prolong dying and be ineffective in ameliorating or correcting all of the infant's life-threatening conditions or be otherwise futile.
- The provision of such treatment would be virtually futile in terms of the survival of the infant and the treatment would in itself be inhumane.

Fig. 3-1. Neonatal ethics (Baby Doe regulations)

single mother just awakening from anesthesia, or a young couple traumatized by the discovery that their baby is suffering from a severe birth defect, make informed and clear decisions?

Most authorities agree that the best interest of the child should be the basis of the decision making in these often tragic cases. Such an ideal is hard to institutionalize. Imagine, for example, that parents see themselves as unable to care for a child with a severe birth defect and regretfully determine not to sign the consent form to perform surgery that might help the child. How can, or should, health care professionals (hospitals or governmental agencies) work to override the express beliefs of the parents? Institutional ethics committees (interdisciplinary panels working within specific care facilities) may be of some service in providing education and support. Should the courts become routinely involved as well?

Clearly connected to this issue is the recognition that treatment of imperiled newborns is extremely expensive. *Newsweek* recently reported on the typical $300,000 baby who survived neonatal intensive care; and prices rise almost daily. The costs of intervention could be reduced by investment in prevention. Social expenditures for prenatal care, for nutrition programs for expectant mothers, and for an educational campaign related to childbirth could save billions of dollars now spent on imperiled newborns. But is a cost-conscious nation, one in which health care costs are the fastest growing element in a deficit ridden budget, going to pay for the needed prenatal care?

Finally, if imperiled newborns do survive their first year or two of life, what services should we provide families facing the rearing of children with severe disabilities? Changes in values and social attitudes have occurred in recent years. Children born with Down syndrome (Trisomy 21) are not routinely warehoused anymore. Some families can find meaning, if not great happiness, in rearing very ill or disabled children. What obligations does society have to such offspring, whose life expectancy now approaches that of other persons born without genetic problems?

■ FIVE ESSENTIAL CASES ■

Case 3-1
Decisions about terminating a pregnancy are always difficult. The values, needs, and desires of the pregnant woman must be ascertained. They cannot be understood in a vacuum.

Ms. M. (age 24) and her boyfriend (age 29) of several years were referred for genetic consultation. They had planned this pregnancy. An ultrasound performed at the patient's request at 20 weeks' gestation revealed an abnormality. The obstetrician, Dr. R., conferred with the clinical geneticist, Dr. S., a physician specially trained in genetic analysis and counseling. The doctors suspected that a lethal fetal dwarfism was the problem. Ultrasound and x rays were hard to interpret, but seemed to show disproportionate limb-trunk length, marked shortening of the extremities, and deformity of the ribs. It seemed that the thorax was contracted and would make normal lung development impossible. There are many kinds of fetal dwarfism; not all are fatal. Dr. S. informed Ms. M. and her boyfriend (the physician asked Ms. M.'s permission first) of the situation. There were several possibilities. If the pregnancy were continued, there could be a spontaneous abortion (miscarriage), a stillbirth, or, if liveborn, the baby might die swiftly due to respiratory insufficiency. True cases of lethal dwarfism always result in infant death. The physicians were *not* certain of the diagnosis.

Ms. M. and her boyfriend discussed the evaluation, and their first response was to elect an abortion. They then asked for some time to think the matter over. Time was of the essence, because the pregnancy had now reached 23 weeks. After 24 weeks some babies can survive birth (with intensive neonatal care). Many physicians and hospitals are reluctant to perform abortions after 24 weeks. The couple also wanted to have more children. If this fetus were brought to term and died, clinical investigations might reveal the source of the problem (it could be a genetic one) and decisions about subsequent pregnancies might be given a scientific foundation. There was a further complication: Ms. M.'s parents and family were very religious Roman Catholics. She wanted to tell her family about her difficulties, and when she did they encouraged her to continue the pregnancy for religious reasons.

After some thought (24–48 hours), the couple decided to go ahead with the pregnancy. Four difficult, nerve-wracking months of uncertainty followed. The two physicians stayed in constant touch, the pregnancy became painful, and at 38 weeks' gestation a cesarean section was performed by Dr. R. The baby was born with the lethal form of dwarfism. The parents decided not to initiate resuscitative efforts or to transfer the baby to the nearby children's hospital for other interventions likely to prolong life. The infant was maintained comfortably in hood oxygen, and the parents were able to spend several hours with the infant as he died.

In any hard-choice medical ethics situation, identifying and discussing the patient's values, needs, and perspectives are indispensable first steps. In this case, such elements are difficult to discern. The desire to have a healthy baby is clear, but this fetus was likely, though not certain, to be born dying. Having an abortion was against the values of the patient's family. Even if a decision was made for elective abortion, timing factors made for difficulties. The decision not to have an abortion was made thoughtfully, but it was a difficult determination to continue the pregnancy.

For the obstetrician, Dr. R., suggesting to the patient that the pregnancy would likely be problematic was no easy task, but fortunately he was able to rely on the diagnostic and psychological skills of his colleague, Dr. S., the genetic counselor. The role of this physician-specialist is, traditionally, a value-neutral one. Genetic counselors are present to provide data, interpret information about risks and outcomes, and offer support for the patient's decision without regard to the content of that determination. Few genetics counselors, however, are unmoved by the kind of decision made by Ms. M.

Other queries emerge: What is the appropriate role, if any, of Ms. M.'s boyfriend? Also what of the influence of her wider family? Their values are not absent from this case. Do any of the parties in this case, including Ms. M., have responsibilities to the fetus and eventually to the child? Do the values of the caregiver have any substantive place in the discussion?

Knowing the results in this case, if you believe that Ms. M. was correct in bringing this child to term, would you believe that she was wrong had she elected an abortion? Had the suspected condition of the fetus been a nonlethal yet serious birth defect (e.g., spina bifida with a high lesion), would your judgment about right and wrong change? The principle of autonomy is the most frequently cited foundation for guaranteeing freedom of choice in such matters. But a principle, which presumes human reason as a basis for effective decision making, is an abstract notion. Emotional and intuitive elements cannot and should not be absent from such considerations.

After the baby was born, he was given comfort care only. His life could have been briefly extended with more dramatic medical interventions. The grounds by which the decision to limit care were made deserve investigation. Could it be seen as neglect to allow this child to die? Or does allowing a child to die who was born dying emerge from considerations of compassion and a desire to limit suffering? Beneficence is a principle that requires physicians and others to help those in need. While the extension of this baby's life was possible within severe limits, the concern for nonmaleficence might instruct parents and doctors to resist intervention in order to prevent further harm.

Case 3-2

Most birth experiences are positive. The doctor-patient relationship, a most intimate one, is rarely interrupted by outside forces. Occasionally, however, other interests, including the State's (through its courts), become involved.

Mrs. C. was brought into the emergency room at City Hospital by her neighbors after her membranes had ruptured. She reported no prenatal care. She agreed initially to electronic fetal monitoring. When data from the electronic fetal monitor (EFM) suggested fetal respiratory distress, Dr. N., the obstetrics resident, advised a cesarean section. Mrs. C. responded in a manner the resident described as "angry and nasty." The patient was told of the risks and benefits of the surgery but continued to refuse the cesarean section. "I've read about you guys," she stated, "you better not mess with me. Most of the time these operations are not necessary anyhow!" Her mother and her cousin, who had come to the labor room, tried to convince Mrs. C. but could not persuade her to change her mind.

Dr. N. asked for a psychiatric evaluation. The consulting psychiatrist evaluated the patient and found her to be cognitively aware of her situation and its risks and capable of rendering an informed consent or refusal. Dr. N. discussed the matter with the attending OB, who told her to call the hospital attorney. The lawyer immediately sought a juvenile court order to compel Mrs. C. to undergo the operation, on the grounds that the fetus was dependent and neglected. The judge came to the hospital and heard the patient's refusal to accept the doctor's recommendations and then asked the physicians about the risks involved. They told the judge that there was about a 75 percent chance of fetal death if Mrs. C. attempted vaginal delivery. They predicted a 90 percent chance of normal birth if the cesarean section were performed. They emphasized that the decision needed to be made "right away."

The problem presented by this case, as in so many medical-ethical dilemmas, is a consequence of the advanced technology that proves so useful most of the time. The increasing ability to diagnose and even treat the fetus (e.g., via prenatal diagnostic and screening techniques and, during labor, with monitoring devices that can register potential risks to mother and fetus during birth) also shifts the emphasis from maternal autonomy toward treating the pregnant woman and her unborn child as a single entity. Legally, posing the dilemma we see in the case of Mrs. C. as a fetal-maternal conflict appears to pit the rights of the fetus against the privacy rights and autonomy interests of the mother. A number of local and state courts *have* ordered cesarean sections.

More generally, concern for the health of the fetus has led to many novel legal and ethical situations for women near term in their pregnancies. In California, a woman was advised by her obstetrician to stay off her feet, not engage in sexual activities, and avoid street drugs. She was told to go to the hospital immediately if she started bleeding. When she did not follow this advice and gave birth to a baby with brain-damage who soon died, the mother was charged under a criminal statute with failing to provide support, a law intended to force men to provide for women they have made pregnant. In the District of Columbia, a court ordered a woman dying of cancer to undergo a cesarean section against her wishes and those of her husband and parents in order to try to save the life of a 25-week-old fetus, even though testimony stated that the operation would shorten the mother's life. The cesarean section was performed before the mother's attorney could appeal. She died and so did the nonviable fetus. An appeals court later said that the original judge acted improperly.

When in apparent conflict, maternal-fetal interests force a balancing act among maternal health, patient autonomy, and fetal needs. Finding a middle ground—seeking the counsel and consultation of experienced specialists—is surely fine advice. It usually works, but, as in the case of Mrs. C., difficult decisions must sometimes be made. If you were the visiting judge, what would be the first questions you would ask on arrival at the hospital? How impressed would you be by the argument sometimes made by doctors that once a woman has gotten pregnant and continued the pregnancy she has assumed a moral obligation to do everything reasonable to avoid harm to the fetus?

Pregnant women have been referred to as "fetal containers." Does this notion influence your judgment about what to do as Mrs. C. continues to refuse the operation? What rights and duties are involved in this case? Is Mrs. C. denying care to the nearly term fetus? If you think that Mrs. C. should be forced to follow doctor's orders in this situation, how far would you go in getting pregnant women to preserve and protect potential life? Some preventive medicine experts would prohibit smoking, drinking, and drug abuse. Obesity and the failure to control diabetes are also risk factors. How far shall we go in prohibiting dangerous behaviors or habits?

One utilitarian concern is that if judges order prenatal evaluations or cesarean sections regularly, it could encourage women to take matters into their own hands, avoid prenatal care, and not deliver in hospitals. The clinical-ethical challenge is to minimize the adversarial relationship (in this case, between obstetrician and patient). Few people want to see courts routinely involved in the delivery room. Encouraging understanding—utilizing a more empathic approach to problem solving—may extend the possibilities of negotiating agreement rather than mandating compliance.

Case 3-3

Seriously ill newborns mandate special care. In law and in common neonatal practice, intense efforts are made to ensure the survival and thriving of such babies. There are, however, limits to what can and should be done.

Baby Paula was born at term and weighed 3300 g. She was severely impaired with brain damage caused by birth asphyxia. A cesarean section had been performed after fetal distress was apparent, but prior to the surgery the umbilical cord prolapsed. Paula's Apgar scores were 1 and 2 at 1 minute and again at 5 minutes. Paula was placed on a ventilator but never demonstrated any spontaneous movement. She had no gag reflex and consequently could not swallow or take nutrition orally.

Efforts to wean the baby from the respirator were successful; she was able to breathe spontaneously after 1 day. Paula was watched carefully for the next 3 days and was given anti-seizure medication. She was not brain dead. The parents, for whom this was a first child, were told that Paula was in a deep coma. There was no certain way of telling if or when her state of consciousness might change. With artificial hydration and nutrition, Paula could survive indefinitely. The parents asked for some time to think over what they would do next.

Based on Emily D. Miraie and Mary B. Mahowald, Withholding nutrition from seriously ill newborn infants: A parent's perspective. J. Pediatr. 113 (2):262, 1988.

The onset of NICUs in the early 1960s had made it possible to coordinate the development of new technologies to save the lives of premature and otherwise ill infants who would have died in the past. Technology—often deemed a morally neutral set of tools given meaning by its use—has also opened up dilemmas and controversies, especially around the subject of so-called handicapped newborns. Paula was in that gray zone often encountered in the NICU; she was not actively dying, nor was she likely to ever develop the functions we usually attribute to healthy children. She could lie in a crib for a long period of time, without a ventilator, but only if she received quite intensive treatment, including tube feeding. The parents' situation is also a common one. They had no reason to anticipate anything but the birth of a vital child whom they would take home after a few days. Instead, Paula was hospitalized, perhaps forever.

The law has had much to say about handicapped newborns. In the early 1980s a set of regulations was developed (commonly called the Baby Doe Regulations) that govern withholding or withdrawing medical treatment from children like Paula (see Fig. 3-1). Since 1985, these regulations have taken the form of rules passed by Congress that require state child protection services to report and investigate medical neglect in the care of disabled infants with life-threatening conditions. Withholding nutrition is deemed a medical treatment and has often received disapproval from federal sources. The federal rules originated in a conscientious desire to prevent parents and physicians from allowing so-called defective newborns to die because they needed surgery or some other treatment that required parental informed consent.

Children are by definition incompetent, and others must make surrogate decisions for them. A competent adult has the legal right, sustained by common law, court cases, and much legislation, to refuse medical care; this is based on the ethical principle of autonomy and on the court-designated constitutional right of privacy. But babies like Paula are different, in law and in practice. Providing nutrition and hydration for Paula could be accomplished in a variety of ways including via nasogastric tube, gastrostomy, and peripheral or central intravenous lines. All would involve some risk to the baby, but without the hydration and nutrition, Paula would surely die in a matter of days. Paula would never be able to take food on her own; this is a given in this tragic case.

The warnings in the Baby Doe Regulations are not without substance. For those who think that neonatologists or parents do not always have the best interest of the child at the center of concern, the regulations protect the interests of those whose handicapping conditions, whether actual or perceived, make them vulnerable to maltreatment. For pediatricians and parents facing an uncertain future, or, as in the case of Paula, a future in which their child will never interact or experience life as commonly defined, the regulations are an impediment. Practices differ in other nations: In Britain and Sweden there is a presumption not to treat infants born weighing less than 750 g on the assumption that their prematurity would condemn them to a life of pain, suffering, or complete cognitive incapacity. In the United States, however, the presumption is to treat such infants vigorously, at least until some greater certainty about prognosis can be discovered.

Legally there are several exceptions to the mandate to treat newborns with disabilities. In three situations medically indicated treatment may be appropriately withheld: (1) from infants who are irreversibly comatose; (2) from infants for whom treatment would only prolong their dying; and (3) from infants for whom treatment would be futile and inhumane (see Fig. 3-1). We need to look at each of these exceptions in the case of Paula.

First, is Paula irreversibly comatose? Here, the axiom that good ethics depends on good medicine surely applies. Getting the best possible data about the patient, and comparing it with the most recent studies of infants in a like condition, is an indispensable first step. Certainty is likely to be achieved in answering this question. Neonatologists and pediatric neurologists can usually diagnose brain death—the absence of clinical evidence of cerebral or brain stem activity and the lack of evidence of intracranial blood flow can be confirmed. If brain death is not conclusive, it is difficult to resolve neurologic uncertainty. Some infants with severe brain damage at birth, like Paula, eventually die. Some enter a vegetative condition (Paula seems headed in that direction). Some survive with profound impairments, including what we call cerebral palsy (an umbrella term) and mental retardation. There is always the remote possibility in Paula's case that she will sustain less severe damage. Therefore, answering the question about her likely prognosis remains difficult.

Second, would treatment prolong Paula's dying? Answering this question (which would allow an exception to the Baby Doe Regulations) presumes we can state, definitely, that Paula is in a terminal state. Certainly, the absence of food and water would shorten Paula's life, but would continuing feeding and other interventions do anything but lengthen her dying? Much of this is also dependent on medical judgment. If she were to show signs of cerebral activity, physicians might recommend a wait and see approach. But for how long? A satisfactory definition of terminal status is notably lacking, and not only in neonatal settings. Again, there is room for interpretation and debate.

Third, would providing artificially supplied hydration and nutrition be futile and inhumane? It might be futile if we have virtually no hope for restoring Paula's ability to function. It would, of course, keep her alive for a while but risks are also involved. Feeding a child without a gag reflex via nasogastric tube can hasten death because of possible aspiration of food or secretions. The concept of inhumane treatment often entails an assessment of the pain and suffering that the infant could sustain. Just how Paula might experience pain is in doubt. Many of us might think that without those areas of the brain that perceive painful stimuli working actively, Paula will never experience pain as we define it.

Important ethical issues are raised in this case. The personhood, the elemental humanity, of patients like Paula needs to be defined. Paula will most likely never be aware of human experience, never know herself as a self, or have the capacity to develop relationships with those who are closest to her. How important is it for the resolution of this case that Paula is unlikely to experience pain subjectively? What are her best interests? How do we define her interests at all?

Assessing the proper weight to be given to parental concern is no easy task. If we focus exclusively on the significance that should be given to the likelihood of Paula's surviving and growing up with profound physical or mental disabilities or both, we may ignore or slight family needs, including financial problems, which surely should be taken into consideration. In pediatric medicine, parents usually make decisions on behalf of their nonautonomous offspring. A compelling reason to make an exception to this norm is found in cases of child abuse and neglect. Does the case of Paula fall into this category?

Finally, what importance should be given to the real and symbolic nature of feeding and giving water to dependent patients? Is a nasogastric tube different from a tube connecting an infant to a ventilator? How does our language influence our choices: Calling the removal of the NG tube starving Paula to death seems very different from stating that her parents are considering withdrawing artificial alimentation. Is it cruel to withdraw the NG tube if we are nearly certain that no pain will be experienced by the infant? As a rule, when the benefit of medical treatment is unclear, the tendency is to defer to parental decisions made after consultation with medical and nursing professionals. If we decide to follow another protocol, we may force physicians and hospital administrators to be literally and unendingly responsible for children they are treating.

Case 3-4

Surgical intervention in perinatal cases is based on the premise that medicine is dedicated to both maintaining life and diminishing suffering. When risks are difficult to assess, however, parents and physicians must make judgments about life and death that are ethical in content.

Baby V. was born at an estimated gestational age of 26 weeks with a birth weight of 820 grams and was ventilator dependent. His problems included pulmonary hypoplasia, respiratory failure, persistence of fetal circulation, and bronchopulmonary dysplasia with frequent episodes of hypoxemia and hypercapnia. After 11 weeks in the NICU, Baby V. was still on a ventilator but was frequently alert, with good eye contact, and was increasingly active. A grade II intraventricular hemorrhage had been resolved and an ophthalmologic examination indicated a progressive retinopathy associated with prematurity; cryosurgery was recommended to the parents.

Before the surgery could be performed, the infant developed necrotizing enterocolitis (NEC), which required a laparotomy for a sentinel loop of bowel. The infant was stabilized after partial resection of the ileum. The parents were overwhelmed by this series of crises. The neonatologists sought permission to go ahead with the eye surgery. The parents were reluctant: They stated, "Enough is enough. Baby V.'s breathing will probably never be normal. He will always be dependent on special care for nutrition. The stress on our lives is overwhelming. We have other children to care for. Another surgery is obviously risky. We don't want to put him through more."

The surgeons and the NICU were divided. They knew that they were working with responsible, loving parents who did not believe that surgery would foster their child's best interests. The physicians were reluctant to give up. The data regarding Baby V.'s survival was, as always, incomplete. The situation was one of uncertainty. Even if Baby V. were eventually to leave the NICU, he would most likely be ventilator-dependent and regularly subject to numerous complications. The cost of caring for this child, in the hospital, and, if such were the outcome, later on would be in the millions of dollars. The physicians referred the case to the hospital's bioethics committee.

Our perspective on what ought to be done in the case of Baby V. is necessarily interpretive, a function of our perspective on a variety of medical and ethical issues. For example, is human life a sacred thing? Does every person, without regard to sickness or disability, have an equal right to life? Should matters of life and death be in the hands of physicians or (perhaps) spiritual leaders? These are fundamental, theologic questions, and, though we often consider clinical medical ethics to be a secular task, it often crosses the border into the realm of religion.

If we eschew such an approach and concern ourselves with the scientific basis of a decision regarding Baby V., we also encounter difficulties. Can there be objective standards in neonatal care? Using statistics from earlier cases or studies can help identify which infants are most likely to benefit from treatment. Using measurable data (e.g., gestational age, Apgar scores, birth weight, and severity of lesions) and survival rates from other surgeries should lead to a clearer notion of whether proceeding is medically indicated. Responsible surgeons will tell you, however, that you cannot always predict an outcome. There are many anecdotes about the survival of babies who supposedly had no real chance to leave the NICU. Even if objectivity (or, even less likely, certainty) is possible, some parents are apt to ask for intervention even if the outcome is potentially fatal. Baby V.'s parents are asking for the cessation of intervention, but not necessarily on the grounds of objective, verifiable data.

The basic concern, so often repeated (without much conceptual scrutiny) in pediatric medicine, is the "best interest of the child." Such a perspective seems quasiobjective and patently utilitarian, assuming that someone can weigh the potential risks and benefits to Baby V. The standard is a useful, but sometimes vague, yardstick. Just what those interests are is hard to determine. Does Baby V. have an interest in being free from pain? In seeing, if the cryosurgery is successful? In having parents who can care for him? In dying without discomfort? In being dependent on a ventilator?

The other commonly heard notion, quality of life, is also notoriously hard to define. Many have argued that raising quality of life issues discriminates against handicapped newborns who are unaware of both their disabilities and what a presumably normal life means. For those who use such a concept in a noncomparative fashion, focus is placed on the infant's degree of illness, capacity for comfort, happiness, pain and suffering, and long-term outlook. Usually, much emphasis is placed on mental capacity. Many physicians and parents are willing to support continuing care for infants who will never walk, but are reluctant to do the same for those who will never think. An emphasis on communicative capacity, relational potential, is another dimension of quality of life. Is there built-in discrimination in this concept too?

Meanwhile, Baby V. is a candidate for serious surgery. The decision to proceed will be made collaboratively, between parents and physicians. Given the medical and perhaps moral uncertainty about what is in this child's best interest, can we find an operational rule that might lead to a useful conclusion? In circumstances of uncertainty, should we defer to parental desires, as long as no punitive motives can be shown? Or should we, as is so often the case in contemporary medicine, "err on the side of life" and, in this situation, attempt another surgical rescue operation?

Case 3-5

Practicing clinical medicine in an ethical fashion, doing the right thing, may not always be enough. For example, telling the truth may be morally required, but crisis situations often demand even more of the physician.

Sarah and Michael were expecting their first child. They had been married for 6 years, were both in their 20s, and in excellent health. Sarah's prenatal care was provided by an OB/GYN, Dr. N., who had been her physician for 3 years prior to her pregnancy. She went through routine office visits calmly, responded (as did Michael) enthusiastically to seeing their baby via ultrasound, and during pregnancy showed no signs or symptoms requiring special care. Dr. N. was in a small OB/GYN group (there were three physician partners, a nurse midwife, and several nurses), and he made sure that Sarah and Michael were acquainted with the entire staff. Arrangements were made for delivery at H. Hospital. The parents-to-be attended childbirth classes, briefly discussed and rejected natural childbirth as an option, and began preparation of a small bedroom for the baby when she came home.

Sarah went into labor at term late on a Saturday evening. Michael and Sarah called Dr. N.; his service reported that he was out-of-town for the weekend but that his partner, Dr. J., was on call. When Dr. J. called back, she told Michael and Sarah to meet her at the hospital. The couple checked in without any difficulty, and routine monitoring did not show any fetal problems. Labor proceeded quite smoothly (at the appropriate time Sarah was given an epidural for pain control) and fairly rapidly. Michael was present in the delivery room. The monitor, which showed nothing remarkable, was turned off during the final phase of delivery. The baby was born with the umbilical cord around her neck, was blue, and not breathing. Efforts at resuscitation did not succeed. Sarah's initial response was to cry and then to remain silent in response to questions by the nurses and her husband. Michael asked Dr. J., "How could this have happened?"

Very few babies die at childbirth. Michael's question to Dr. J. was a medical and moral inquiry that can be answered by the same response. Dr. J. simply has to tell the truth. If she does not know it (if further investigations are necessary in order to find a cause of the baby's death) then she must say, "I don't know right now. We will try to find out and will tell you immediately." Sarah can say virtually nothing. She needs some time to recover from both the shock of the stillbirth and the impact of the medications she has received during the birthing process. She will surely have questions later.

It appears that doing the right thing is singular; Dr. J. should be honest and open with Sarah and Michael. She should not try to hide any facts nor be concerned with future problems, such as potential litigation. Things are not so simple, however, when a person dies, perhaps especially during birth. The psychological climate provided by the physician and hospital during the patient's stay after stillbirth has an ethical dimension as well. Perinatal loss, and the grieving process that surrounds it, call for medical and ethical interventions, not all of which receive much discussion among practitioners. One immediate choice that must be made in the delivery room concerns what to do with the baby. Should the parents be encouraged to hold the child, to take a snapshot, to verbally express feelings about the dead infant? Offering this option is a most sensitive task: Parents are very suggestive at such moments. Sophisticated OBs realize that the grieving process is a long-term agenda: Is it helpful or harmful to begin it right away? Consulting an experienced OB nurse can be useful.

In order to meet the parental request for information about the death of their baby, and in order to be able to give advice about subsequent pregnancies and deliveries, an autopsy will have to be performed. In most jurisdictions, the county coroner's office must be notified of an unexpected death in the hospital, but unless public officials mandate an autopsy, parental consent must be sought by the attending physician shortly after the stillbirth. Dr. J. naturally will feel a need to discuss the matter in a sensitive manner with the parents. Michael and Sarah are likely to respond positively to such a request; it is certainly a rational and appropriate next step. If they do have an objection, even an irrational one, how can this be dealt with? Are these parents being given a choice? If they consent to the autopsy, who will pay for it? Insurance policies do not cover such procedures, and the cost could be substantial.

Can a physician even begin to know how to speak with Sarah and Michael without probing the background of their story, without being sensitive to their hopes, expectations, disappointments, and angers? Parental grief after stillbirth was once treated in an almost cavalier fashion. The assumption was that not talking about it would help the family to get over it. Sometimes, physicians or nurses said, "Well, at least you can try again!" The support of friends and relatives was assumed to be sufficient to get the couple through the time of crisis. Today, health care professionals know that much more is required.

The doctor-patient relationship and its ethical substructure does not dissolve after the initial consultation. Sarah and Michael will have many questions and may want to continue their connection to Dr. J.'s group of practitioners. Certainly giving factual, current, and straightforward medical information is a first step. In order for the parents to make sense of this tragedy, much more is required. The father must be reassured that his wife is in good medical health at least. The mother must know that the stillbirth was not her fault. Physician's responses to parental grief symbolize trust or the lack of it in the healthcare delivery system for the parent. Should bereaved parents be given the option of a private room away from the maternity ward? Should sedatives be prescribed for the mother, who may be both fatigued and incapable of sleeping? Will such drugs mask the grief?

Clinical ethics in practice demand more than cogitation, reflection, or the resolution of issues. The very words of the physician matter enormously. If Sarah and Michael say to Dr. J., "Well maybe this wouldn't have happened if Dr. N. had been available," many responses may be evoked. Simply telling the truth will not be enough. A truthful statement would be, "Such surprise stillbirths happen rarely, and Dr. N. would not have been able to do anything different from what we did."

Reacting nondefensively in a human and humane fashion means going beyond truthfulness. Stating that, "at least the baby died before you got too attached to her," is perhaps honest. It also obscures deeper truths: that physicians are also disappointed; that not everything works out all the time; that birth is still something of a mystery, notwithstanding our technologic powers. A statement by the doctor such as "I know how you feel," is not useful because it is patently false. A more basic and more honest response might be, "I am so sorry that your baby died." This validates parental feelings and may help Sarah and Michael feel less isolated. Learning how to listen, even to unpleasant emotions such as anger, can be more than therapeutic. It can provide a milieu in which the resolution of ethical issues blends gradually and naturally into a psychologically useful (even satisfying) enrichment of the physician-patient relationship.

■ PRACTICE MODEL CASE ■

O. C., aged 23, was admitted with vaginal bleeding to the emergency department of a small, rural community hospital. Her husband accompanied her. She told the staff that she was more than 20 weeks pregnant but that she had not received prenatal care because she could not afford to go to the doctor. Her husband told the nurse that he was an outdoor laborer and that his wife stayed at home. O. C. said that her family was Roman Catholic and that she had been raised in a conservative farming community. They have no close friends in this small town. Her obstetric history was quite unusual. She had had five previous pregnancies. Three of them ended in spontaneous abortions, and two yielded live births. One of those was a premature delivery at 29 weeks' gestation. The child, Linda, is now 3 years old and has significant mental retardation (MR) and "lung problems." The second child, Billy, was a term delivery and, at age 1 year, seemed to be developing normally.

The OB gave O. C. a complete physical examination and diagnosed an incompetent cervix, with a high probability of premature delivery. The doctor then advised her about possible courses of care or treatment for the balance of the pregnancy: (1) bedrest restriction; (2) performance of a *cerclage* (a stitch through the cervix to prevent premature dilatation), which might increase chances of a term delivery; or (3) letting nature take its course. The first choice seemed unlikely: With two small children at home and without resources for respite care, bedrest was hardly an option unless O. C. were hospitalized. The couple conferred and decided to proceed with the cerclage. O. C. consented in writing. The procedure was performed without complications, and the patient returned home.

Three weeks later, O. C. was readmitted to the hospital. She had seen a doctor—her gestational age was determined to have been 22 weeks at the time of her emergency department care—and now she was experiencing uterine contractions. Her physician, an OB/GYN, thought that labor was imminent. He told her that for the fetus (now 25 weeks' gestational age) to have any significant chance for survival she would need to be transported to a hospital with an NICU; the closest such facility was more than 200 miles away. He also explained that there would be a risk of abnormalities in the birth of such a premature infant.

Again, there were several choices. The cerclage could be removed and nature might take its course. Just when the patient might go into labor was unpredictable. Once labor commenced there would be no choice: The cerclage would have to come out to avoid the risk of uterine rupture. O. C.'s obstetrician could deliver the baby at the local hospital, but in this rural setting the only pediatrician available was away and her duties had been assumed by a general practitioner with very limited neonatal experience. It was likely that immediate delivery of a premature infant would result in death. The couple did have the option of transfer to the distant tertiary care center with an NICU. There the chance of survival for the baby would be about 10 to 20 percent. The C.s did not have insurance that would reimburse transportation costs, but they were concerned about more than financial costs. The emotional burden of another "defective" child was also considered.

Based on Angeline Bushy, J. Randall Rauh, and Bernard F. Matt, "Ethical Principles: Application to an Obstetric Case." J. Obstet. Gynecol. Neonatal. Nurs. 18:3, 207–212, 1989.

Patient

A miscarriage is the loss of a pregnancy at a stage before a fetus is born alive. Most miscarriages take place during the first trimester and are due to a defect involving the fetus or the placenta in the early development of the fertilized egg. Occasionally miscarriage occurs because of an acute or chronic illness of the mother. Most later miscarriages result from a structural problem with the uterus: It is unable to retain the pregnancy until term. Most such miscarriages are not the result of an inherited defect, but some are and O. C. is in a high-risk category. Her history suggests structural difficulties.

A so-called incompetent cervix can be responsible for spontaneous abortion between weeks 16 and 28 of gestation. (This archaic terminology is unfortunate and could be regarded as another example of blaming the victim.) An incompetent cervix may be due to soft stretchy tissue in the cervix, rendering it incapable of resisting the normal contractions of pregnancy. It could also be due to damage by a previous miscarriage, termination of a pregnancy, or a normal or forceps delivery. These causes of incompetent cervix matter little in this case. O. C. agreed to the cervical cerclage, which entailed reinforcing the internal os by circling the cervix under general anesthesia with nylon or dacron tape or thick sutures. Bleeding, cramps or ruptured membranes indicate that the cerclage sutures should be removed promptly. Uterine contractions could result in lacerations; delay in expulsion of the uterine contents could result in serious infections. Not much time is available for a decision in this case.

Psychologically, the couple is not totally surprised by these complications. Earlier pregnancies have been difficult. This one has required emergency intevention. Their history weighs heavily on them. They have few financial resources, and the possibility for community support is also minimal. Their experience with their retarded child, Linda, is another influence. How the couple sees the 25-week-old fetus is central to their decision. Their perspective will surely depend on many factors, including the nature of their own relationship. Their religious convictions may also be important, but they certainly need further exploration.

Relationships

The C. family, though limited to a single generation, is a complicated entity. Mr. and Mrs. C.'s individual and mutual concerns are filtered through their experience of several miscarriages and a problem delivery. Their life with their children has been unusual and not simple. We must not assume, however, that having a child with MR is an entirely negative experience. Some families, particularly religious ones, report a sense of challenge and fulfillment from raising children with disabilities. Because the decision about this imminent birth will be made by O. C. (presumably with the support or contribution of her spouse), the projection of future relationships within the family will also be considered.

O. C. now has a fiduciary relationship with her OB. It is a new one, but it is important enough for her to want this doctor to continue to render care. This physician, aware of the headlines, of the legal vulnerability, and of high malpractice insurance premiums for OB/GYNs, may be cautious in agreeing to deliver what might be a stillborn or severely defective baby. Her fidelity to the patients is a fact of this relationship. How it evolves is not predictable.

Advocacy

To advocate means to struggle on behalf of another. Who is that other in the case of O. C.? She is, presumably, a competent, autonomous adult patient and can accept or refuse treatment on the basis of the information provided her. O. C.'s self-determination takes precedence, all other things being equal. From the advocate's viewpoint are other things equivalent? Could the fetus, statistically capable of viable, though assisted, existence outside the womb, be regarded as an incompetent patient? Does the parental concern for an adequate quality of life for their fetus and for themselves impede the future autonomy of that entity?

A strenuous advocate for the fetus might argue that there is a maternal obligation to provide the best possible care for that unborn baby. Others with a less rigorous but perhaps more realistic point of view might claim that parents must pursue all available treatment, which in this case might include big city NICU care or even flying in a specially skilled pediatrician.

Certainly, anyone wishing to discover the rights and duties in this case would have to inquire: What impact did the initial decision to have the cerclage have on the decision now being pondered? Did the original agreement, in effect, create a commitment to do almost anything to save the life of the fetus? Or was it a time-limited experiment that failed after a few weeks?

Conflicts

The most apparent conflict, characterized rather harshly as a fetal-maternal dispute, centers around deciding whether or not to attempt an NICU rescue of the fetus. A determination about transportation amounts to a resolution of this dilemma. Earlier cases of conflict between mother and fetus have sometimes been resolved by what the Roman Catholic church calls the doctrine of double effect. A pregnant woman, for example, who has uterine cancer and whose uterus is removed in the interest of preserving her health is not regarded as morally despicable even though the results are disastrous (i.e., fetal death). The effects are unintended consequences. The doctrine states that some actions have both good and evil results. If an act's motivation is good or pure and the secondary effect is one that is harmful to another person, the original act may still be morally virtuous. This is ethics of motives. Consequences, though not ignored (the good results must be proportional to the evil ones), do not prohibit or justify such actions.

Seeing the C. family case purely in terms of a single or simple conflict may be misleading. The cerclage would not be removed for the purpose of improving maternal health. Running the risk of letting premature labor progress may not be focussed solely on the goal of benefitting the unborn child. Anxieties about financial burdens and subsequent psychological trauma for the family if the child survives neonatal special care are also implicated. O. C. has never, intentionally or otherwise, sought to harm her fetus. She has not used drugs, alcohol, smoked cigarettes, or engaged in dangerous behavior. On the contrary, she has wanted to have a baby and without complicating problems.

Treatment or Nontreatment Options

The options are obvious. O. C. can ask to retain the cerclage (it will be nearly impossible to force her to submit to the procedure required to remove it) and run the risk of bleeding, infection, or permanent damage. Retaining the cerclage is not an option at all because the danger would be too great. If O. C. consents to have the cerclage removed then the fetus will most likely be born, in great (probably irremediable) distress at the local hospital, attended by a physician with a paucity of experience in such cases.

There is also the possibility that O. C. could agree to be flown to the large urban hospital. There, she could wait and see. Gestational age of the fetus is a crucial element in any outcome. Most likely, her labor will progress and she will deliver a fetus who would be taken to the NICU. If the result is a stillbirth, an effort to resuscitate the fetus will likely be made in the delivery room. Once the child is born and is taken to the NICU, results are unpredictable. Federal regulations and hospital policy and practice are likely to govern (see Fig. 3-1). All the choices involve matters of autonomous choice, beneficent concern for the dual patients, and economic issues of cost and access to the health care system, and they must be decided right away.

Interests

All parties would like to have a healthy child be the result. Maternal interests and future interests for the baby are identical, in this view. But a medical crisis — organically based, but ethically complex — has created an impediment. The interest of the parents must take into account the financial realities, the needs of their other children, and the problems of being in a geographical area where only limited medical services are available.

The interests of the fetus or child require determination. Do third-trimester fetuses have an interest in being born? Do 26-week-old premature infants have an interest in long-term survival? Some authors think that such questions are unanswerable. Certainly neonates without severe brain damage have an interest in being free of pain and in being kept warm and nourished.

Do the local physicians and hospital administrators have identifiable interests as well? How much should the reputation of the institution matter? Will the local general practice physician suffer a loss of esteem if, as expected, he fails to provide needed neonatal services? Does the community itself have an interest in helping those in grievous need? How can this interest be asserted? Is there a justice claim in this case: Those who argue for a kind of medical affirmative action might say that preferential treatment ought to be given to those with the greatest need. Does the C. family fall into this category?

Consequences

In the short term consequences of any of the treatment or nontreatment options are hard to predict. If the cerclage is removed and the fetus is born at the rural hospital, it is still remotely possible that survival might occur. (Even the best dating of gestational age is an estimate, and there are exceptions to all but the most absolute statistics.) Death at birth or within minutes after birth is more likely. The meaning of this result for the parents is hard to imagine. We cannot know results in advance. Statistically there is no reason to expect a child with birth defects to be born. If autopsy reveals that the child was severely or profoundly handicapped, then Mr. and Mrs. C. may feel in the midst of their overall grief that much pain and suffering was prevented. We cannot know this.

If the parents follow the recommendation of going to the city hospital and the child is born alive and is placed in the NICU, consequences are also hard to prophesy. The child could die, swiftly or slowly. She could live for a few weeks or a few years. She could leave the hospital after several months and come home. Her growth and development are unpredictable. Statistically she is likely to have many problems, due to low birth-weight and prematurity. Not all such babies require long-term institutionalization. Many go to public schools through mainstreaming programs and live with their families. Again, we cannot be sure what level of impairment might be sustained.

The longer-term consequences are interesting. What will be the nature of the marriage, no matter what the results for the fetus, of Mr. and Mrs. C.? What are the responsibilities of the local health care providers in this small rural town to this family? If the child survives who will fund the social services she may desperately need? (If she enters the school system, the cost of providing speech and hearing services for this one child could equal the price of all extra-curricular activities for the entire school district.) What are the consequences of flying every at-risk mother 200 miles for a procedure and rescue operation with unknown benefits?

Ethical Principles

Virtually every basic principle in clinical medical ethics is present in the case of the C. family. Certainly the commitment to autonomy means that in a hard-choice situation the views of the principal patient (here, O. C.) receive priority. In order to be touched, transported, or taken to surgery she must consent. The capacity to consent means the right to refuse care. For those who claim that fetal rights are established in this case, O. C.'s autonomy may interfere with those rights. To force her into a course of action however, would abridge her autonomy.

Beneficence, promoting the well-being of patients, can take many forms. Helping O. C. understand the nuances of her situation can be most helpful, and it will also nourish the doctor-patient relationship and promote the principle of veracity. Determining what is in her best interest can move even the most supportive and intelligent doctor into the realm of paternalism. If O. C.'s liberty is limited—if a guilt trip about her ostensible responsibility to the very premature infant is enunciated—then beneficence can come into direct conflict with autonomy.

The other side of the coin mandates health care professionals to avoid harm, to practice nonmaleficence. Protecting persons from pain and suffering and from danger is an inherent obligation of physicians and nurses. Pain can be variously described and understood. A local delivery might reduce the family's emotional pain and having a mentally retarded child can also cause collective suffering, but such predictions are notoriously inaccurate. Avoiding harm as a principle depends on who is the focus of such a noble motive. Certainly there is great potential harm if the fetus is born with severe, perhaps fatal and painful, birth defects. Statistically (again, a dangerous territory in making moral judgments), this is the likely outcome if O. C. is taken to the tertiary care hospital.

The principle of justice tells us that fair and equal treatment of patients must be pursued. It also takes us outside individual cases and into the realm of social policy, with particular concern for the allocation of scarce health care resources. The C. family is needy in many ways. Some needs could be alleviated. (Providing respite child care earlier in the case might have allowed the pregnancy to proceed with fewer difficulties.) Flying in a neonatologist to the rural hospital might influence the choice. But who will pay for this unusual, some might say preferential, treatment? Will this serve as a useful precedent when other, similar cases evolve?

■ CASES FOR DISCUSSION ■

Case A

Rachel Allan is a third-year medical student (who has never been pregnant) beginning a clinical rotation in the OB clinic at a large urban hospital. Among her limited responsibilities is talking with pregnant women who have come in for alpa-fetoprotein (AFP) screening. This blood test is usually done between 15 and 18 weeks from the last menstrual period. It measures a substance that, if markedly lowered or elevated, may indicate problems with normal growth and development of the fetus. Among the birth defects that can be detected by AFP testing are spina bifida and Down syndrome. It is quite possible for the AFP test to yield false-positive results. Further screening (including a second blood test, ultrasound examination, or amniocentesis) is usually recommended if preliminary findings are significant.

One day in the OB clinic, Ms. Allan is interviewing a 19-year-old-woman pregnant for the first time. The medical student explains the nature of the test, emphasizing that 95 percent of babies with neural tube defects or Down syndrome are born to families without a history of these disorders, and tells the patient that taking it is completely voluntary. The patient asks, quite sincerely, "You are only a few years older than I am. I hate having blood taken from me. Do I really need this test? Would you do it if you were me?"

Questions

1. Considering the nature of the information provided to the patient, in what sense do you understand the medical student's statement that taking the test is "completely voluntary."
2. Who is the most appropriate person to talk with a pregnant woman regarding pregnancy screening?
3. How do you interpret the patient's effort to press the medical student for an opinion regarding the test?
4. How should Ms. Allan respond to this inquiry? What should her purposes be if she chooses to answer?

Case B

Dr. P. is an OB/GYN in private practice with admitting privileges at two tertiary-care hospitals. Twice each month he works in the OB clinic at C. Hospital, serving patients without private doctors. Most of his work is providing prenatal care. He often recommends prenatal diagnostic studies and, on occasion, he refers patients for genetic counseling. During the past 3 months he has been seeing Ms. R., a 23-year-old single woman with a boyfriend who lives with her; she is pregnant for the first time. She revealed to him on their first meeting that she was abusing crack cocaine. More recently, he has detected a detached placenta. Last month, after consulting about Ms. R.'s condition with several colleagues, he told the patient two things: (1) Cease using the illegal substance and (2) abstain from sexual intercourse because of the placental irregularity.

Yesterday, at another routine clinic appointment, Ms. R. told Dr. P. that she was continuing to use the drugs. "I'll stop after the baby is born," she said, "right now I really need the stuff." Regarding sexual intercourse, the patient volunteered that she had "cut down" and reported sexual activity "no more than three times during the past month." Dr. P. has read that prosecutors have recently been trying (with some success) to indict women who have given birth to infants testing positive for the presence of illegal substances. The physician tells his patient that she is risking great danger. He wonders how far he should go in attempting to protect the fetus.

Questions

1. There are estimates that the health care costs of treating and caring for drug-exposed neonates may be as high as $3 billion per year. Should the total economic impact of this problem influence Dr. P.'s determination about what to do with regard to the behavior of Ms. R?
2. Dr. P. has learned that the patient is engaging in illegal activity. What are his moral obligations in this matter?
3. If Dr. P. offers to help his patient enroll in a voluntary drug treatment program and she refuses, should he make an effort to mandate treatment via legal methods?
4. What are the most important interventions for Dr. P. to consider regarding Ms. R.'s continuing to engage in sexual activity contrary to medical advice?

■ THINK PIECE: BIRTH ■

Getting pregnant is sometimes difficult. Infertility is always more than a medical problem. Most cultures teach that women should reproduce and that men should have heirs. The norms demand that children be biologically related to their male and female parents. Other kinds of families, though tolerated, are seen as alternative (e.g., lesbian couples who utilize artificial insemination, single males or females who adopt, or heterosexual couples who provide foster care).

New reproductive technologies, including the use of potent fertility drugs, in vitro fertilization, gamete intrafallopian transfer (GIFT), and carefully designed surgical procedures, are available to help couples who cannot achieve pregnancy readily. One obvious and predictable complication of these novel medical interventions is an increase in multiple pregnancies. The use of fertility drugs, for example, may produce more than one ovum and result in multiple gestations. Implantation of several embryos (recommended to increase the likelihood of getting pregnant) may also produce twins, triplets, or quadruplets. Multiple pregnancies may present risks to both the mother and the fetuses. One or more fetuses may be found, through ultrasonic imaging or other methods, to be handicapped or at substantial risk for a genetic disorder. Reducing the number of fetuses in the uterus can also increase the chance of survival for one rather than risking losing all.

Advanced maternal age (over 35 years old) can contribute to the problems encountered in achieving a viable pregnancy. Many couples try for a decade before seeking specialized medical help. When a multiple pregnancy occurs, the focus of the ethical debate may become very pointed: Should selective termination of one or more of the fetuses be undertaken? The situation can be distinguished from many abortion choices where pregnancy is not wanted. In fertility clinics, pregnancy is a strong desire, a product of (sometimes) years of trying, hoping, and wishing. Motives for selective termination may vary, but most such women do not want their bodies invaded or their fetuses destroyed.

Selective termination in multiple pregnancies has been done when one of a set of twins has been found to have a chromosomal disorder (e.g., Turner syndrome, Down syndrome), genetic diseases (e.g., thalassemia major, hemophilia A, Tay-Sachs disease), and developmental abnormalities (e.g., spina bifida, microencephaly). Selective reduction of the number of fetuses has been used in pregnancies resulting from the unintentional multiple implantation of drug-induced ovulation. In situations with more than 3 fetuses, the recommendation for reduction is routine. Efforts to reduce the number of fetuses can sometimes result in miscarriage and the end of the pregnancy. Add to this difficulty that women with multiple pregnancies have often visualized the fetuses via ultrasound and are bonded to them emotionally.

Selective termination presents many ethical challenges. What arguments can be given for the termination of so-called normal implanted embryos or fetuses because of excessive numbers; how should the risk of damage to surviving fetuses be assessed; what is the impact of such a procedure to the mother both during pregnancy and after the birth (if successful)? What weight should be given to the assertion that continuing a multiple pregnancy increases the risk of preterm delivery, early and lengthy hospital stay, and serious complications during birth? The fact that multiple pregnancies increase the risk of premature delivery, low birth weight, and birth defects (including mental and physical retardation) cannot be ignored. But how are decisions about selective termination to be made, even taking into consideration the data?

Behind the micro-choice (do we keep the triplets or terminate two of the three fetuses?) are many macro-assumptions. These cultural-social bases also need scrutiny. Why should women try to get pregnant? Why is it so hard for triplets or quadruplets to be raised in our society, especially if one or more is disabled? Who should choose selective termination? Is the new reproductive technology one that has developed ahead of ethical awareness of its prospects and its problems?

■ VOICES: NURSE-MIDWIFE ■

What led me to become a nurse-midwife was my experience as an obstetric nurse in a large city hospital. I got to know women just before they were about to give birth. I saw them at a critical time in their lives and never again. I was really frustrated. I wanted to see them during the course of their pregnancies and to get to know their families. The doctors, mainly residents, who delivered these babies did good work; they worked long hours. But they had a hard time caring about what was happening. They found the technology fascinating but spent little time with the woman in labor; they were there to check things out, to rupture the membranes, or to do a cesarean section if required. As a nurse on the unit I wanted more interpersonal contact. I craved relationships. So I became a nurse-midwife.

There are still frustrations, however. I do both home deliveries and in-hospital care. Hospitals represent rules for me and for the woman giving birth. You always have to accommodate the policies. You can't always give the couple the birth they want. C. sections are always disappointing to these women. I work with lay midwives as well as nurse-midwives.

Last year our practice supervised 140 births: 70 were in the hospital and 70 at home. I prefer home births for appropriate, low-risk candidates. It's hard to develop rapport and relaxation in the hospital. At home you are treated like an individual. I know that there are criticisms of home delivery: that it's unsafe or even child abuse. Complications are sometimes encountered, but midwives are trained in both normal and difficult births. We deal with them capably. We monitor the heart tones at home; if there's any indication of difficulty, we get transportation to a hospital immediately.

I think that continuous electronic monitoring is misleading. Checking heart tones is accurate. Things change swiftly, I know. I am willing, if necessary, to insert that internal monitor into the baby's scalp very carefully. Overall, we do just fine checking heart tones on a frequent basis. Giving birth is not really a medical procedure. It's a natural event.

I worry about dividing fidelity between mother and the baby. These days, with all the possibilities for treating the fetus, there is a split developing. I resist it. What's good for the mother will be good, most of the time, for the baby. If we can let things proceed naturally (letting the mother move around as she wishes) even in the hospital, things will usually turn out fine. Squatting in bed is the most common position for delivery in the cases I take. I resist the dichotomy between mother and fetus and try to set a climate where they are seen as a unit. If the baby is in distress, the mother wants the best thing for her baby. Mom can hear those heart tones—we share our knowledge with them—and they pick up quickly on what needs to be done, often before we do. My goal is always to explain as much as possible about what's going on as we near the end of labor and begin delivery. We all go through the prenatal period together so that we know how to communicate; we trust each other. We're not strangers. So even if we have to go for a c. section, it emerges from a close relationship.

One of my current ethical dilemmas is a family that refuses to go to the hospital even when I think it's indispensable. Sometimes the grounds for saying no is religious. These are very religious people and I respect their desire and beliefs, but I am torn. What if you go into labor early, I may say to the woman. Sometimes this does happen. If the mother resists going to the hospital, I have to show my fidelity to the fetus. I will not abandon the patient. I will not drag the woman to the hospital. I will call the paramedics and offer to accompany the family to the hospital. If they refuse the paramedics, then I leave it up to those professionals. We stay with the case until we are told to leave.

It's hard to say if third trimester fetuses have rights. I have not really resolved this issue. When I was practicing in another state, a couple was tried for murder when they refused hospital delivery and the baby was born dying. I really can't understand this couple's attitude. On those occasions when I have to press parents to go to the hospital, I am not terribly happy. But it's the right thing to do, so I do it.

We don't do home births for women who smoke or drink or use other chemical substances. Home delivery is too high risk, for both mother and the baby. I don't see a lot of such patients. In some ways, persons who drink or smoke *need* midwives. We could give them the education and counseling they obviously require.

There is a political dimension to being a nurse-midwife. I don't want to be a doctor: They are concerned with pathology. My interests are with women dealing with the experience of pregnancy and childbirth. It is a feminist statement to be caring for women and to be providing an individual level of care so that they can have the birth they want. I don't think of a woman, as some obstetricians do, as "the hypertensive" or "the cesarean." For me empathy and understanding are ethical things, moral obligations. My politics are such that I sometimes think that male physicians have no place working with women in normal labor. Women have always helped in deliveries, and in the majority of the world women are attended by midwives. Doctors should be available for pathologies. Other than that women should be cared for by midwives. I don't think men can relate to persons who have wombs. I might be getting radical here, but I think that men act as obstetricians by using their dominance. They actually think that they are delivering the baby. In reality, the physician is receiving the baby. Some OBs are women, but they have gone through a regimented medical education that makes it hard for them to emerge from medical school as whole persons. I don't have many conflicts with physicians these days. I think this is because I am a patient advocate. I press the doctors at times. If they say, "Let's go for a c. section," I might respond, "Let's wait a few hours," and they usually agree. They know that I know the patient. My advocacy is clearly a political statement. I worry that if I am not around, there will be no advocates. In private hospitals, especially, staff nurses can't raise issues easily. They have to please the doctors and keep them happy. This makes it harder to effectively advocate for women in labor.

These days, doctors and nurses in the hospitals are much more receptive to my presence. My credentials as a nurse-midwife are seen as valid. I do think that attitudes are changing slowly. The importance of being a midwife comes not from delivery, but from the developing relationship. I have attended the births of four children of one mother. I have known the family for years. This is very rewarding. I feel a sense of responsibility. On those rare occasions when the baby needs neonatal intensive care, I will stay with the mother for as long as I am needed. It might be a matter of months but I will be in touch with the parents and visit the family when I can be of use.

We have had babies die. It's usually in the hospital, though the birth may have begun at home. It's terrible! I always have incredible guilt. I wonder what more I could have done. It is hard for the couple and hard for our practice. These moments are unforgettable.

I have had experience with so-called nontraditional families. I have helped lesbian couples get pregnant by means of artificial insemination. I can get frozen sperm in the mail, ordered from a catalogue. I like opening up the process to women. I have taught women how to inseminate themselves; it's not a hard thing to do. I have no objection to such alternative modes of getting pregnant. I have helped those in solid relationships and also single women who want to be pregnant. I don't see why either category of women should be denied access to sperm.

RECOMMENDED READING

Bayles, M. *Reproductive Ethics.* Englewood Cliffs, NJ: Prentice-Hall, 1984.

Frohock, F. *Special Care: Medical Decisions at the Beginning of Life.* Chicago: University of Chicago Press, 1986.

Hull, R.T., ed., *Ethical Issues in the New Reproductive Technology.* Belmont, CA: Wadsworth, 1990.

Murray, T. and Caplan, A., eds., *Which Babies Shall Live?* Clifton, NJ: Humana, 1985.

O'Neill, O. and Ruddick, W., eds., *Having Children: Philosophical and Legal Reflections on Parenthood.* New York: Oxford University, 1979.

Weil, W.B. and Benjamin, M., eds., *Ethical Issues at the Outset of Life.* Boston: Blackwell, 1987.

▪4▪

Primary Caregiving: Ethics in Family Practice

"Who's your doctor," seems an innocent, almost innocuous question. It isn't, and its answer can be quite complicated. For nearly one-sixth of adult citizens of the United States, the answer is quite clear: "I have no physician." The medically indigent and underserved (mainly poor persons or those with no or inadequate health care insurance) cannot identify a primary caregiver. Their medical problems take them to hospital emergency rooms for long waits, often only after a disease or disorder is well-developed. The clinician they see in the ER is unknown, unless they have interacted with this same doctor at some time at the hospital.

For those fortunate enough to have financial resources, the answer to the question is also not so simple. If one is enrolled in a health maintenance organization (HMO) or preferred provider organization (PPO), a primary care physician is either chosen or assigned to the patient or family. This doctor is often a family practitioner, a local pediatrician, sometimes an internist, or for some women an obstetrician/gynecologist. These physicians act as gatekeepers for the patient, screening for diseases, referring for tests, and recommending other practitioners specifically skilled in dealing with particular problems (e.g., a gastroenterologist for irritable bowel syndrome).

Other patients choose a primary care physician on the basis of convenience ("his office is near the shopping center"), reputation ("they say she is a careful listener"), rumor ("he'll give you tranquilizers without asking a lot of silly questions"), or custom ("she treated my mother, so she's just right for me"). None of these reasons is outlandish, but because the relationship between a patient and his or her primary care doctor is the foundation, the entry mechanism into the world of medical care, the nature of that connection is patently important. Primary care physicians, family doctors especially, need to know their patients well in order to serve them effectively.

Primary care is often seen as the work of skilled medical generalists who are the first contact for patients in need of medical services and who provide continuity of care for individuals and sometimes families. Primary care is usually offered to persons who are ambulatory and able to function at home. When patients need acute or long-term institutional intervention, the primary care physician is frequently the manager. The immediacy and intimacy found in the primary care relationship entails psychosocial approaches to patient management, with emphasis on communication between doctor and patient regarding problems that may be biologic, behavioral, or social or any combination of the three. Primary care doctors are there for the long haul; they are also referral specialists.

Because other chapters (see chapters 3, 5, and 6) address the concerns of primary practitioners in OB/GYN, pediatric and adolescent medicine, and internal medicine, this chapter will focus on family medicine as a fundamental primary care delivery system. Family medicine traces its origins to the old notion of the general practitioner. Today, family medicine is well-established with its own residency programs, academies, and professional organizations. Efforts have been made to differentiate family medicine from family or general practice. These are often distinctions without a difference. We use the terms interchangeably to designate those primary care providers who see patients across the age spectrum and who provide continuing, comprehensive care (including health maintenance) for any and all persons or families.

Although not all family practice physicians care for entire families, many do. There are fundamental, and often unstated, assumptions about family life that inform ethical judgments in family care. Examining these value assumptions presents an opportunity that, if sustained, can lead to the resolution of ethical difficulties in patient care. For example, families are assumed to have mutual concerns and interests. The reciprocity of individual development and collective well-being defines family structures. Families come together around issues of health management. Taking the baby or another family member to the doctor is a family responsibility and a ritual. Families influence health, for better or worse, in important ways (e.g., a family with a single smoking member can often influence behaviors leading to cessation). The family perspective is often an intimate one: Having lived together for perhaps generations, families know the views, preferences, fears, and dreams of one another. And although unanimity is rare, families do share values and ethical perspectives on controversial issues. Even if agreement is unreachable, the family forum for discussion of such matters as euthanasia or abortion may be a secure space for the elaboration of such viewpoints (a "haven in a heartless world," is how the social critic Christopher Lasch has described the family).

Families also present ethical difficulties to their caregivers. Conflicts abound! Disagreements about financial matters ("Why should we waste all this money on the last days of Dad's life?"), family responsibilities ("Who's going to take Momma if we don't put her in a nursing home?"), religious values ("If you listen to this guy you're sure to go to hell."), and appropriate decision-makers ("Well, maybe Pop used to know what's best, but now he can't find his way to the bathroom.") are very common. The family physician, often aware of the history of such conflicts, knows that trivial choices can inflate swiftly into full-fledged crises.

Even benign family desires can have an impact on the area of confidentiality. For a competent patient, the family might have a sincere interest in discovering from the physician the patient's condition or prognosis. Should the doctor reveal details at all, or only with permission? Telling an adult son or daughter about the patient's colostomy, in order to ensure that the parent will have adequate nutrition while recovering from surgery, might be a violation of confidentiality, if offered without explicit permission from the patient. Can, or should, family physicians request such a waiver each time information is requested?

Family doctors, in their brokering and gatekeeping roles, must often mobilize medical, social, and community support for patients in need. They must make use of the strengths families can provide to patients ill or recovering from treatment. The authority of the doctor is rarely questioned, but that legitimated power can sometimes be abused. A simple glance at a daughter who is reluctant to undertake the at-home care of an aging, demented parent can "guilt trip" the daughter into acceptance of an enormous responsibility. Family physicians worry both about having too much and too little authority.

All physicians have limitations. Psychiatrists, for example, are rarely called on to give thorough physical examinations. Remembering all of the signs and symptoms from medical school or their internship is virtually impossible. Specialists whose work requires exquisite attention to detail (e.g., ophthalmologists who specialize in laser surgery) may have little opportunity to keep up with innovations in cardiology. Family physicians, as generalists, may try to be all things to all patients, but in reality no person can provide every medical service. For example, some family doctors do offer obstetric care and deliver babies. But high-risk pregnancies, involving numerous investigative tests and sophisticated prenatal interventions, are usually outside the purview of family practitioners. In the inevitable nexus between family doctors and specialists to whom they refer patients can be found a rich variety of ethical problems.

■ FIVE ESSENTIAL CASES ■

Case 4-1

Knowing a patient well, establishing a good doctor-patient relationship, is indispensable to responsible family practice. Some patients, however, are unusually demanding and call on physicians to tread the borders of unethical practice.

Mr. C. was a very independent 70-year-old farmer with controlled hypertension and mild osteoarthritis who came into the family practice office for a routine blood pressure evaluation. He had a thick chart, having made many visits for arthritis pain control and hypertension, and the office staff was glad to see him. His usual doctor was on vacation, so Dr. H., a new member of the practice who had met the patient on one previous occasion, strolled into the examination room to do the blood pressure check.

A fit, young appearing man, Mr. C. rose as Dr. H. entered the room. He angrily cut the young doctor's introduction short as he waved a newspaper under Dr. H.'s nose. Jabbing at the doctor with a finger, he said: "It says here that everyone has to wear seatbelts, but you can give me an affidavit so I don't have to wear one." Mr. C. believed that the arthritis in his hands and shoulder prevented him from fastening his seatbelt. He also wanted a handicapped sticker for his car, "so I don't have to walk so far with my groceries. People with hardly nothing wrong with them can park up close to the store."

The physician had spent substantial time in the ER during his years of training and had seen many traumatic results of motor vehicle accidents. He certainly did not want to give Mr. C. what he requested. Dr. H. dealt with the parking sticker first, by referring him to the state motor vehicle agency. He told him that, as a doctor, he could not bend the truth for Mr. C.'s convenience. As he concluded the brief examination, Mr. C. again demanded an affidavit and a statement that would get him handicapped parking privileges. Dr. H. asked the patient if he were angry, or if he were feeling that nobody was paying attention to him. The patient rose and scowled. "No, I've already taken enough of your time," he said and walked out muttering, "To hell with seatbelts!"

Based on Charles Margolis, Theodor Herwig, Ellin L. Bloch, John R. Kues, and Terry M. Perlin, "To Hell with Seatbelts": Changing Confrontation to Collaboration, Humane Medicine 4 (1):54–56, 1988.

Mr. C. is not the typical difficult patient. Many patients who give family doctors grief exhibit noncompliance ("forgetting" to take medications; missing scheduled appointments; continuing to smoke against medical advice). Such challenges to physician authority may present a dilemma of care for the family practice doctor. The patient who has a history of ignoring his antiseizure medication, and who has applied for a job as a long-distance truck driver, presents the conscientious doctor with a real difficulty.

Mr. C., however, isn't forgetting or neglecting: He's demanding! Patients like Mr. C. are not frequently encountered; they can be scary, especially for residents or physicians in practice for the first time. Mr. C. is demanding and negative: He challenges physician authority by attacking state rules (i.e., motor vehicle bureau). He also asks Dr. H. to violate his own duty of professional conduct by asking for an inappropriate exemption. Frustration with patients who are demanding, nasty, or whose behaviors (e.g., substance abuse) are morally objectionable is common among family doctors. Doctors are often involved in the enforcement of laws (i.e., reporting suspected child or elder abuse; notifying public health authorities regarding sexually transmitted diseases; testifying in guardianship or custody hearings; providing information to courts deciding about the involuntary civil commitment of mentally ill patients [see Chapter 7]).

Mr. C.'s challenge to Dr. H. was a direct one. The patient would not accept the family doctor's assessment of his best interest. Clearly, the physician was concerned about patient health and safety. Was he also worried about Mr. C.'s emotional response? Was his desire to protect the patient by insisting in effect that he wear seatbelts built on a solid foundation? Did Dr. H. act protectively to a fault and thus behave paternalistically? The physician's earlier experience with automobile trauma surely influenced his behavior. Was he worried not only about injury to the individual patient but also about avoiding unnecessary health-care costs to society? In affirming society's needs, Dr. H. may have aligned himself with the authority that the patient held in contempt.

From Dr. H.'s perspective, in granting the exemption he would have to lie, exaggerate, or be duplicitous. Many physicians, when pressed, would agree that sometimes lying may be in the best interest of the patient (e.g., expressing hope and optimism to a seriously ill person, when it is not fully warranted by clinical evidence). Family physicians have been known to falsify diagnoses in order to gain approval by insurance companies for tests deemed necessary but not likely to be covered. For example, many companies do not pay for routine mammographies, but if the doctor writes suspicion of small mass on the test referral, even if nothing palpable has been found, the mammogram will be paid for by the insurance company.

On occasion, doctors may act duplicitously on behalf of patients for their benefit. Does Mr. C.'s case fall into this category? Or should steadfast refusal to give the patient what he thinks he needs be the appropriate tactic? Will Dr. H.'s saying "No!" secure the patient's compliance with the seatbelt law? This is hard to predict, but if Mr. C.'s resistance to the rule is symbolic, if he is saying that his freedom to choose is on the line, then the fact that the doctor will not support his cause is unlikely to induce conformity.

Would Mr. C.'s original physician have handled the situation differently or better? What strategies could be devised to keep the dialogue going? What model of doctor-patient relationship would allow the family physician to hear the patient's expressed and real wishes in order to find a mode of collaborating rather than conflicting? Is the physician's role in the doctor-patient relationship best structured as:

Medical Scientist: The doctor investigates, diagnoses, prescribes, or refers in a rational and authoritative fashion. Her principal function is scrutinizing the patient's illness and making every effort to restore the unwell person to maximal levels of health.

Confidant/Counselor: The doctor is a skilled listener, available to the patient for advice and for solace. His main job is to provide a safe space in which the patient can discuss matters of health and illness, both physical and psychological.

Proponent/Advocate: The physician works for, and with, the patient to help create a path through the complicated and bureaucratic system of contemporary health care. Her basic task is to discover resources and to mobilize necessary medical and psychological aid for the patient.

Collaborator: The doctor works with the patient to resolve any sort of problem that emerges in the course of care. His fundamental duty is to provide an atmosphere of trust and honesty that will allow both parties to devise strategies to improve patient health.

This list is far from exhaustive. Most family physicians provide a combination of these models for patients, emphasizing one over the other depending on doctor inclination and patient "style." In the case of Mr. C., which model would have been most efficacious? What is the extent of Dr. H.'s duty to help this gentleman who seems so angry at authroity and determined to reject physician advice? On what grounds should he "bend" in order to maintain the doctor-patient relationship? The flexibility needed to come to some middle-ground solution has ethical implications: Dr. H.'s fidelity to his principles — veracity but especially beneficence — may have an ironic impact. By sticking to his sense of what is best for Mr. C., he may win the fight over seatbelts or parking privileges but lose his patient as a result.

Case 4-2

Family physicians may see patients over the course of years and develop a truly trusting relationship. The revelation of certain patient behaviors can affront the values of the physician. Such lifestyle differences can sometimes precipitate ethical soul-searching for the primary care practitioner.

Ms. S. is a 29-year-old married woman who has been a patient of Dr. L. since she was a young child. This family physician has had a close and frank relationship with Ms. S. since her teenage years. He attended her wedding 5 years ago. One evening, Ms. S. calls her family doctor and says that she is experiencing some unusual vaginal bleeding. Dr. L., a conservative 56-year-old physician who provides obstetric and gynecologic services as part of a group family practice, meets the patient at the local hospital's ER; examination reveals several vaginal lacerations. The injuries are sutured and pain medicine is administered.

When Dr. L. asks Ms. S. how she sustained the cuts, he is told that it happened during sexual intercourse. Dr. L. seems surprised, he has never seen such damage caused in this way, and says as much. Ms. S. then admits that her husband sometimes asks her to "do things." Dr. L. asks her to be more specific. She says that her spouse "ties me up really tight with some old cloths. He asks me to 'beg for it,' and when I refuse he sometimes uses a vibrator or even a metal tube. He inserts it into me until I pretend to have an orgasm. Once in a while I really do have the orgasm."

Dr. L. asks the patient to see him the following week at the office. There, after a brief examination and discussion of her recovery, Dr. L. tells Ms. S. that he is perturbed by what she told him about the cause of her injuries. Ms. S. is puzzled, "Look, it was just an accident. I got cut. It's no big deal." Dr. L. asks her how often she engages in this kind of sexual activity. "Well, whenever we make love. About three times a week." Dr. L. asks her if she undertakes these activities willingly. Ms. S. replies, "Sure, I guess. I mean, I love him and all. And except for this last time I've never been hurt. It's true that, lately, he seems to be getting rougher. Once in a while there are some bruises. But I know what I'm doing. It's a turn-on for him. And he's real nice to me the rest of the time. I have no complaints about my marriage." Dr. L. is deeply chagrined by this statement and wonders what sort of response or intervention is now appropriate.

By asking questions about his patient's sexual behavior and, particularly, about the level of voluntariness in her relationship, Dr. L. has gone well beyond medical matters. Is this an appropriate area for scrutiny and concern by a family practitioner? Does Dr. L. assume that there is a problem here? In pursuing the options available to both doctor and patient we need to sort out the real or potential value-biases suggested by Dr. L.'s inquiry from his legitimate anxiety about his patient's well-being. The risk of physical injury is only one factor in this case. The physician's sense of the propriety of Ms. S. and her husband's practices must also be considered.

Doctors are committed to the health and safety of their patients. The broader the definition of health and disease, the more likely it is that the doctor will become involved in lifestyle management. Smoking, excessive alcohol use, abuse of prescription and non-prescription medication, risk-taking behavior (e.g., participation in demolition derbies, compulsive overeating, extramarital sexual activities, involvement in abusive or neglectful relationships) all come to the attention of doctors every day. When the relationship between an individual behavior and a clear health danger can be established (e.g., between heavy smoking and the appearance of a spot on the lung) the physician's responsibility to intervene seems clear enough. Few lifestyle matters, however, are so clearly related to health risks or disease development.

Ms. S.'s sexual activities seem strange to her doctor. Are they also morally objectionable to him? If so, does this alter the nature of Dr. L.'s responsibilities to the patient? Physicians who entertain principled opposition to, or reservations about, patient behaviors or requests do have alternatives. For example, doctors who are opposed to abortions on religious or secular grounds certainly do not have to perform them on request. At the same time, physicians cannot simply refuse, or abandon, patients in need. A family doctor who is, for example, a Mormon and refuses to drink alcoholic beverages may feel revolted by a patient who has become an alcoholic. Should the doctor's viewpoint inform her analysis of the problem and her recommendation for treatment?

The tendency among health care providers is to attempt to remain value neutral when dealing with controversial behaviors. Historic lessons of physician bias and prejudice abound. A recent illustration is the antihomosexual attitudes of American physicians, at least prior to the American Psychiatric Association's 1973 statement that removed active homosexuality from the official list of psychiatric diseases. (Yet bias and discrimination against gay patients remain in this era of AIDS.) Medical training in family practice emphasizes an open-minded tolerant attitude toward patients who appear to be different.

Dr. L. has two related tasks. First, he must explore his own sensibilities. He needs to try to separate his natural concern as a physician for a patient who has been injured, from his sense of propriety and responsibility in matters of sexual intimacy. Dr. L. may wish to seek some help in this regard—not help for the patient but for himself in clarifying his subjective response to the story told by Ms. S.

Second, he has to come up with a plan that both respects patient autonomy and provides careful follow-up for Ms. S. How blunt should Dr. L. be? Should he tell this young woman that "your sex life seems pretty dangerous. Have you thought about future risks? Would you like me to refer you and (if you wish) your husband to a qualified sex counselor?" Or should the family doctor be as nonjudgmental as possible, stating, "I believe that you engage in these practices because, as you say, they give your spouse and you real pleasure. If any medical problems come up, I hope you will give me a call." Are they *any* circumstances in which a family doctor can bluntly tell a patient, "I think that is disgusting. You should stop it, for your own sake and for the sake of decency?" Such statements are often made outside of medical practice (we can imagine a member of the clergy speaking such a rebuke). Does this absolve the physician from making a value judgment?

Case 4-3

Family practice physicians must act as "brokers" for patients and their relatives when medical crises emerge. Advocating a perspective reflecting patient's interests can situate the family doctor in the midst of conflict among patient and family views and the objectives of other professionals.

The health care team gathered at the bedside of Mrs. V. in the intensive care unit (ICU) was a large one. Dr. F., the attending physician (a family practice doctor), Dr. C., a pulmonologist who headed the ICU, three medical residents, a geriatric nurse, and a psychiatric social worker were present. Mrs. V., a 74-year-old woman whose husband had died a year earlier, was in the hospital for the third time in 2 years after a major myocardial infarction (MI). There was not much left of her heart, functionally speaking. Her ejection fraction, indicating a traumatic decrease in the heart's pumping capacity, was 17%. On admission, she was very ill, suffering persistent ischemic pain and showing signs of significant renal failure.

Mrs. V. was not in much pain today; earlier she had been on a good deal of morphine and on a nitroglycerin drip to relieve the painful angina. She was not a candidate for either coronary artery bypass surgery or a heart transplant: Her heart and her other organ systems were so weak that the consulting cardiologist felt that even a less invasive procedure (i.e., investigative angiography) could be life-threatening. Mrs. V. was dependent on dopamine to keep her alive.

The physicians were divided about what to do for this patient. All agreed that Mrs. V. would never recover her capacity for full function; she was, in fact, expected to die within a few months. The pulmonologist thought that Mrs. V. should be "allowed to die. There's really nothing we can do for her. We shouldn't keep her in this ICU bed." This doctor regarded Mrs. V. as an apt candidate for hospice care: She should be "allowed to die." Her family doctor disputed this viewpoint. His first questions was: What did Mrs. V. think about her future? A discussion 2 months earlier had evoked these words from the patient: "I know I've had some bad heart attacks. But as long as you people can keep me ticking and breathing, I intend to be here. I ain't ready for the Lord, not by a long shot."

The team entertained the idea of approaching Mrs. V. in the ICU to probe these matters. In a preliminary staff discussion, Dr. F. asked team members about their experience with the patient. "When she was in the ER 5 days ago I asked her about code status," said a second-year medical resident. She said that she wanted to live and that she wanted everything done for her. Her husband had been very ill and had been kept alive on "one of those breathing machines," Mrs. V. had said.

The patient's family consisted of several children. According to the social worker, only the oldest daughter, Olivia, was "with it." The other off-spring, all adults, were regarded as insufficiently capable of understanding the gravity of Mrs. V.'s condition. A brief talk a few days earlier with Olivia resulted in her asking the doctors to "do all you can for my mom." When the suggestion was made that a family discussion about code status be attempted, Olivia said "No." She did not want her mother upset and she knew that Mrs. V. would insist on resuscitation, no matter what.

The ICU director and the family physician discussed the case several times. Moving Mrs. V. to a general, medical-surgical floor, with the hope of eventually getting her home seemed unlikely. Her condition was so perilous that she would likely die outside the ICU. Raising these issues with the patient was a delicate matter. She was weak, though clearly competent; the strain of such a discussion might prove dangerous. The pulmonologist and some of the ICU nurses agreed that Mrs. V. might not understand or participate fully in a lengthy discussion of DNR orders or comfort measures. Dr. F. continued to insist that Mrs. V. be kept in the ICU. His sense was that she would want to be kept alive for as long as possible.

This case raises many difficult questions that family physicians face when their patients enter an acute-care facility. Because he has to defer to other doctors (specialists, consultants) and has to keep a continuing relationship with a hospital, Dr. F. may feel obligated both to be an advocate for his patient and to be realistic. He knows that Mrs. V.'s condition is terminal. He has also provided services for her, her deceased husband, and for family and friends in the community. His reputation for faithful care is at stake. So is his need to do what seems best for his patient.

Fortunately, other members of the team are available. The social worker can be asked: Did the patient have any religious views about her future? Did she say anything about dying? Was Mrs. V. capable of talking about such difficult subjects or would such a discussion be too upsetting in her condition? The team already agreed that, today at least, Mrs. V. was very aware. She had the mental capacity to understand her situation. She was also a very likeable patient. Other caregivers can be interrogated. In fact, one resident reported, "She's a granny. She's very Appalachian: lively, funny, engaging."

The geriatric nurse, who had talked with Mrs. V. twice, was asked what the patient understood. Did she have a visual picture of what an in-hospital resuscitative effort would look like? The team was equivocal. "She did have a husband on a ventilator," the nurse said. But that is not the same picture that someone who knows what CPR entails—chest pounding, the insertion of catheters and tubes, even the possible use of an electroshocking defibrillator—would have. Dr. C. noted that few patients or family members know what CPR entails. He argued strenuously against even offering CPR to this patient. "We all know the statistics. Even if she survives resuscitation, there's about a zero chance that she'll ever leave this place alive. Why put her through this torture?"

Should Mrs. V. be aproached for a discussion of these matters? Without her agreement, a cardiac arrest will be met with a full resuscitative effort. Some very concerned doctors might argue that even asking the patient's opinion could be life-threatening. Which physician's viewpoint should predominate? What do the other perspectives (e.g., of her daughter, the social worker, the nurse, the medical residents) suggest? We may lament that treatment options were not presented to Mrs. V. prior to her hospitalization. This crisis is frequently encountered, even in those states with living wills or durable power of attorney for health care options.

Dr. F. feels strongly that Mrs. V. should stay in the ICU: How hard should he push his determination? No matter what the politics of the situation, as the primary care physician and case manager, Dr. F. may have to remind the ICU staff that a DNR order is not equivalent to "do not treat." Resuscitation aside, if Mrs. V. remains in the ICU she is entitled to all available intensive care services. The temptation to "go slow" on patients in her condition is often present. Dr. F. has a great deal of work to do monitoring Mrs. V.'s condition.

A persuasive case can be made for removing Mrs. V. from the ICU. A bed in that facility can cost thousands of dollars per day. There is only a slim possibility of restoring her to useful function. Her death in the ICU will be slow and lingering. Her resolution to stay alive "no matter what the price" has metaphoric power, but who will pay the literal bill? Beyond cost concerns, ICU bed space is scarce. Shouldn't her bed go to a person for whom it would be more useful? Is she creating a problem for another person by insisting on inappropriate medical treatment? Does Mrs. V. *know* what she is demanding? How realistic is her sense of her own future? How much patient education has been provided for her by her family doctor or by the nursing staff caring for her?

Supposing that all these arguments were met—that sufficient funds were available for Mrs. V.'s care; that there was *no* competing demand for ICU space; and that the patient was fully informed and competent while making this request—could Mrs. V. stay in intensive care indefinitely? Though we might agree that Dr. F. should support his patient by advocating her wishes "until the end," is the family doctor's commitment eternal? It is hard to predict the actual moment at which treatment plans are altered—some estimates indicate that 60 percent of all hospital deaths are "negotiated" through withholding or withdrawal of treatment—but at a certain point (unless Mrs. V. dies first) some modification is likely.

Case 4-4

Because family physicians must refer their patients to specialists, the control of information can become a significant issue. When violations of standard ethical practice by other doctors are suspected, caution as well as concern should be exercised.

Mrs. T. is a 72-year-old woman who has been followed by a family practice physician, Dr. A., for 7 years. She has experienced chronic obstructive pulmonary disease (COPD), bronchial asthma, and chronic mixed anxiety and depression. On her most recent visit, she reported general malaise, poor appetite, and a decrease in her ability to work around the house due to a feeling of restriction in her left leg. She reported pain on walking as well. An x-ray showed Mrs. T. to have mild scoliosis of the lumbar spine and partial sacralization of L5. She was referred to an orthopedic specialist, Dr. B.

This physician performed x-rays as well as a bone scan and diagnosed probable metastatic disease to the hip, based on a positive bone scan of metastasis to the calvaria, ribs, and vertebra. Dr. B. did not tell the patient or the family physician of his preliminary assessment. Instead, the orthopedist referred Mrs. T. to a specialist for further workup. She was not told that the doctor to whom she was referred was an oncologist; she was only given the physician's name. She met with this doctor, who immediately ordered a CT scan of her chest and a mammogram. Mrs. T. became suspicious and asked several pointed questions about cancer. The oncologist avoided all discussion and told the patient that her family physician would get a report. She was not told the probable diagnosis by the oncologist, even though he noted in his records a 2-cm soft tissue subpleural lesion located posteriorly in the right lower lung. This was not regarded as an absolute confirmation of a primary cancer site. There was no radiographic evidence of a mass in either breast. The oncologist reported by mail his findings to Dr. A. The cancer specialist noted in his letter to Dr. A. that "the patient has a history of depression and seemed both depressed and anxious after examination."

Mrs. T. returned to Dr. A. and expressed her concerns about possible cancer and her frustration in "getting anything" from either the orthopedist or the oncologist. Dr. A. had not yet received the letter from the oncologist. So, the family doctor phoned the oncologist, who verbally reported his preliminary finding. Dr. A. was advised not to inform Mrs. T. about the initial diagnosis, at least until the primary lesion could be identified. The oncologist recommended that the next step be a needle biopsy of the lung.

■ ■ ■

This case seems, at first review, terribly obvious and clear-cut. The oncologist is failing to communicate vital information to the patient, even after repeated requests. This doctor, we may presume, resists telling Mrs. T. about the real possibility that she has cancer not from malice or a desire to find some sort of advantage. The oncologist, we have reason to be sure, wants to postpone any discussion until absolutely certain that the identity of the site of the primary tumor has been confirmed. The duty to practice veracity, it seems, has a temporal dimension: It will have to wait. Seen in a wider context (family practice) there are a variety of ethical problems.

First, Dr. B., the orthopedist, failed to tell either the patient or the referring doctor anything. What should Dr. A. do about this? (He wants to maintain his relationship with Dr. B.; he respects this physician's skills and wants to be able to send future patients for care.) Should Dr. A. fuss and fume; or should he let it go? What is the nature of Dr. B.'s offense? The rules of etiquette in referral relationships usually require an orthopedist such as Dr. B. to, at the very least, inform Dr. A. about sending the patient to another specialist. As for failing to tell Mrs. T. that she was being sent to a cancer expert, this was surely an error of omission, not commission. The family practice physician should think long and hard before speaking with Dr. B. What should be said?

The oncologist also presents several ethical challenges. Is there ever a good reason for withholding the truth? Does the legal and ethical doctrine of informed consent figure here? Statements of medical condition and descriptions of potential treatments are rarely matters of certainty. Physicians, formally and informally, have long believed in an exception to the doctrine of informed consent: the practice of *therapeutic privilege* (see Fig. 2-5). This means that if the information about to be given the patient is likely to cause grave harm, then waiting is neither legally nor morally erroneous. Has the oncologist misused this fundamentally humane concept? Physicians often delay giving the truth, or shade it in ways presumed to be in the best interest of the patient.

Can we assume that a major justification for evading Mrs. T.'s inquiry is the oncologist's awareness that she has a history of depression and anxiety? Oncologists routinely see patients who are dramatically upset by hearing the news of cancer or suspected cancer. Many become very upset and, occasionally, threaten to commit suicide. No studies sustain the likelihood of following through such threats. The folklore of medicine contains numerous anecdotes about patients who "just couldn't take the news."

Still, in this case the problem is compounded by and might be alleviated by the presence of the family practice physician as a primary care advocate for Mrs. T. Family medicine is never practiced in a vacuum; referral to a variety of specialists is the norm. Family practitioners are often gatekeepers, making referrals and doing follow-up in acute-care hospitals and long-term care facilities. Such work is real, but delicate. Turf wars are often the norm: for example, who is responsible for the patient in the ICU—the intensivist, the pulmonologist, the oncologist, or the family physician?

No reasonable person would expect an ER physician to tell a patient in the midst of a major MI, "You're having a heart attack, and there's no reason to expect you will survive." This would be honesty with malice and would serve no identifiable purpose other than meeting the barest requirements of the law. In less obvious situations, however, can physicians withhold the results of their investigations legitimately?

On Mrs. T.'s behalf, the family practice physician has made the appropriate referrals, first to the orthopedist, then to the cancer specialist, in order to get a specific diagnosis for his patient. Now, given the message delivered to him by the oncologist he has several choices:

Wait: The oncologist wants to proceed with a needle biopsy of the lung. The family doctor could finesse Mrs. T.'s questions and let the oncologist proceed, awaiting the results.

Tell: The family physician could speak the truth to Mrs. T. His knowledge of her history of mood and personality disorders would be an important element of the judgment. He could tell Mrs. T. that cancer is suspected and that further tests are in order.

Advocate: The family physician, running the risk of alienating, perhaps permanently, his oncologist colleague, can insist that the truth be told by the oncologist or, with Mrs. T., demand that the results of the preliminary tests be revealed. If the oncologist refuses, the family doctor can tell the patient.

Counsel: This difficult case requires a great deal of balancing and could call on the family practice physician to exercise a needed skill: psychological counseling. Mrs. T. is going to require support no matter what the outcome of the present quest for data. Beginning this process by hearing her fears and frustrations is an alternative.

What is the role of the primary care physician, in this case the family practice doctor, when patients see several specialists in the pursuit of a diagnosis? As gatekeeper and advocate Dr. A. has pledged fidelity to the interests of Mrs. T. But doctors must operate in the "real world," one in which collegiality and referrals are valued. Dr. A.'s response as a practicing family physician depends, in some measure, on his ties to the oncologist, with whom he has had good relations in the past and to whom he will surely send many patients for studies and treatment in the future. Will he pursue utilitarian self-interest or will he "make waves" without regard to the potentially difficult consequences?

Case 4-5

If lying to patients is wrong, can shading the truth ever be acceptable? When a patient's own goals are in conflict, the physician may have to choose a course of action with the smallest amount of harm.

Dr. W., a family physician, had been taking care of Mr. D. for 30 years. The patient, a widower 78 years of age, was now confined to the local nursing home. He was a favorite resident in this long-term care facility, and many of the nurses and nursing aides had developed a rapport with him. But Mr. D. was very sick. Liver cancer, with widespread metastases, was fully developed, and Mr. D.'s life expectancy was less than 6 months. No family or friends were available locally. Mr. D. was well aware of his prognosis. His only daughter, Linda, was an international business executive whose work took her to the Orient on a regular basis. At present she was spending 2 months in Hong Kong. On one of Dr. W.'s visits to the nursing home, Mr. D. told his physician that his fervent wish was to see his daughter "once more before I die." When the doctor asked his patient what he wanted to communicate to Linda, Mr. W. said: "Well, we were never that close. She preferred her mother, and I respect that. I wasn't always around. But now, when my time's up, I want to tell her how proud I am of her and how much I love her."

The physician arranged for the nursing home's social worker to contact Linda in Hong Kong. She said that she could visit her father in 3 weeks, and suitable arrangements were made. Two weeks later and a few days before the scheduled visit, Mr. D.'s pain increased dramatically. He was given narcotic medication (morphine) that relieved his symptoms but that left him confused and drowsy. He began to ask for more and more medication. Dr. W. was not concerned about addiction with this terminally ill patient. He also thought that Mr. D. would be unable to communicate with his daughter if he continued to receive ever more powerful doses of painkillers. So he decided to try, for one day, using a placebo. He told the patient that he was going to try a "different pill for your pain." Mr. W. did not notice the difference, but later he remarked, "I feel a little better today, not so sluggish." Dr. W. felt uneasy about using the sugar pill but felt that this was preferable to continuing to give Mr. D. the morphine. He also thought that if he were to tell the patient that he was using a less powerful drug, Mr. D. might ask for an increased dose of the narcotic.

■ ■ ■

Patients speak to their doctors in many voices. When Mr. D. asked for pain medication he was speaking as a person in need of immediate relief. When he told Dr. W. of his moving desire to have a last visit with his daughter, he was speaking of ultimate goals and life purposes. Dr. W. perceived these needs as being in conflict and acted accordingly. If Mr. D. discovered the duplicity, what might be his response? Certainly patients rely on their physicians to give them real, biochemically active medicines. Though the perception of pain is surely subjectively understood, Mr. D.'s experience was not false, psychosomatic, or imaginary. He had real pain that originated from a diagnosed disease. His first responses to the morphine, pain relief and sleepiness, were quite routine.

Placebos are often prescribed. Patients who come to a doctor and reveal no organic disorder after examination and rigorous testing do not always accept the family doctor's judgment. They may continue to have headaches, stomach aches, lower back pain, or other complaints. If the family doctor dismisses such ailments with a strong dose of truth ("Now look, there's nothing wrong with your body"), she may still pursue the presumably psychological underpinnings of the complaint. Counseling may be in order. So may referral to a psychiatrist. These are complicated, and often expensive, interventions. Physicians, however, are well aware of the placebo effect. Clinical drug trials and physician experience testify to the fact that some patients either get better or feel better using nonactive substances. For patients who suffer from no organic disorder, the prescription of a sugar pill, some argue, cannot hurt and could help.

Dr. W. believes that Mr. D. is an apt candidate for a placebo, given his special circumstances. Do the usual objections to using placebos apply in this case? One argument stresses that patients who receive placebos only postpone their problems, which are usually psychological in nature. They should be encouraged to seek counseling, not given phony drugs, but this does not describe the situation of Mr. D. A second argument points out that deception, no matter how benign, deprives the patient of his or her autonomy. It also violates the principle of veracity. The patient is prevented from exercising authentic choice. If the patient does not seem to be physically ill, this does not give the caregiver the right to dupe by means of placebo. Dr. W. believes Mr. D. is very ill. The placebo is administered, he believes, in accordance with the patient's true wish. Given Mr. D.'s location in the life-cycle, the anticipated visit of his daughter may be a most significant moment, one whose value transcends the normal requirements of veracity.

The dangers in prescribing placebos extend beyond the care of the individual patient. If the physician becomes an omnipotent shaman, unreasonable expectations will be encouraged. If family doctors give placebos with success for "good" reasons in limited cases, a precedent may be set that will encourage using such substances in situations that are less justifiable. The discovery by a patient that a placebo was used can also prove problematic. Individual doctors and the medical profession as a whole would not want to be known as fraudulent, even with pure (or mixed) motives.

Can a compelling case be made by Dr. W.'s giving Mr. D. a "drug" that will allow him, probably for a few days, to stay relatively pain-free and also to be alert enough to have the final meeting with his daughter Linda? If we choose the more ethically steadfast approach—perhaps by trying no drugs, which will likely result in Mr. D. asking for a great deal of morphine, thus rendering him incapable of seeing his daughter—whose interests are we serving? Does fidelity to principles have an inherent value, even when a patient in grave need can be helped by crossing the border and temporarily loosening one's standards?

For a family physician, concern and compassion for patients in the family is an often-heard maxim. What does Dr. W. owe Mr. D.'s daughter Linda? Presumably they have never met. His view of this person is filtered through her father's remarks. The family doctor's goal is to keep his patient alive long enough so that the father-daughter meeting can proceed successfully. Dr. W.'s use of the placebo is rationalized by this seemingly noble goal. If, for example, Mr. D. dies soon after seeing Linda, should Dr. D. tell the daughter of his prior action? Should he seek a kind of retrospective absolution? Or should he remain silent about his use of the sugar pills?

■ PRACTICE MODEL CASE ■

Mrs. Roberts, a 73-year-old widow, was taken to her family practice physician, Dr. M., by her married daughter, an only child with three young children. The patient lived at home alone in the suburbs of a major metropolitan area. She had been experiencing a decline in memory functions and symptoms of mental confusion for about 2 years. Her problem was now so substantial that she could not perform simple tasks such as keeping the house clean or going to the grocery store. The daughter, who resided about 6 miles away, looked in after Mrs. Roberts every day and made certain that she was eating enough and was keeping clean. Mrs. Roberts seemed quite at ease during Dr. M.'s examination. When he asked her if she had been having any trouble recalling things, she stated, "Well, you know how it is. When you're my age you have so much more to remember."

Dr. M. arranged for Mrs. Roberts to be seen at a nearby geriatric clinic. The interdisciplinary team there, led by a geriatrician but including nursing and social work staff, ruled out other causes of the patient's cognitive loss and diagnosed the problem as senile dementia of the Alzheimer's type (SDAT). The geriatrician both called and sent a written report to Dr. M. with the diagnosis and with the recommendation that the patient be placed in adult day care with a live-in assistant for her time at home. If this were impossible, the recommendation was for nursing home care.

The family physician, who had taken care of Mrs. Roberts for two decades, called the daughter with the news. Her first question was, "Couldn't this just be depression?" When Dr. M. assured her that Alzheimer's disease was the problem, she asked a very direct question: "How much responsibility do I have to take for Mom? As it is, I spent 3 hours a day dealing with her needs." Dr. M. invited the daughter to his office to discuss the matter. Mrs. Roberts, at this point, had not been told of the diagnosis or about possible living arrangements. When the daughter came to the office, her first remark to Dr. M. was, "My husband says that we should put her in the home. She'd be safer, and we'd all be better off."

Dr. M. wonders what to do next. What should he tell Mrs. Roberts? The daughter says, "I don't think we should say anything to Momma. It will only scare her. What good can it do her in her condition? I really don't think I can give her much more than I do right now. Let's just do our best to make her happy and comfortable." Dr. M. ponders what he should recommend to the daughter and to her family. He is inclined to work with them, because they are the main sources of support for his patient.

Based on Diana E. Meier and Christine K. Cassel, "Nursing Home Placement and the Demented Patient: A Case Presentation and Ethical Analysis," Ann. Intern. Med. 104 (1):98–105, 1986.

Patient

Mrs. Roberts is suffering from SDAT, a progressive disease with unknown etiology (though recent research is promising) and without cure. Her neurologic function will continue to deteriorate visibly, but the rate of her decline remains uncertain (the course of the illness may range from 3–20 years; average length is 6–10 years). During the final stages of the disease, she will lose most of her verbal abilities; her motor skills will deteriorate, and she will require total care. Eventually, she will be unable to interact meaningfully and will become bedbound. This could be several years away. At the moment, Mrs. Roberts can speak, move about, and experience the world, but she is certainly difficult to manage.

A common complication of SDAT is dramatic mood swings, often presenting as outbursts of anger (perhaps due to frustration). Agitation is frequent—here Mrs. Roberts seems an atypical patient. Wandering, sleeplessness, anxiety, and apathy are also frequently observed in SDAT patients. There is no efficacious drug therapy for the disease, although major tranquilizers such as halperidol are sometimes prescribed to control agitation. The side effects of these high potency agents can be very powerful. Mrs. Roberts' problems with memory loss and confusion suggest that she is between stage 3 and stage 4 on the global deterioration scale (GDS) for SDAT. Stage 3, mild cognitive decline, is characterized by clear-cut deficits and objective evidence of memory loss, with decreased performance in social settings. Stage 4, where Mrs. Roberts is headed, shows more substantial cognitive problems and an inability to perform tasks, thus requiring assistance in daily activities. The comprehensive assessment by the geriatrics clinic is not absolute. Certainty of diagnosis can be attained only after death through examination of brain tissue during an autopsy.

Mrs. Roberts' subjective status is very difficult to assess. Many SDAT patients are able to mask their confusion by routinizing behavior and by simply smiling in response to difficult questions. We can also assume that Mrs. Roberts knows that *something* is problematic. The fact that she has had a thorough diagnostic assessment, which includes tests of memory function, has told her that she is in need of some kind of intervention.

Relationships

Mrs. Roberts does have a caring daughter who has already demonstrated her involvement in the case and, to date, a willingness to support her mother. We know of no other resources available to Mrs. Roberts, but we can assume, given the recommendations of the geriatrics clinic, that social services are available locally. We know little about the patient's financial status. The only certainty is that, although she is over 65 and likely receiving Social Security and Medicare benefits, such payments will not cover the costs of nursing home care, at least in the beginning stages of SDAT, which do not require skilled nursing interventions.

That Mrs. Roberts is a widow and that she has chosen to live independently tell us that she is like most Americans in her position. Only a small portion of older people are institutionalized. Mrs. Roberts has grandchildren who live in the same community. Her connections with other members of that community—friends, congregants of her religious institution, members of societies she has joined—will have to be explored.

She also has a long-standing relationship with her primary care physician. He cares for her and, presumably, about her. He has taken an appropriate first step by referring Mrs. Roberts to specialists who can assess her condition. In communicating the diagnostic results to the daughter first, he has said that his relationship with the patient is compromised. He has bypassed her, for reasons that bear exploration.

Advocacy

Both daughter and physician seem obliged to look out for the best interests of this patient. They have begun to do so by initiating a conversation about Mrs. Roberts. Their concern for her is surely genuine, but it could present an ethical issue. Is it premature?

Although both Mrs. Roberts' daughter and family physician want to help her, could they be squashing her rights? Can advocacy slip unnoticed into protection and, then, to paternalistic denial of this woman's opportunity to make choices?

If Mrs. Roberts lived completely alone, without help or supervision by her daughter, her case might have come to the attention of public authorities (i.e., the health department, a social service, or an adult protective service agency). A common signal to such authorities is a report by a neighbor that an older person has been wandering about the neighborhood. A visitor may also report that there are signs of small fires in the kitchen or that the older person has let his or her house become filthy. When such reports are filed and a social agency becomes aware of the case, an advocate from within the bureaucracy (e.g., a social worker) is appointed to "case manage" the problem. Such a person is distanced from the affective dimensions of the case. The professional is unlikely ever to have met the older person. Does this present, from the perspective of advocacy, an advantage or a disadvantage? Does Dr. M.'s and the daughter's closeness to Mrs. Roberts guarantee that they will advocate more responsibly than someone for whom it is a professional task?

Conflicts

The case is still at a preliminary stage. No one has approached Mrs. Roberts and asked *her* opinion. She seems a potential candidate for involuntary placement in a nursing home. If she is put into long-term care, the decision is likely to be irreversible and can be stigmatizing for a patient like Mrs. Roberts, who will *know* where she is, against her will. To pose the ethical conflict in conventional terms as a dispute between voluntary and involuntary decision-making—will we be violating the autonomy of Mrs. Roberts if we move her out of her home?—may be naive.

There is already a conflict because Mrs. Roberts has become the *object* and not the *subject* of this case. This patient's SDAT diagnosis is her property: It is on her medical record. Yet she is in the dark about it. By acting paternalistically, the daughter and family physician, no matter how benign their motives, have decided that Mrs. Roberts' condition requires doling out the truth to her because they doubt her ability to process that information. Should SDAT patients, at this stage of the disease, have a right to know the nature of the disorder and its likely future course? Or will presenting such data to Mrs. Roberts further confuse her, lead to profound depression, and at the very least make her care much more complicated?

Within the daughter's family there is apparently conflict as well. Nursing home placement can become a symbolic as well as a very real issue. The role of women as caregivers for their aging parents has been a traditional one. This uncompensated, and often unrecognized, activity may be voluntary, or a result of guilt, desperation, and even coercion. Mrs. Roberts' daughter comes to the physician's office with a strong statement from her husband: He demands the institutionalization of his mother-in-law. What are the fundamental questions that should be asked? Some are clearly psychological: Placing a parent in a long-term care facility can be commonly seen as a sign of failure. On the other side of the coin, continuing to care for a parent whose demands accelerate can be seen as a demonstration of familial, even moral, reciprocity: "She diapered me when I was a baby; the least I can do is keep her dry."

Assume that Mrs. Roberts is much worse off, that she completely lacks decisional capacity, and a decision must be made about keeping her at home or moving her to a nursing facility. What are the appropriate grounds for such a decision? Patient medical status? Patient perception of well-being? Family needs? Economic factors? Physician availability (few doctors make house calls; most family doctors visit nursing homes routinely)? Future prospects (placing the patient now means that she will be routinized at the facility so that her dementia can be more easily managed when it gets worse)? The list could grow.

From the conflict perspective, what is missing is a fundamental question: What does Mrs. Roberts want? How can we know this without asking her?

Treatment or Nontreatment Options

In the immediate future, options for Mrs. Roberts include:

Staying at home, with her daughter continuing to provide whatever aid she can, perhaps supplemented by home health services.

Adult day care, usually available on weekdays, with either a family member (why not ask for a service contribution by the son-in-law?) or a professional providing the balance of the help.

Moving to the home of her daughter and family, with appropriate support services, including respite care.

Placement in a long-term care facility, on a trial or permanent basis.

Remaining at home seems to be the least restrictive alternative. But is it the best, the safest, the most useful? Once again, choices depend on *who* should decide. Mrs. Roberts may accede to several of the recommended courses of care. Or she may adamantly refuse all, save the first. Must we respect her judgment, given the medical determination that her cognitive capacity is impaired? Does a person with diminished mental status lose all, or some, of her rights?

In the long run, many other treatment options will have to be determined. Will Mrs. Roberts require a guardian when she can no longer speak coherently? Will that guardian necessarily make the right choices? Who will really decide about her medical care? Guardians usually defer to physician judgment, so Dr. M. will still be authoritative in the care of Mrs. Roberts. If the court-appointed surrogate decision-maker errs, who is to guard the guardian?

When Mrs. Roberts is unable to swallow readily, should she be given a feeding tube? If she becomes ill (e.g., a urinary tract infection) during the final stages of her disease, should she be treated vigorously with antibiotics or should she be given measures designed to keep her comfortable? If she develops an intercurrent disease (pulmonary complications are frequent for patients who spend most of their days in bed) how aggressive should interventions be on her behalf?

Embedded in the conflict about even telling Mrs. Roberts the SDAT diagnosis is the kernel of an important question. Is this patient one who could tell us, right now, before nearly total decline of her brain functions, how she wants to die (see Chapter 8)? Could she execute a living will or durable power-of-attorney for health care document? Can we evoke from her a sense of *her* moral principles and perhaps religious values, which will allow us to act on her behalf not by using our standards, but by following her express wishes?

Interests

From a legal standpoint, the assertion of best interests concerning Mrs. Roberts will perhaps best be settled by a court hearing. If she is determined to be incapable of making sound decisions, then a court-appointed guardian will determine her significant interests. Should this be a once-and-for-all decision? Some studies show that reassessments of patients with primary or secondary dementia demonstrate that about half the patients show improvement in their level of confusion and interpersonal tensions. Pragmatically speaking, a guardian for Mrs. Roberts is unlikely to have her reevaluated.

What, indeed, are this patient's interests right now? Does she have an interest in hearing the diagnosis and in collaborating in care plans made for her? If Dr. M. and the daughter never ask her, can they be sure that she will accede to their determinations? Could Mrs. Roberts have an interest in giving up her residual autonomy: For example, would designating her daughter as the principal decision-maker serve the patient's needs most effectively? Can there be a compromise that will allow Mrs. Roberts some decision-making authority while granting to others the right to make determinations about managing her finances, for example?

In the future, Mrs. Roberts will presumably have an interest in remaining as free of pain as possible. She will want an environment that is clean and caring, and that permits her the maximum possible freedom. (Some long-term care facilities have developed special wings for people with Alzheimer's disease, with specially designed architecture and furnishings that allow considerable patient mobility.) She will also want assistance with the activities of daily living. When Mrs. Roberts can no longer communicate, will her interests be enshrouded in her disease? Not necessarily, if we can elicit from this patient the present sources of her pleasure. Some SDAT patients who lack speech are noted to smile when hearing soothing music. Others enjoy being out of doors. Advance planning, beyond the formalities of treatment options at the end of life, can include a listing of patient preferences in very homey and simple ways.

Consequences

We already have a sense of the options available for this patient (see Treatment or Nontreatment Options). The immediate consequences for Mrs. Roberts entail either independent living, institutionalization, or some blend of the two. The consequences from the ethical perspective are a bit more complex: *Who* chooses will dramatically affect the personae in this case. Mrs. Roberts can maintain some decisional authority; this may enhance her sense of effectiveness and competence. Were she to choose to live at home, however, the realistic results are eminently unpredictable. Patients with SDAT sometimes harm themselves (starting fires has been noted) and others (those who continue to drive an automobile can be quite dangerous). Knowing Mrs. Roberts' future is impossible, but it is a fair bet that nursing home care for her, while perhaps defeating her desire for independence, will be safer than staying home alone and being visited infrequently.

For the daughter and her family there are consequences, too. Nuclear families have been sacrificed on the altar of service to a parent. Women are often trapped in the middle, unable to balance a job outside the home with child rearing and parent care-taking responsibilities. Somewhere in the calculation of decision making in this case, we must figure the costs, as well as the benefits, of asking Mrs. Roberts' daughter to keep her mother either at home or with her own family in theirs.

For Dr. M. there are also ends worth scrutinizing. These can be long term. His decision—whether or not to accede to the daughter's request to keep the diagnosis from Mrs. Roberts or not—will influence his subsequent attitudes and practice. And not just toward his patients who have SDAT. The family doctor, because he prizes communication and continuity of care, needs to speak the truth (bluntly or gently) in order to maintain credibility. If Dr. M. takes the paternalistic route in this case he will do so for good reasons, but confronting a sick patient with bad news will always be difficult— and this applies to persons with cancer or AIDS or emphysema or kidney disease—and each episode of shading the truth may have an almost invisible impact on Dr. M.'s interactions with future patients.

Ethical Principles

Mrs. Roberts' autonomy is the ethical center of this case. Assessing her competence, of course, is a complex task (see Chapter 2). Her dementia is an impediment, but is it so debilitating that she cannot understand in clearly presented descriptions the nature of her condition and the likely course of her disorder? Because immediate decisions will not be life threatening (no one is about to place her on a ventilator), how demanding should we be in determining her decisional capacity? Must she be completely rational and articulate? Or is awareness of her problems and an ability to dissent or assent to recommendations sufficient? Whatever standard is utilized, and for whatever reasons, the veracity expected of Dr. M. is on the line.

Daughter and doctor, in their desire to preserve Mrs. Roberts' well-being, are acting from a motive of beneficence. They want to keep her from worry, depression, and further confusion. Her daughter is asking Dr. M. to help in devising a care plan that will, presumably, give Mrs. Roberts as much freedom as possible, within the limits of a safe environment. In initiating this discussion behind the patient's back, beneficence can easily be converted into paternalism. One solid question that could help clarify the motives in this situation is: Which "fear" is paramount, the anxiety that Mrs. Roberts will react to the news of SDAT with self-destructive behaviors or the concern that simply telling such news will make ultimate decisions such as nursing home placement more complicated for the caregivers?

Preventing harm to Mrs. Roberts (i.e., practicing nonmaleficence) is not quite the same as trying to benefit her. Harm varies remarkably, from the patently physical to the distantly psychological. Dr. M. must keep such a pledge in perspective, for he is a family doctor with a long-standing relationship with this woman. He must see her as she is: embedded in a history that includes family obligations and personal values. While not ignoring the importance of the daughter's and son-in-law's wishes, Dr. M. must ask himself, "How can I discern Mrs. Roberts' own sense of what harm she wishes to avoid?" The cliches about senior citizens (e.g., they are inherently conservative; they become more child-like as they grow older) are generally false and should be resisted. Dr. M. has a true judgment call to make: Can he summon the strength to do the best for this patient during her years of inevitable mental decline?

■ CASES FOR DISCUSSION ■

Case A

Mr. Zinn is a 71-year-old widower and has severe chronic obstructive pulmonary disease (COPD); he has been admitted to the hospital by his family physician, Dr. Y., twice in the past year for difficulty breathing. He is currently on the common COPD medications, as well as prednisone and Lasix. Mr. Zinn has a long, continuing pattern of tobacco and alcohol abuse. Dr. Y. has asked the patient many times over the years about his wishes regarding resuscitation should he stop breathing or have a cardiac arrest. Mr. Zinn has never made a decision about this issue. When the patient is admitted to the hospital again, this time for pulmonary insufficiency, a determination is made by patient and physician *not* to place a DNR order in the chart. "I still need some time to think about it," Mr. Zinn tells Dr. Y.

Mr. Zinn, during the same discussion, rejects the possibility of connection to a mechanical ventilator. "No machines!" he tells his family physician. Early the next morning, on rounds with a resident and medical student, Dr. Y. enters the patient's room and sees that Mr. Zinn is not breathing. Vital signs are absent. He decides, there and then, *not* to "call a code" or begin resuscitative efforts. When a nurse enters the room she conveys her uncertainty about the situation. Dr. Y. tells her that, "Mr. Zinn would have wanted it this way. He's better off now." The nurse does not describe her anxiety to Dr. Y; instead she tells her nursing supervisor the story.

Questions

1. Does the long-standing relationship between physician and patient give Dr. Y. a basis for *not* attempting resuscitation, even though the patient lacks a DNR order in the chart?
2. What weight if any should be given to Mr. Zinn's decision to reject ventilatory support?
3. The values and concerns of three others—the resident, the medical student, and the nurse—are implicated in this case. What are Dr. Y.'s obligations to them?
4. If the nurse does report this event to nursing and other hospital administrators, what should Dr. Y. do?

Case B

Rebecca M., the 4-year-old daughter of Mr. and Mrs. M., was struck by an automobile and was taken to the ER of the nearby hospital, where she was pronounced dead on arrival. The social worker in the ER called the parents as well as Dr. P., the family physician. They arrived at the hospital simultaneously and met briefly with the ER director, Dr. F., who told them that the child has died. Dr. P. discovers that the coroner has already seen the body and has ordered an autopsy. When the family physician states to Dr. F. in private that he believes Mr. and Mrs. M. should have a chance to see their daughter, the ER director says, "No, she's a real mess. They would be hysterical! Let's let the funeral director 'fix' this one first!"

Questions

1. Is there a sound ethical foundation for the ER director's determination to prevent the parents from seeing their daughter's body?
2. Given the traumatic circumstances, should the family physician press the ER doctor on behalf of the parents?
3. What should Dr. P. say to Mr. and Mrs. M., who are waiting in the ER lobby, when he sees them next?
4. Whatever the outcome of the present conflict, what action if any should the family physician take in the near future with regard to the ER director?

■ THINK PIECE: FAMILY PRACTICE ■

Addressing the needs of a family can be an all-encompassing task. Complete expertise is unlikely. Family practice and primary care physicians provide services across the life cycle. For the family practitioner, medical needs are notoriously hard to define. Taking a systems view, seeing families as existing not just here and now but also across the generations—these are great and substantial challenges. Physicians are often seen as more than medical authorities; they are also viewed as experts, giving moral permission to acts deemed controversial by families. Difficult questions emerge all the time.

For example: A married couple with several children have been patients of a family practice group for decades. The couple has a child, living at home and also a patient, who is moderately mentally retarded. Should this child, who has the usual teenage interest in sexuality and who wants to live independently from her parents, be encouraged, discouraged, or prohibited from having children of her own? Do persons who are physically able to become parents have the right to *be* parents? Because mental retardation is associated, in some cases, with an inheritable disorder, should conventional practice prohibit reproduction by persons defined as retarded? More than scientific accuracy is at stake here: Economic issues and questions of social policy are also on the line.

In 1927, U.S. Supreme Court Justice Oliver Wendell Holmes, in approving the sterilization of Carrie Buck, an ostensibly mentally disabled young woman, wrote that "three generations of imbeciles are enough." These harsh terms are often decried today. The questions opened by this patently eugenic phrase have not withered: Do families and their caregivers want to encourage parenting by persons labeled retarded? Does the presumed fact of retardation increase the likelihood that parenting will be seriously deficient? From a legal perspective, does the state have an interest that could justify intervention designed to prohibit reproduction on the grounds of mental retardation?

We know, medically and psychologically, that people who are called mentally retarded share no single physical or intellectual characteristic, common set of symptoms, or psychological property. Retardation is often grouped into four categories: mild, moderate, severe, and profound. IQ distinctions based on these rankings have been standardized. Such constructs are both mechanical and misleading, however, for they tell little about the specific skills, or life contexts, of persons being so measured. Still, assuming that there are some persons called mentally retarded who are disabled in important ways, trying to make reproductive decisions presents a difficult problem.

In order to recommend, in a single discreet case or on the policy level, whether or not to impede reproductive freedom in such cases, one would need an adequate definition of parenting, itself the subject of controversy. What abilities are required, at a minimum, for a person to qualify as a potential parent? What skills of intellectual analysis, physical skills (e.g., meeting the needs of a neonate), planning capacity (e.g., to help in avoiding health and safety problems for the child), or psychological attributes (e.g., warmth, empathy, concern, love) are indispensable? Which are optional? Do we require them in *all* parents, not just those who seem to be suspect due to mental disability?

We do know that, in most places, social agencies (the legally responsible state institutions) treat MR parents differently from parents who are not retarded. Agencies value rationality and devalue passion; they emphasize economic efficiency measured in utilitarian terms over the value of moral equality. Child protection agencies legitimately work to protect the welfare (health as well as safety) of vulnerable children. Do we know if these ideals are discerned objectively? Or does *difference* itself make caregivers (e.g., MR parents) suspect?

The issue goes beyond reproductive rights. Some states forbid the sterilization of MR persons; others permit it. Whether or not MR parents can keep their offspring will also be of importance to the family practice doctor who is involved in such decision-making. Many statutes say, often without definition, that a diagnosis of mental disability or mental incapacity or developmental disability is enough to deem MR parents as incompetent to retain their children. Even when such children are allowed to stay with their natural parents, the burden of proof for continuing the relationship falls to the MR parent and his or her advocates. Quite frequently, children are seized, placed into foster care, and parental rights are terminated.

Where does the family practice or primary care physician fit into this scheme? What sort of expertise is needed to give advice to both the parents of a MR person and to the person herself? Does the family doctor act as an advocate if requested? Should a physician push a social service agency not to order the termination of parental rights but rather to try to extend rehabilitation efforts to ensure good caregiving by the MR parent? Knowing that the world is imperfect, should the family physician discourage or encourage an experimental attitude towards child rearing by MR persons? What obligations are owed to the children? What rights should grandparents retain in such situations? If mental retardation is grounds for the termination of rights usually granted others, what ethical justifications can be found for such practice? What are the duties of physicians who take exception to standard social policy or practice?

■ VOICES: SOCIAL WORKER IN FAMILY PRACTICE GROUP ■

Young doctors have so much to learn! I work with family practice physicians and residents in both in-patient and office settings. I emphasize as much as possible the behavioral aspects of medicine—for me families are the primary "reality"—and the psychological dimensions of illness. When the residents or attending physicians see individual patients, however, they often see illness in isolation. Even in a family practice, there is a tendency to treat symptoms in the body of *that patient* who presents today. Concern for context—most ethical decisions are made with a variety of needs in mind—has to be encouraged and I try to do so. Otherwise important data will be neglected.

For example, a woman is post-partum, feeling "blue" and reporting headaches and stomach pains. The family practice doctor will naturally order a whole bunch of tests and try to find the cause of the problem. They might, eventually, prescribe some pain medication. Do they ask, "Who's taking care of the baby? What are your family resources? How are you getting on with your husband? Are the bills getting paid now that you have stopped working outside of the home?" I am always asking, "What else do we need to know?" Because if the so-called patient has to make a significant choice, we need to understand her in every possible aspect. We shouldn't be throwing medicines at people. Family practitioners, who may want to find a quick fix, say that they don't have the time to pursue such issues. This isn't true. If you've ever seen a really gifted family practice doctor integrate the psychosocial and the biologic, you'll remember it as a great piece of work.

Family practitioners do a fine job. They generally respect their patients. They make real efforts to maintain confidentiality. (This doesn't always work; I see too much talking in the hospital corridors.) I do think that our doctors treat patients of various ages fairly and appropriately. Age discrimination is rarely seen. Teenagers, of course, get complicated because of the family practitioner's responsibility to the parents. With young adults, many residents tend to identify with the patients and can get very involved and very upset with particular cases.

Physicians sometimes refer to patients as "difficult" or even "hateful." I prefer the term "challenging patient." Some people out there present facades that are scary or ugly or impenetrable. We have to find the person behind the mask.

I see striking differences between male and female doctors. The domination of males, white males particularly, in the profession is obvious. I think that female residents, for example, have better relationships with their patients. They are more empathic and want the inside story. When it comes to informed consent, you're likely to have a more successful dialogue with a female doctor and, as a result, more likely as a patient to understand a forthcoming procedure. I also think that women patients are more satisfied with female physicians: They feel better understood. Many women report terrible interactions with male doctors. I still think that male doctors *can* treat all patients very well, but a lot of education needs to be done.

As a behavioral medicine team member of a family practice group, I do have some ethical worries. Is it fair for me to care, much of the time, more about the residents than about the patients? I see their growth and their dilemmas as most immediate. In some respects, the residents are my patients. I also wonder about my role when I see mistakes being made—medical mistakes not revealed to patients. Doctors talk privately every day about their errors—they're only human! What is my duty when I hear about such problems? I guess I've accommodated myself to the system. I'm not a whistle-blower. I do make suggestions and do raise questions such as, "What are you going to do about this?" But if the doctor lets it slide, nothing is going to occur.

RECOMMENDED READING

Bok, S. *Lying: Moral Choices in Public and Private Life.* New York: Pantheon, 1978.

Brody, H. *Ethical Decisions in Medicine* (2nd ed.). Boston: Little, Brown, 1981.

Christie, R.J. and Hoffmaster, C. *Ethical Issues in Family Medicine.* New York: Oxford University Press, 1986.

Mappes, T. and Zembaty, J. (eds), *Biomedical Ethics.* New York: McGraw-Hill, 1991.

Smith, H.L. and Churchill, L.R. *Professional Ethics and Primary Care Medicine: Beyond Dilemmas and Decorum.* Durham, NC: Duke University, 1986.

Veatch, R. *A Theory of Medical Ethics.* New York: Basic Books, 1981.

▪5▪

Parents and Children: Ethical Issues in Pediatrics/Adolescent Medicine

Most young persons live long and prosper physically: Few get terribly ill or suffer serious injuries. When they are in need of significant, interventional health care, they present special challenges. To see a child in pain often causes suffering in families and among health care professionals. We think of children as being "special," but such special qualities make medical decisions in the best interest of the child or adolescent difficult.

There is a long-standing legal requirement that someone else speak for a minor. We refer to children as pediatrics cases prior to the age of 13; from 13 to 18 (and sometimes 21), we refer to them as adolescent cases. Not all 16 year olds are alike, however, and the same could be said of 12-year-old children. Many acute care hospitals that treat this population have come to refer to the patient as "the child/adolescent and her family." Thus the conventional doctor-patient relationship becomes complicated: How can a physician have a private conversation based on mutual trust with a teenager when the adolescent knows that significant revelations may be reported to the parents? The more optimistic side of this unique status for the patient, of course, results from the natural advocacy that parents provide for their children in need of health care.

The responsibilities parents must exercise on behalf of their children are considerable. (The decision to bear and raise children is one that few can take lightly.) Everyday decisions in infancy and early childhood regarding nutrition, sleeping habits, personal cleanliness, and schooling have a substantial impact on a child's health and well-being. Parents choose a pediatrician and speak for the child. This does not end with adolescence. Paternalism, a concept that suggests undue influence or even limitations on the autonomy of another person, derives linguistically from the Latin term for father (parent). Thus, paternalism with regard to one's children seems justified. Conflict, however, often emerges over choice-making and responsibility for health-related matters, especially with older children and adolescents. For example, 17 year olds with behavioral disorders can be involuntarily institutionalized in acute or long-term mental institutions with parental discretion, against the will of the patient. Courts have generally sustained this power, on the presumption that mothers and fathers would not act contrary to the interests of their teenaged children.

For infants and very young children, however, seeing the child as embedded in the family and in need of parental decision-making and advocacy seems a reasonable and realistic approach. Small children cannot give informed consent; their refusal is also assumed to be less than rational (see Chapter 2 concerning informed consent). This can also present problems for caregivers. For example, when parents disagree, or when a surrogate decision-maker (e.g., a court-appointed guardian) has authority, complications often arise. Must both parents consent? Are there limits on parental agreement to treatment: For example, can a mother or father say yes to a dangerous experimental drug trial? If we agree that parents or their legal surrogates are the appropriate decision-makers, what weight, if any, do we give to the desires of the pediatric or adolescent patient? Does the perspective of a 12 year old shift sufficiently so that at age 17 we can hear her opinion with greater credibility? And if she turns 18 during the course of treatment, do we automatically (following the letter of the law) assume that she is now the decision maker?

Several other factors make pediatric/adolescent medicine and its ethical dilemmas especially interesting. Our desire to protect the vulnerable is a powerful emotion; young persons seem in need of such aid. We also grow angry at those who either neglect the care of children or, worse, physically or psychologically abuse young persons. In recent years there has been a growing consensus about the need to protect such children. Pediatricians and specialists in adolescent medicine are assumed to have a social responsibility to detect child abuse and neglect and to, at the very least, report it to the appropriate authorities. This has not been a traditional role for physicians.

Younger patients need labor-intensive care in hospitals and in outpatient settings. Their physical problems are usually, though not always, overlaid by psychologic and behavior problems. Sick children are sometimes aggressive, have school problems, display anger at authorities, and are dependent on adults for basic needs. In acute care hospitals, pediatric cases entail a lot of nursing care. The responsibilities of nurses are considerable, but the rewards are significant. In pediatric and adolescent medicine, nurse-physician relationships are filtered through a concern for a unique population. This presents real challenges.

Though reliance on chronological age is a useful guide, the law in most states and conventional practice (for reasons of public policy) make an exception to the requirement that responsible adults must give consent to care on behalf of minors. The *emancipated minor* is a young person who is self-supporting and who lives independently. (Being married or serving in the military are other criteria in some states.) Some young patients are deemed to be *mature minors*, usually 15 to 18 year olds who show rational intelligence and significant sophistication in understanding their medical conditions. Legally children and adolescents have authority to consent to medical care regarding sexual behavior and reproductive decision-making. For example, in most states, a 14 year old does not need parental permission to be tested for venereal disease.

■ FIVE ESSENTIAL CASES ■

Case 5-1

Parents are the preferred decision-makers for children who need health care, but the demand for parental autonomy is often a challenge to practitioners of pediatric and adolescent medicine.

Dr. J. is in private pediatric practice. He is accustomed to treating contagious childhood infections. He has seen about 30 school-aged children with a common viral infection this week. When Mr. and Mrs. W. bring 6-year-old Jason into the office to see Dr. J. they seem very upset. (Dr. J. has been Jason's pediatrician for 3 years.) Four months ago Jason had a painful ear infection and antibiotic therapy helped him. Today Jason is cranky: Even in the office he is crying. He is also fever-ish. The examination shows all the classic signs of having the viral infection.

The parents want some kind of medicine for Jason. Their past experience with drug therapy has been positive. Dr. J. explains that the infection will work its way through Jason's system and that medicine can do no good. Acetaminophen and fluids, with lots of rest, are the best treatment, Dr. J. states. Jason's mother and father are adamant, however, and insist on a prescription. They have friends, who see other pediatricians, who have received medications for the same symptoms. The parents imply that they will go to another physician if Dr. J. refuses to satisfy their demands. Dr. J. feels uncomfortable about writing a prescription, though he tells himself that no real harm would come of it.

■ ■ ■

Jason, clearly, cannot speak for himself. He is too young and perhaps too ill to express more than a desire to go home and watch television. His parents, we assume, have no desire to see their son in discomfort; their motives are quite pure. But in making what Dr. J. deems an irrational demand, they have precipitated a minor crisis between physician and patient/family. Parental autonomy is almost universally taken to be indispensable in pediatric health care. In a true emergency, a pediatrician might contradict a parental determination, but Jason's illness is not critical. Surrogate decision-makers in pediatrics cases "speak" for the child, but this speech is not based on Jason's thoughts. Family members who make health care choices for older adults who are presently incompetent usually do so because they have previously heard or seen documented the prior expressions of the patient. But Jason—crying and body language aside—has had nothing to say over the course of time regarding antibiotic therapies, so if we leave decision-making authority in the hands of parents we do so as an act of faith.

The doctor-patient relationship is complicated by Dr. J.'s sense that Jason should not take a drug for his presumed viral infection. Dr. J. has several reasons: (1) While the antibiotic will do little harm in the short run, giving it will encourage the use of unnecessary medications in the future; (2) for Dr. J. to write the prescription he will, in effect, have to lie to himself; this is an odd consequence because he has certainly been truthful with the parents; (3) Dr. J. thinks that he knows better than the parents what is in Jason's best interest in this case. Medically he does, but he is not the principal caretaker of this child.

If Dr. J. remains firm with the parents they may respond by going elsewhere. (Though Jason's case has a special feature—a minor who cannot give consent or have a meaningful discussion with the physician—the role of the surrogate seeking unnecessary intervention is not limited to this parent-child situation. Fifty-year-old children with a moderately demented parent have been known to be similarly demanding.) They may, in fact, get the prescription they desire from another physician less principled than Dr. J. He knows this, and he wants to maintain a relationship with Jason and his family. So he is more than a bit stuck about what to do next.

The case at hand seems relatively basic, if not simple. Dr. J. has a choice. But our method of deciding the rights and wrongs in Jason's case has implications for other, perhaps very serious, situations. For example, in several states parents, rather than demanding care, have sought alternative treatments and therapies, often religious in nature. Christian Science families have refused to bring their ill children to mainstream physicians, preferring to use the services of religious healers or practitioners. Some of these children have died, and the parents have been prosecuted. If Dr. J. was aware of such a child (e.g., a former patient or a friend of his own offspring) would he have a moral obligation to intervene? What are the limits of parental autonomy? On what ethical grounds can physicians "invade" the ostensibly sacred territory of family integrity?

In situations of disagreement such as this, who is the appropriate decision-maker? What are Jason's rights, if any, here? Dr. J. may take the high road and tell the parents that he will not acquiesce, but will the physician benefit anyone but himself if he refuses to write the prescription? Principles beyond parental autonomy are at stake here. They include concerns for beneficence and nonmaleficence: Helping Jason, or at least not harming him, is at issue. Cost factors (antibiotics are not cheap; prescribing them may mean a follow-up visit for Jason) may also influence our view of this case. One way to ponder the case in a wider, social and economic context is to ask: If Dr. J. does write the prescription, and you were his partner in private practice, what would you say to him when he reviewed the case with you?

Case 5-2

We want to give ill children every chance to survive. But knowing if, or when, to stop treatment involves ethical, psychological, and sometimes economic considerations.

H.C. is 13 years old. She was diagnosed with leukemia/lymphoma at 4 years of age and has had a difficult, prolonged course of medical treatment. Her leukemia has repeatedly recurred in the brain, requiring radiation and many doses of chemotherapy delivered directly into the cerebrospinal fluid. She has experienced many episodes of confusion, erratic behavior, depression, and anxiety. Her psychologic and psycho-educational tests show considerable dysfunction. A CT scan of the head reveals changes in the brain, most likely due to her therapy.

Despite the massive treatment she has received, H.C. has had a relapse of her leukemia, with central nervous system, abdomen, kidney, and breast involvement. So serious was her condition that the physicians told her parents that the only option that would give her a chance to survive would be bone marrow transplantation (BMT), with her 16-year-old (minor) sister serving as donor. The standard regimen for BMT would be too toxic for H.C.; a new, experimental combination of chemotherapies was chosen. (The hospital's institutional review board—the committee that serves to protect human subjects in medical research—gave its approval.) The parents and the child were told of the risks of the BMT: bleeding from the bladder, mouth sores, infections, graft versus host disease (GVHD), and further brain damage. The parents signed the complex consent form.

The patient received her chemotherapy and bone marrow infusion from her sister without complication. Two weeks after the transplant she began to experience minor internal bleeding but could not tolerate platelet transfusion, despite receiving many from different sources. H.C. was a difficult patient for the nursing staff: Her behavior problems worsened. Physically, her platelet problem persisted for many weeks. The donated bone marrow did not show signs of "taking." Her parents insisted on being included in virtually every minor decision regarding her care. It was decided to give H.C. back her own bone marrow, which had been stored as backup, despite the risk of returning leukemia cells to her.

Soon afterward, H.C. experienced a large hemorrhage into the brain. She was exhausting the supply of platelets at the blood bank and such material had to be shipped in from other parts of the country. Because of the bleeding into her brain, she had to be put on a respirator along with other modes of support in the pediatric intensive care unit. Her bone marrow did not seem to be recovering.

The physician team approached the parents and suggested that no further efforts be made to prolong H.C.'s life. The parents did request that no CPR be done but wanted to continue her present level of care. H.C.'s mother had been staying at the hospital during the entire hospitalization and was an active spokesperson for her daughter's medical and psychologic needs. The father, who visited regularly, was nurturing and supportive and accepted his spouse's advocacy role. H.C. was unconscious but did respond to painful stimuli, and there was no suggestion of brain death. Her leukemia seemed to be intractable, but the parents continued to insist that she be given blood products and that she be kept alive unless she had a cardiac arrest.

Although the precise protocol followed in H.C.'s bone marrow transplantation was experimental, BMTs even for children are no longer rare. At least 5000 have been performed since the early 1980s and more than 60 BMT units in the United States treat children in this manner for certain leukemias. Mortality rates for patients (children and adult) who undergo BMT for acute myelogenous leukemia are almost 60 percent; for those with acute lymphoblastic leukemia it approaches 70 percent. Survivors of BMT often suffer long-term effects: chronic GVHD, endocrine disorders, and secondary malignancies; children experience physical growth problems and impeded neurologic development; intellectual function may be permanently compromised.

We can look at the case of H.C. as it emerged. She lived with leukemia for 9 years, at times functioning well, most often in pain and with difficulty for herself and her family. During the course of her chemotherapy and radiation treatments, many decisions were made on her behalf. Clearly a single value predominated: saving the life of this child. Eventually, however, the cancer caused systems problems too massive to control. BMT was offered as a last ditch effort to achieve a remission. When the parents signed the informed consent agreement for the research study to use the new drug combination as preparatory for BMT, what were they told?

The informed consent process made them aware that the standard regimen was too dangerous, given H.C.'s clinical situation. They were told that the experimental preparation gave the best chance to control the lymphoma and that high-dosage chemotherapy kills both the malignant cancer cells and the normal cells of the bone marrow. The parents were given a precise description of the procedure and of the conditions of recovery (e.g., details of diet, antibiotics, other drugs, blood products, anesthesias, and the insertion of lines) and follow-up. Benefits (i.e., a better chance of curing the lymphoma than with traditional dose chemotherapy) and burdens (e.g., risks in administering the drugs, side-effects, potential lung damage, GVHD, neurologic damage, recurrence of the cancer) were detailed. Finally, the parents were given the option of rejecting the experimental procedure and trying the conventional chemotherapy. They elected the experimental approach. Psychologically, can parents who have spent nearly a decade trying to find a cure for their daughter's grave illness really refuse any experimental treatment? Can they give a full and informed consent?

A 13-year-old patient is at the chronologic border between pediatric and adolescent health care. In a strictly legal sense, a 2 year old and a 17 year old are both minors, and the authority for permitting or rejecting medical procedures resides with parents or designated surrogates. But many 13 year olds can think, reason, express opinions, understand problems, and imagine futures. Was H.C. given a chance to participate in this most important decision, whether or not to go ahead with the experimental preoperative chemotherapy before the BMT? Did she have an opportunity not to *consent*, but to voice her perspective and her concerns, perhaps to *assent* to the intervention? She did not. She was too sick and, significantly, too confused and dysfunctional due to previous treatments.

Suppose H.C. had been "with it." Suppose she had said, "I don't want to go through with this thing. I'll leave it in the hands of the Lord." Would you respect such an expression? Should her parents give credence to this viewpoint? Beyond the consent issue there is the question of how much should be tried using experimental therapies in children. The uncertainty of outcome was a given in this case. What forces were at work in recommending the protocol to H.C.'s family? How do the values of patient care and the consequent hope for a remission or cure balance the values of research (and finding a new chemotherapy that will benefit future patients and offer data for other, improved interventions) and teaching (at this hospital, residents, nurses, medical students and staff would learn through the efforts of H.C. and her family)? How does anyone begin to decide the best interest of this patient at the time of deciding whether or not to go with the experimental protocol?

A related ethical question revolves around the donation of bone marrow by H.C.'s minor sister. How should medical personnel "test" whether an organ donation is voluntarily given (a BMT is an organ transplantation)? It was parental discretion that permitted this donation to go forward. Bone marrow donation is not without its complications, though it is not a very painful or dangerous procedure. Everyone would want to know just how this agreement to donate was reached.

The last stage of the case introduces two related further issues: the massive use of scarce resources (e.g., platelets) and, finally, a conflict with the request by the doctors to stop treatment and to let H.C. die. Health care resources involve more than equipment or fluids or intensive care technology. Nursing and physician time are also expensive and in short supply. H.C.'s hospitalization utilized an extraordinary amount of these commodities. Some argue that there should be an imposed limit on such scarce resources. The platelets, obviously, could be used to aid others with a more reasonable hope of recovery.

Finally, can or should physicians contradict parental autonomy? Should the doctors—who, with almost as much intensity as the parents, hoped for positive results from the BMT—state that their sense of H.C.'s best interest meant stopping transfusions? In an experimental therapy, a decision about when the experiment is over is based on a calculation of costs and benefits. Even when benefits are minimal or nonexistent, the actual decision to stop treatment is reached through a delicate balancing act between institutional protocol and parental need.

Case 5-3

The religious views of parents are constitutionally protected. But when they stand in the way of providing medical care for a child, legal authorities and practitioners' values can supersede the family's wishes.

Seven-year-old Robby presented at the hospital with a 4-week history of intermittent left upper-arm tenderness and swelling. There was no history of weight loss, anorexia, or fevers and he had otherwise been in good health. Radiographic scans revealed very extensive bony involvement up to the joint capsule of the left shoulder with a significant invasion of the soft tissues. A biopsy revealed osteogenic sarcoma.

Treatment plans recommended to the family included a chemotherapy regimen consisting of a 2-month course of preoperative chemotherapy and surgery, followed by several more months of chemotherapy. Due to the extensive involvement of the tumor in the left arm and shoulder, the surgical procedure would need to be a fore-quarter amputation. The parents sought a second opinion; the consultant concurred with the original plan. Prognosis for long-term survival with appropriate chemotherapy *and* the definitive surgical procedure could approach 60 percent.

Robby is the oldest of three siblings. His mother works at home and his father is a salesman; both are educated and articulate. Both maternal and paternal grandparents live close by and have been involved in Robby's care. The parents acknowledged feelings of grief to the staff after the diagnosis. Robby's father said, "We have strong faith and will accept whatever happens." The nursing staff encouraged the parents to talk with Robby the next day about the diagnosis using such words as cancer and tumor. They acknowledged that they would do this.

Robby's parents consented to the treatment plan, and he was readmitted a week later to begin preoperative chemotherapy. His mother was very teary eyed about the prospect of Robby's hair loss. Both parents alluded to the difficulty that they were having talking to Robby about his illness, the treatment plan, and side effects. The nursing staff observed the parents withholding information or minimizing the impact of what they told Robby about procedures and the discomfort that might be involved. The parents also seemed reluctant to allow hospital staff to intervene to help support and prepare their child.

A meeting with key nursing staff was held during this admission to explore with the parents ways to help them support their son and give him the necessary information to facilitate his coping. Robby's mother verbalized that she was still hoping a miracle might happen and all the tumor would disappear. His parents stated that they would talk with Robby about everything after discharge at home.

As the 2-month period of preoperative chemotherapy drew to a close, the parents expressed their hesitation about going through with surgery and decided to postpone the surgery indefinitely. Over this 2-month period Robby had become more anxious and agitated with each hospital admission, worrying over daily procedures, verbalizing that he hated the hospital.

His parents contacted a religious advisor, the pastor of the New Age Christian Church in a suburb near their home. The pastor told them that prayer could cure Robby and that the entire congregation would marshal its spiritual forces if the family requested such intervention. Robby's parents had long been fervent in their religious faith. They asked the pastor to help them and he agreed.

The parents then requested a meeting with the oncologist, the orthopedic surgeon, and Robby's primary nurse. His father stated that he and his wife felt the surgery to be unnecessary, that Robby "would be healed by the Lord." After future exploration—including meetings with the legal staff—a decision was made by the hospital to seek court protection for Robby.

■ ■ ■

Robby is incompetent according to legal definition. He is a minor; dependent on parents and caregivers, he lacks even the rudiments of autonomy. This is not unusual for a 7 year old who is ill. But this case presents a very special feature: Freedom of religion, a zealously guarded public value, is at stake. The responsibility of health care professionals to the child is emerging into a full-fledged court battle.

Robby's medical condition is very serious. The tumor is extensive and has invaded the shoulder, muscle, and surrounding soft tissue. Osteogenic sarcoma (one of the most common malignancies of childhood and adolescence, exceeded only by leukemia, brain tumors, and lymphoma) is treated most effectively by limb amputation and chemotherapy. Further progress of the tumor makes surgery substantially more difficult, if not impossible. Chemotherapy alone usually does not work: Almost all children with this disease who are treated with drugs alone die within 3 years. For osteogenic sarcomas involving the leg, en bloc resection of the tumor as an alternative to amputation is sometimes recommended. This option was not available for Robby.

Most ethical issues are enacted for patients, families, and medical personnel on a psychological substructure. The usual process is plain, if not simple: Physicians diagnose and recommend treatment. Patients or their surrogates agree and treatment progresses. But family complications frequently infiltrate clinical ethical decision-making. Here, Robby's parents may be assumed to be responding to their son's illness with agitation and concern. Fear is normal among parents who think that their children might die. So is some form of religious crisis. (Many very religious families ask, "Why us?" and renounce faith; others find solace and inspiration in religious counseling, ritual, or reflection.) Robby's parents are presumably sincere in their belief that faith will heal their son, but they could be in error.

There is a temptation, especially in pediatric cases, to define eccentric parental behavior as damaging or dangerous to the interests of the child. Legal precedents can be found in cases involving parents who are Jehovah's Witnesses who refuse blood or blood products for their minor children or in prosecutions of parents who are Christian Scientists who provide alternative health care to children who might benefit from conventional treatments and who are thus placed in life-threatening situations. Such efforts at interposing society's will against parental claims are based on the interest of the state in the well-being of children.

This interest has sometimes, via court order, transcended parental autonomy: Blood transfusions have been ordered for children in life-threatening circumstances, against the professed wishes of their parents, often supported by church officials. More recently, Christian Scientists have been prosecuted for refusing traditional medical care for their children. After a child died of a reversible bowel obstruction when the parents failed to take him to a conventional physician (preferring Christian Science healing instead), the couple was found guilty of manslaughter and sentenced to 10 years probation.

The perspectives of physicians and nurses demand attention. Robby was a patient in a famous research hospital. This very modern and sophisticated institution had a perspective dramatically different from that of Robby's family. The doctors believed that they could save the child's life with amputation and chemotherapy. They would also learn from Robby's case: This kind of osteogenic sarcoma, because it involves a preteenaged child, and because of its difficult location, is rarer than most. Surgeons and hematologist-oncologists, their residents, and fellows, would profit intellectually from proceeding with the recommended treatment. Nurses at the hospital were frustrated by the family's unwillingness to acknowledge their offers of support. The parents' hope for divine intervention was seen as a rejection of the nursing staff's psychosocial support.

The hospital authorities, supported by physicians and nurses, decided to seek a court order. This step was not taken lightly. Hospitals have reputations to preserve. Forcing surgery on a child (and family) could be seen by the public in two divergent ways.

Some might see the court process as demonstrating institutional concern for children in need of protection. Others might be alarmed by the hospital's request that, in effect, Robby be taken away from his natural parents and placed in the hands of a court-designated guardian who would go along with hospital desires.

Many issues are raised by this case that go beyond the specifics of the situation. Are all religious rights in pediatric cases subject to veto when a child's life is at stake? Suppose that the parents refused treatment for another reason (e.g., the statistical promise of a 60 percent recovery rate is pretty close to a 50-50 chance). Robby's parents could have said that they were unwilling to take such a risk. If the court were to order care for Robby, we would have to admit that such an act was purely paternalistic. Is this a useful precedent? State interests in such cases are usually limited to four important goals: (1) the preservation of life; (2) the prevention of suicide; (3) the protection of innocent third parties; and (4) the maintenance of the ethical integrity of the health care professions. These are powerful ideals. If courts continuously intervene in medical emergencies—or, as in Robby's case in situations of parental disagreement with medical protocols—is the health care system improved?

This case certainly is legally significant. It pits freedom of religion against the state doctrine of *parens patriae* (which justifies seizing the child when the state is forced to act as parent). It also opens up questions of medical and moral uncertainty. Where is Robby in all of this debate? Time is certainly not on his side: Such cancers develop rapidly, metastasize swiftly, and grow ever more virulent and life-threatening. Placing the decision in the hands of a judge (usually a person with no special medical nor, for that matter, religious expertise) is not the best possible solution. But it is one that is sought more and more often.

Case 5-4
Nurses and physicians sometimes have different perspectives on the ethical issues facing parents whose children are very sick. Advocacy for the child can entail both benefits and problems.

Ricky, the first child of Connie and Tim, is born in January. This is a planned pregnancy, and Connie has arranged for 2 months off from her managerial job when the baby is born. All grandparents live nearby and are very supportive. The problem is that Ricky was not due until March. He weighs 2½ pounds. Connie and Tim are stunned. They are able to see the tiny infant for a few seconds before he is rushed to another hospital for intensive care. Connie sees how perfectly Ricky is formed and feels his little fingers around hers. Tim is proud of the way Ricky moves around and seems eager to fight to live.

The doctors are communicative and supportive. The nurses are very encouraging to the parents. Ricky does well on the ventilator. The first 2 weeks are the roughest, but time flies by. By mid March he is off the breathing machine. He still needs extra oxygen on occasion, but doctors say he will outgrow his lung problem. Ricky appears to be developing normally. Tests of his brain, vision, and hearing are normal. He opens his eyes and looks around. He turns his head from side to side. Connie knows he recognizes her, and she and Tim hold the baby once a day. Feeding is a major problem. Connie continues to bring in her breast milk. Ricky is tube fed and refuses to take a bottle. He has x-rays to see why he spits up his feeding so often. Weight gain is slow, and Connie and Tim give permission for a surgeon to place an IV near the heart to give extra nourishment for growth.

In May, a physician calls in the middle of the night. Ricky has spit up his feeding again, but this time he has choked on it, and his heart has stopped beating. He has received CPR and "several rounds of meds." He had no heartbeat for 30 minutes. He is now stable, but back on the ventilator. Connie and Tim rush to the hospital, but the situation is worse than just being put on the ventilator again. Their son is back in the neonatal special care unit, but he is the oldest and most mature child there. Most of the cases involve complications due to prematurity. Ricky needs some of the same kinds of interventions, even though he is physically and chronologically mature.

Ricky doesn't move or open his eyes when they touch him. During the next few weeks, the news is all bad. Ricky has continual seizures, and his tests show little brain activity. Medicines and time make no difference. His vision and hearing tests show almost no responses. When Connie holds Ricky his eyes are closed and he feels stiff. In June, Ricky's lungs are the major problem. He choked on his milk, got pneumonia, and is on the ventilator. The pressure and the oxygen from the ventilator are causing progressive damage to his lungs. Connie and Tim are told that he may never get off the ventilator. Connie stops bringing breast milk, and she goes back to work.

In July the problem is nourishment. Ricky weighs 5 pounds (the same amount as in April). Many tests are ordered. Special nutrients are added to the formula and the deep IV to make Ricky grow. Tim receives a notice from his medical insurance company advising him that Ricky has used up the "lifetime benefits" of his policy. The hospital will bill Connie's insurance company until these funds run out. In August, the problem is infection. Many tests and x-rays are done. Ricky is on antibiotics the whole month, sometimes three at a time. His lungs are getting worse. Tim hardly visits any more. Connie comes in twice a week, but Ricky is attached to so much equipment, she only gets to hold him once.

In September, the baby's heart begins to be damaged by the work of pumping blood through his damaged lungs and by the low level of oxygen in the blood. The cardiologists do tests and add medicine. Ricky now receives all his medicine and nourishment intravenously. The nurses in the intensive care unit have begun to talk to one another privately about Ricky. They have provided continuous care for the child. The medical residents change each month, but Ricky has had only a few primary nurses during his long hospitalization. The nurses question continuing interventions. Ricky is getting more and more medication. His cognitive status is hard to determine. The nurses are not sure if he can feel pain. They believe that he will never leave the hospital alive. They see the family as growing distant, perhaps due to the stress of so many months of illness. When they mention, gently, to the residents that the family might be approached about limiting or withdrawing treatment, they are "not heard." The young physicians on the unit seem to the nurses to be interested in Ricky for teaching and research purposes, not as a child who is dying. Meanwhile, Ricky's lungs are getting worse and worse; his oxygen level is raised routinely.

In clinical medical ethics, value assumptions may not be everything, but they count for a lot. The cliche "When there is life, there is hope," founded on scientific optimism as much as religious or secular hope, underpins the care of young children like Ricky (conventionally, we do not apply the phrase to 89-year-old persons very often; see Chapter 8). Just as the legal system works with so-called *burdens of proof* (i.e., a person is innocent until proven guilty, and that must be shown beyond a reasonable doubt), so the medical system has a built-in balancing weight: Always err on the side of life (breath, brain activity); even if chance of recovery or restoration of function is slim, it is better to persist than to cease treatment. This set of assumptions is not limited to physicians or other health care professionals. Patients and family members share in the pursuit of hope. Clinicians, anecdotally, insist that optimistic patients get better, or get better faster, than those who have given up. At most children's hospitals, the value assumption takes the form of an unstated policy: "For sick children we always give a full court press!"

A less strident version of this supposition suggests, "We'll treat now and see what happens later." When Ricky was born prematurely, initiation of ventilatory support was, of course, immediate. Optimism was realistic. Five months later, Ricky was still in the hospital and aspirated. After resuscitation, though he had no heartbeat for half an hour and his brain surely received insufficient oxygen for a long time, again every effort was made to sustain his life. Continuing support (ventilatory and nutritional) does not help very much—though it does keep the baby alive—and in fact can be harmful. Ricky's lungs are damaged by his ventilator dependency.

In Ricky's case there are other factors that led to continuing treatment, even beyond the point of rational expectation of recovery. The law, or its adversarial image, is a powerful force. Physicians are afraid of being sued if they do not offer every possible intervention, suggest every test, and try every orthodox and sometimes experimental surgery. Hierarchical issues on the wards are also influential. Even physicians concede that asking the question "Can't we withdraw treatment" is more often initiated by nurses than by doctors. But saying such a thing aloud, while consonant (at times) with the nurse's role as patient (and family) advocate or educator, flies in the face of the physician's self-image as curer. Tensions often linger beneath the surface on the wards because raising the issue about continuing treatment cannot be expressed readily in a nonthreatening environment. Most medical units—certainly intensive care units, whether for children or adults—depend on interdisciplinary team cooperation. What are the ethical implications of the empowerment of one perspective (medical) over another (nursing)? This question is not political, *per se*. Rather, it asks: If the fundamental concern is for the best interests of the patient, how does hierarchy influence life and death determinations?

Timing has remarkable influence on facing and resolving clinical ethical problems. As infants like Ricky grow older, questions emerge about who will be responsible for the child and who will pay for his care. Parents must get on with their lives: Emergencies do not last forever. Visiting becomes more difficult. Insurance companies some-times call hospital units (they are permitted to do so when policy-holders waive confidentiality) and ask about treatment decisions, cost being their fundamental concern. In Ricky's case, the father's insurance ran out; the mother's eventually will. The months of Ricky's life could cost more than $1,000,000.

Were Ricky to survive on the ventilator, at 10 years (as opposed to 10 months), he would look very different. When newborns are encountered for the first time and show signs of abnormality, they are sometimes referred to in private, by house staff as funny looking kids (FLKs). This observation suggests two things: Such children are "abnormal" and are in need of clinical, perhaps genetic, studies. But the notion of anomaly pervades medical ethics well beyond the birth of a child with a rare genetic disorder. We speak of how some premature children will "always be retarded" and about how chil-dren with spina bifida are "permanently handicapped." Anomaly implies stigma. Mental disability is often deemed worse than physi-cal incapacity. The fact that Ricky, if he lives, will most likely lead a very limited life may influence a decision to withhold or withdraw care. A purely utilitarian assessment of costs and benefits may seem cold and calculating. Principled alternative viewpoints include a concern for pain and suffering from the perspective of beneficence.

Case 5-5

Pediatric and adolescent medicine providers can be caught between older teenagers and their parents. Fidelity to certain ideals (e.g., confidentiality) can be both noble and difficult.

Sue is a 17-year-old student in her third year of high school. Her boyfriend Cal, 22, attends a nearby technical school and lives in his own apartment. Sue tells her pediatrician (she has made this appointment on her own with Dr. G., who has seen her since she was 11) that she intends to move in with Cal in about 5 months at the end of this school year. She expects to finish her final year of high school and, in fact, wants to go on to the local community college. The patient's plans seem well formed and quite rational. Dr. G., as always, inquires about her family and gets a polite, though brief, response from her.

Sue asks the physician for information about birth control. She says that she does *not* want a prescription but just needs to know about these things. She is aware, in a general sense, of the risks of sexually transmitted diseases, including AIDS. Sue tells the physician that she sees nothing morally wrong in having sex with the guy she loves. Dr. G. asks Sue if she has discussed these matters with her parents. She says, "No, they wouldn't understand. I'm not rushing into this, but I don't want to get grounded!" Dr. G. expresses his concern for her well-being and for her judgment. He wonders to himself: "Should I inform Sue's parents about our conversation?"

■ ■ ■

In the strict sense, Sue is not Dr. G.'s patient. She is a minor, legally unable to make health care decisions without parental consent. But, pragmatically, Sue is a mature young woman, only months away from her eighteenth birthday. She does not appear to lack the abilities necessary to make an informed decision: She is rational, purposeful, and understands the consequences of her actions. The very fact that she is talking with the physician suggests that she is *not* impulsive. In addition, in many states there are statutory exceptions to the parental-decision model of pediatric care. In the areas of birth control, pregnancy, and sexually transmitted diseases, physicians are sometimes not required to talk with parents. Legally, Dr. G. may be protected. Ethically, his fidelity may remain split between parent and adolescent.

Sue presumably goes into the appointment with Dr. G. with the full expectation of confidentiality. Pediatricians have many roles; one of them is to act as advisors to their patients. The aid Sue is requesting is of a medical nature. It is also a life-style choice she is contemplating. The physician feels torn between his loyalty to his young patient and to the implicit promise of privacy made by discussing this topic in the confines of his office, and his obligation to her parents. They, after all, have been the principal caretakers of Sue for as long as Dr. G. has known the family. There is an important contextual element in this ethical dilemma. The level of prior family involvement in Sue's health care is a factor. Some parents want to know everything; others are content to give their teenagers an abundance of independence.

Do the facts that Sue will soon leave home, presumably after she is 18 years old, and that her parents cannot legally prevent this move, make a difference? If Dr. G. does tell Sue's parents, one could argue that his duty to treat Sue fairly has been violated. Perhaps some alternatives available to the practitioner (e.g., the recommendation of counseling agencies or consultant psychotherapists) are more viable. But referrals can only postpone the physician's accepting or deferring responsibility. The basic question remains: Should Dr. G. inform Sue's parents about her proposed course of action?

Sue's own behavior must be considered. Were Dr. G. to say that he intends to speak with her parents, she may take any number of actions. If she chooses to see another doctor or health care professional (Dr. G. may even refer her to a colleague less troubled by such cases), this action itself may cause the "beans to be spilled." The very personal content of this problem complicates matters. The patient's request for information about birth control and her anticipation of sexual activity may add a dimension of responsibility for the physician in this case. If Dr. G. tells Sue's parents a very limited truth ("Your daughter came into the office this week and we had a very interesting conversation."), he may be trying to finesse the situation. Doctors who provide services to adolescents must be prepared to "continue the conversation," often without being able to prophesy the outcome.

■ PRACTICE MODEL CASE ■

Jamie is a 16-month-old male whose infancy was perfectly normal, according to his parents. Three weeks ago he became ill with an apparent respiratory infection. His mother found Jamie in considerable distress and called the paramedics. The family lives in a rural county; by the time Jamie was transported to the local community hospital he seemed not to be breathing at all. He was given prolonged CPR for over 40 minutes. The helicopter from City Hospital, a tertiary care facility 50 miles away, transported him to their emergency room. Jamie was stabilized and was placed on a respirator. When his mother and father asked about their child's prognosis, the ICU physician said she was unable to make a definitive prediction.

A CT scan was ordered and results were normal; the physicians felt that it was too early for any substantial brain injury to be obvious. After a few days in the ICU, Jamie was removed from the respirator and was able to breathe on his own. A week later he was transferred to a general medical-surgical floor in the pediatric division. At no time did he regain consciousness or demonstrate any awareness of his environment. His parents told the doctors that if Jamie stopped breathing again, they did *not* want him revived. Accordingly, a DNR order was charted. Jamie was being fed by nasogastric tube. The neurology consultant felt that any future mental development was unlikely, due to the severity of the brain damage. Jamie's EEG showed marked slowing with marked seizure activity. CT scans were repeated and showed multiple areas of gray matter abnormality. Jamie was clearly *not* brain dead, but the level of his neocortical function remained unknown.

The parents demanded answers about their child. Their response to medical uncertainty was anger. They stated that "nothing should have been done when Jamie died the first time." The parents felt that the hospital was not telling them the truth about the likely outcome. The father did most of the talking. Yesterday he made the following requests:

1. No further medications should be given to the child, including seizure medications.
2. No antibiotics should be administered; no suctioning should be done.
3. No laboratory tests, including blood work or x-rays, should be ordered.
4. Permission was given to allow feeding and hydration of the child.
5. The parents said that they did not want to bring their child home to die again.

As of this date, Jamie has no swallowing mechanism. He cannot see, though there is pupillary response. There is no way of knowing if he can hear. He shows some jerking of the left arm, some spasticity, and perhaps some spontaneous movement of the lower limbs. Jamie's major response is "quieting to sound," his primary nurse says.

Patient

Jamie is the recipient of recent advances in medical technology and health care delivery. No one would have expected him to be so sick, based on his first 16 months of life. He was healthy and thriving until a sudden and apparently virulent infection caused him to stop breathing. He was taken immediately to the nearby hospital. CPR was administered (this procedure is itself relatively new) at great length. Forty minutes without the restoration of heartbeat and pulmonary function is unusual. He was flown to a major hospital and given intensive care, including ventilatory support, until he could breathe on his own. Had Jamie arrested without a witness to call for help, he would have died rapidly. Emergency medical help made it possible for him to reach City Hospital alive. Now he has been deteriorating steadily there.

His medical condition has changed. The initial statement, that Jamie's prospects for recovery were uncertain, is both true and frustrating. The common cliche that when in doubt, err on the side of life, seemed applicable at the time. Three weeks later Jamie can breathe spontaneously; other principle functions are limited. He gives no sign of being able to see or hear. The extent of his brain damage is under investigation, but it seems clear that the damage is considerable and that Jamie will most likely be profoundly mentally retarded if he survives. (He retains sufficient residual brainstem function so that he can breathe spontaneously.) He will probably never achieve consciousness of himself or others. He suffers from seizures, which can perhaps be controlled by medication. He could arrest again at any time. Jamie cannot swallow and is being hydrated and fed by nasogastric tube.

The physicians can state with conviction that Jamie will never be restored to the status he had prior to the CNS insult. He is neither brain dead nor in a persistent vegetative condition. He is breathing on his own. He does seem to experience pain. Just what meaning should be attached to the fact that he calms down when comforted is hard to discern. Of course, we cannot know what Jamie's internal experience might be. (Can he dream? Is he really soothed or comforted by tactile contact?) There are both unknowns and knowns. One of the latter suggests that Jamie will stay alive with medical support but that his capacity to experience that life may not exist. Another is that if treatment is withdrawn (e.g., suctioning or antibiotic therapy is stopped), Jamie will probably die in a few weeks.

Relationships

Psychosocially, Jamie's parents are likely to report something like the following:

This is not our son, the cute kid who played all day long and half the night. He was never sick before. When he stopped breathing back home, they should have known that reviving him would make him this way. They never asked us what we wanted. They just took command. Now they want to give us back this nearly dead child who will never know us, or himself, again. The hospital doesn't give us the truth. They tell us what they are doing for Jamie medically. Most of the time they ask us to wait and see. Well, we've been doing this. Now, the best information we get says that Jamie has been stabilized and we can bring him home. They say he'll get home care and every effort will be made to find the money for it. But what about our lives? What about Jamie? We know that this is no life for him. We will always feel terrible about what has happened to our son. But we are his parents and we have to make the decisions.

Jamie's relationships with his family are derived from past experience. He is already a memory for his mother and father. His hospital caregivers are beginning a relationship with him based on his grave illness and mediated by the tubes and monitors that sustain his system and measure his status. But the nurses care about him and are very interested in his response to pain. They are also concerned about the suffering of his parents.

Advocacy

Jamie's parents may be presumed to be his most fervent advocates. They not only care *about* him; they are the ones who are ultimately responsible for caring *for* him. But their assertion of rights and their expectation that caregivers do their duty is complicated by the fact that doctors and nurses may have a sense of Jamie's best interests. Their perspectives do count; as the attending physician can tell us:

Our patient's medical situation is somewhat ambiguous. It is clear that Jamie will never be restored to the status he had prior to the CNS insult. His brain has been traumatized and his mind will forever be diminished in its capacity to interact with the environment. But we are sure that Jamie is neither brain dead nor in a persistent vegetative condition. He shows signs of awareness, if minimally so, that he senses the presence of others and he is breathing on his own. What's unclear is just what this means to Jamie and what the future holds for him. If we withdraw treatment, as his father wants, however, we can be pretty certain that Jamie will be uncomfortable (with no suctioning or antibiotics infections are likely in the coming weeks) and that he will probably die, though not from starvation.

Jamie's primary nurse can become an advocate by stating:

One system problem in this case is due to the absence of any primary care physician to look after Jamie. In our hospital, attending physicians change every month. Jamie was admitted at "change-of-month" time and has already had two attendings responsible for his care. Such doctors rarely know the family or the patient and have little opportunity to establish much rapport.

As his primary nurse I have had a lot of contact with Jamie; I admit that this contact is pretty much one-sided. But when he is trembling or shaking I can relax and quiet him. I am sure he knows that I am with him. When his mother comes to visit she also spends time holding him and stroking his head. It's very hard to figure out what is in the best interest of this patient. Surely anything we do to limit his pain is desirable. But his family thinks that he is not the son they once loved, the child with promise whose growth they welcomed. Now Jamie just lies there, hooked to tubes and monitors. The nursing staff wants to support the family, but their involvement seems to be diminishing. The parents are adamant about not bringing their child home. Is this a case for the hospital's bioethics committee? The choice seems to be centering around either continuing to treat Jamie or providing only comfort measures. But I thought this was only possible if a patient is really dying. Is Jamie terminal? The nurse is supposed to be an educator as well as an advocate, but I feel that I need an answer to this question before I can do so effectively.

Conflicts

Jamie was not born with a disability; he is also not an infant (see Fig. 3-1.). He is a profoundly ill child, and questions about the quality of his life are obviously influencing his family, or at least his father as spokesperson. The conflict in this case emerges while trying to create a treatment plan (one that takes into account different circumstances) for the patient. The family is saying that Jamie should get only very limited care and that, if he were to die, it would be because of his underlying medical condition. Only hydration and nutrition would be maintained. All other forms of support (Jamie does not now require a ventilator) would cease. Were Jamie to have a cardiac arrest, develop a fever, or suffer a seizure, no intervention would be permitted.

The health care team (especially at City Hospital, a first-rate facility with available technical resources) may be reluctant to let Jamie go. He is not dead; he is not in a persistent vegetative state. He does show minimal signs of consciousness, and he is calmed in response to comforting touch. Reasonable physicians or nurses could resist the parental decision to stop treatment.

Treatment or Nontreatment Options

Is there a difference between withholding and withdrawing care? If the request made by Jamie's father is followed, future interventions will be withheld. Removing the nasogastric tube, which is hydrating Jamie and providing him with artificial alimentation, moves into the realm of withdrawing care. Courts, and most clinical medical ethicists, have said that there is no significant difference between these two acts. Physicians and nurses, however, say that "pulling a tube" (i.e., withdrawing care) is much more difficult, both physically and psychologically. Practitioners often feel as if they are causing the death of a patient when a ventilator or feeding tube is taken out. (See Chapter 8 for further discussion.)

Within the realm of treatment choices there are many options. Suctioning could be provided, if all agreed that painful choking might be the result of failing to remove secretions from Jamie's lungs. If the child were to spike a fever, antibiotics might be utilized, on the grounds that a high fever could cause undue suffering. But there are limits to such alternatives. If antibiotic therapy prevents or treats the pneumonia that could strike Jamie, his life could be extended for a very long period. This would contradict the parental decision. Jamie has a DNR order written in his chart. All parties presumably agree that CPR should not be exercised. What differences are there between that form of intervention and other, perhaps less dramatic, steps that might lengthen Jamie's life?

Interests

Medical uncertainty always entails moral uncertainty. Is Jamie dying? Is he being subjected to burdensome treatment only because, in a literal sense, he is still alive? A utilitarian measure of this patient's interests would require stating and perhaps comparing the benefits and the burdens of care or its cessation. What benefits would Jamie experience if his parents' recommendations were rejected and he received ICU care? Would he ever know that he is being treated in this way? Is there an interest in life *per se*? Perhaps Jamie, sick as he is, retains an interest in dying as peacefully and in as little pain as possible.

The burdens of treatment (as a measure of what is in Jamie's best interest) are also hard to project. If he is so cognitively impaired that his responses to pain are unregistered (i.e., if he is not conscious of his condition), then he is not burdened by suctioning or intubation or even dying slowly. But were Jamie to have the minimum of brain activity that would allow him to feel some pain, our sense of the burdensome nature of care would necessarily shift. Waiting may be the best plan: Perhaps later, as a result of further deterioration, we will be able to tell more definitively just how Jamie is, or is not, experiencing his environment.

Consequences

The end for Jamie remains uncertain. Just as no one expects him to recover useful function, few would anticipate immediate death. Jamie, whether treated or untreated, will probably die soon. How he dies is at issue in this case, and projecting various scenarios (e.g., as we did in weighing treatment options) may appear gruesome. But they are not intended to devalue this young patient. They are offered as a way to find the best possible consequences for him.

Others involved in this case have short- and long-range needs and goals. The parents will eventually mourn for Jamie. Their grieving (as we have seen in other cases of pediatric death) is likely to be related to the kind of dying their child experienced. The hospital team also cares about consequences. Does agreeing with this father set a precedent for the care of other impaired children? If doctors and nurses disagree in their estimation of what is best for Jamie, will the wounds of the dispute heal satisfactorily? As in many pediatric cases, the results for the relatively silent parent, Jamie's mother, need to be considered. Statistics show that after the death of a child marriages are in jeopardy. We may wish for a stronger sense of Mrs. D.'s role in this case.

Ethical Principles

A brief checklist may suffice: Parental autonomy (if we are satisfied that the father speaks for the couple) could be validated if all parties agree that Jamie should be allowed to die. Such a decision would have to be rooted in the principles of beneficence and nonmaleficence: It would rest on the conviction that there would be no benefits from continuing to provide intensive care for Jamie and that keeping him alive against all hope of recovery would be harmful.

The actual list of treatment options requested by Jamie's father needs to be explored in light of these ethical principles. In particular, physicians need to ask the parents (with sensitivity) to give their *reasons* for approving certain kinds of care (e.g., hydration and nutrition) or rejecting others (e.g., medications, including antibiotics). If the reasons offered seem plausible and demonstrate true concern for the child, they can be validated. But if they are rooted in fear, or misunderstanding, or seem terribly inconsistent, then perhaps referral to supportive services or the institution's bioethics committee is in order.

■ CASES FOR DISCUSSION ■

Case A

B. R. is an 11 year old who was diagnosed with acute nonlymphocytic leukemia. The course of chemotherapy sustained by B. R. lasted about 10 months and left him weakened and vulnerable to infection. It also failed to secure a remission of the cancer. B. R. now has a DNR order and is suffering from a progressive fungal disease that was first diagnosed in the pulmonary tissue. In the hospital the patient is being maintained on IV antibiotics, IV antifungal and hydration fluids (which contain electrolytes). For 2 months he was able to ambulate in the hospital halls and even left on weekends to visit his family. Now he is unable to eat: Any foods he takes into his stomach are vomited immediately. He cannot be sustained by IVs for very long; he will require the insertion of a feeding tube within a few weeks.

Questions

1. What does the fact that this patient has a DNR order written into his medical records indicate about other treatment options?

2. What arguments can be made for continuing to give B. R. antibiotics?
3. If the patient is sustained via tube feeding (either a nasogastric tube or a gastrostomy), he will live much longer than he could without such support. What ethical justification can be given for inserting a feeding tube?
4. The cost of care for this patient is more than $1000 per day. Should B. R.'s family be encouraged to make provisions for him to leave the hospital?
5. In attempting a benefit/burden assessment of treatment or nontreatment options for B. R., what weight should be given to the *family's* anxiety and stress over the many months of hospitalization?

Case B

G. R. is a 16-year-old high school student with a 3-year reported history of anorexia nervosa (self-starvation). She has been seen by a pediatrician and a child psychiatrist for 2 years for the condition, has been in group therapy for 7 months, and presently is 5' 3" tall and weighs 81 pounds. When her parents discover that she has been exercising fervently because, as G. R. says, "I'm just a blob!," and that she has lost 3 pounds during the past month, they take her back to the pediatrician. After a brief conversation with the patient, the doctor recommends to the parents that G. R. be hospitalized for tests and serious behavior modification treatment. When G. R. is told this recommendation, she is resistant and refuses to go to the hospital voluntarily. Her parents place her in the family car and take her into the admitting office of the hospital. She reluctantly agrees to go upstairs and, after a brief history and physical examination, goes to sleep in her hospital bed. The next morning she tells the pediatrics resident that she intends "to get the hell out of here as soon as I can. But you better not tell my parents what I just said."

Questions

1. As a minor, does G. R. possess the right to accept or refuse treatment?
2. What ethical principles apply to this patient's situation, both outside and inside the hospital setting?
3. Should the resident seek an independent advocate for G. R.?

4. Is the resident obliged to tell others, including the patient's parents, about her expressed, though possibly ambiguous, intention to leave the hospital?

■ THINK PIECE: PARENTS AND CHILDREN ■

Who "owns" children? What is an acceptable level of risk in caring for minors? What are the responsibilities of physicians (pediatricians or other primary care doctors) whose clientele include vulnerable younger patients? Are social and cultural expectations changing in this subject area? What is child safety?

Some data and situations demonstrate these questions more precisely. About 1.5 million children were abused and neglected in 1986, the most recent year for which data is available. The reported incidence of sexual abuse of children has tripled since 1980. Seventy-eight percent of deaths among youths in the United States are caused by accidents, homicide, or other violence. The United States and Australia have the highest child-poverty rates: 17 percent each.

A mother repeatedly overdoses her small child with ipecac. Hospital authorities suspect maltreatment but do nothing. Eventually, an overdose proves fatal. The mother pleads guilty, but to involuntary manslaughter, claiming that *she* was suffering from a Munchausen's Syndrome. Neonatal, infant, and toddler homicides are caused primarily by family members. The most common means are strangulation, drowning in a toilet or bathtub, or being struck with a blunt instrument. In a notorious case in New York City a father was tried for habitually beating his 7-year-old daughter; his final act was to throw her on the floor and fracture her head, killing her.

Less obvious, but not necessarily less ubiquitous, are cases of psychological abuse. A young child is threatened by a parent who says, "If you don't behave, I am packing up and leaving you." A parent responds to a depressed child doing poorly in school, by saying: "You must be stupid. I can't wait until you're 16 so we can take you out of school." More active abuse involves making sexual threats to a child, isolating the infant from contact with others, verbally bullying the teenager, perhaps in front of friends. Some parents have encouraged antisocial behaviors, including alcohol and other substance-abuse and demanded sexual activities with the parent and others.

There is a fragile line between parental autonomy and medical beneficence. Families in our society count for a great deal and are delegated both respect and responsibility. Pediatric medicine, however, means more than the physical care of young children; it is a psychosocially informed primary care field. Ironically, medical advances may have led to the present family problems of the children we are discussing. More premature infants and children who need repeated surgeries for long-term survival are living at home today. They are frequent subjects of abuse and neglect. The increased lifespan of children with chronic illnesses such as leukemia, sickle cell anemia, or cystic fibrosis places enormous psychological strains on families already burdened by poverty, unemployment, alcoholism, and drug abuse. Social support services have increased for such families, but clearly not in accord with demand.

Pediatricians and other physicians encounter severe abuse of children. This can often be diagnosed in the office or clinic when the child has massive subdural, subarachnoid, or retinal hemorrhages or multiple fractures. A statement such as "he fell off the couch" may be made. Reporting to the criminal or civil juvenile justice system may be in order. Most cases, however, are not so overt and involve not apparent physical violence but less obvious assaults or parental neglect. What are the responsibilities of caregivers? What ethical obligations—to the child *and* to the family—do pediatricians incur when they offer medical services? How far should they go in identifying and investigating possible trouble? Should we encourage the creation of a pediatric police force or team? What rights and duties can be ascribed to parents? What should be the locus of attention— criminal prosecution, family support, economic changes leading to a diminution of poverty? What are the dangers of over-involvement? When does beneficence convert to paternalism? What risks are taken in trying to manage the unmanageable?

■ VOICES: CLINICAL NURSE SPECIALIST/PEDIATRICS ■

I think that the nursing viewpoint can only be heard if we realize that there is a difference between medical care and health care. Physicians intervene to diagnose and, if necessary, fix medical problems. Health care professionals, including nurses, deal with a great diversity of ethical issues—there's almost nothing outside their purview. Nurses have to worry about families, about poverty, and about social change as well as lab values.

The fact that I serve children (I include my patients from age 0 to age 18 in this group) makes for ethical difficulties. Decisions about when to start and stop treatment, and how far to go, are different when you deal with kids. We tend to idealize children and sometimes to trivialize their viewpoints. In pediatric settings, the child, whether 13, 12, or 2, has to be talked with in the presence of others. We have to filter care through families or surrogates and *their* value systems. Kids sometimes object to procedures—who wouldn't; they can be painful. But such objections often freak out their parents. Since establishing relationships is so important for nurses our job is very tough, because we have to do so with many people, not just one patient. Questions of confidentiality emerge immediately when we work with older kids. Getting parents to talk with their children who *can* understand their medical problems is very difficult.

Now, of course, parents do care enormously for their children. We treat this as an assumption. When it's not a reality, we tend to impose our middle class values on parents who don't meet our expectations. Nurses, and sometimes doctors and social workers, try to get parents to come around to our way of thinking. Parental autonomy is an ideal, and sometimes it's a dream. What doctors want is usually what they get. If physicians think parents are caring, then all goes smoothly. But when there are economic and social class differences, doctors tend to condemn parents who are not "like us."

This is an authority issue and it has implications at both ends of the economic spectrum. Parents with a background of poverty who do not obey orders are characterized as uneducated and their views are often written off. They are seen as incapable of exercising their autonomy. But even when very rich, educated parents disagree with medical advice, they are viewed as attacking physician authority and are considered suspect by pediatricians.

Many ethical issues challenge me to examine my own beliefs. When a parent who is a Jehovah's Witness speaks, I often ask myself what my spiritual values are. I don't always get a sense that the child is the center of concern for parents who present religious objections to pediatric treatments. Such moments force me to confront my own sense of what's right and wrong.

Doctor-nurse relationships, especially in the hospital setting, are often centered around value concerns. I've been in nursing for 15 years in a fairly conservative environment. Things are certainly different today. The quality of a nurse-doctor relationship is still almost totally dependent on the individuals involved. Much of it is just vibes or simple courtesy. Nurses are more assertive these days—more verbal and more questioning. Doctors sometimes welcome active nursing participation in making choices about such decisions as stopping care for patients with cancer when it seems untreatable. The turf issues, however, haven't really changed.

We still do most of the patient care. The doctors and the residents in a teaching hospital are certainly there to take care of the children. But for them it's a teaching or learning experience, and of course there are research tasks too. Around July 1, when the new residents start, nurses around the country take a deep breath and ask, "Am I ready for this?" Just showing these young doctors how to get things done falls mainly to the nurses and sometimes to the children. As for research values (and I am not talking about official research protocols), at teaching hospitals, the learning process means that things (such as new drugs) tried on a specific child are done not for the child but really (we hope) for future generations. I am not opposed to such research strategies, but I wonder if the parents really know what's going on and why. Their child may have to be sedated, may have to hold still for an hour, may have to undergo a spinal tap, may have to have blood tests three times a day—these little things add up. I don't know if patient care is the primary value in such activities.

Private practice doctors don't always like having nurses question them. They can be quite conservative, and their interactions with house staff (i.e., attending physicians and residents) are sometimes problematic. It's hard for these private doctors to keep up with the latest studies and procedures. How could they; they have so much else to do! But they still want to feel like they are calling all the shots when they admit a child to the hospital. But they can't stay overnight like the residents. They can't really provide intensive care for the child; they have to be observers. They complain about turning over control. You can't have it both ways.

Chronic illness, especially in teenagers, presents very special difficulties. Facing the imminent death of a teenager is the toughest of all. Sometimes we offer experimental care and give hope, but at great risk. When teenagers have been treated as infants by their parents in the past and at the age of 16 have to face surgery, enormous control issues arise. It's hard to figure out from adolescents just how much they really want to decide for themselves. As a nurse-advocate I often feel trapped in the middle. Just getting doctors to take the time to deal with these complications is really difficult. In the area of ethics, we often bring people together to talk.

Some of what we call ethics in health care is a reflection of male-female differences. I believe that women (most nurses are female) are more comfortable dealing with emotional distress. They tend to be empathic and attuned to listening. (Not all women are like this; some try to out-guy the guys.)

Technology in pediatrics is very powerful and very seductive, and the glitz and glamour often blind us. Many little babies are sick because we spend money on neonatal intensive care rather than on prevention and prenatal care. Sometimes I think that the flashiness of science gets in the way of our humane instincts. Nurses often speak out *against* the new machines, but in reality what they are speaking out *for* is returning the child to the center of our concerns and for a more sensible allocation of scarce resources.

RECOMMENDED READING

Forman, E. and Ladd, R. *Ethical Dilemmas in Pediatrics: A Case Study Approach.* New York: Spring-Verlag, 1991.

Gaylin, W. and Macklin, R. eds., *Who Speaks for the Child?: The Problems of Proxy Consent.* New York: Plenum Press, 1982.

Goldstein, J., et. al. *In the Best Interest of the Child.* New York: Free Press, 1986.

Holder, A.R. *Legal Issues in Pediatric and Adolescent Medicine.* 2d edition New Haven: Yale University Press, 1985.

Koocher, G.P. and Keith-Spiegel, P. *Children, Ethics, and the Law: Professional Issues and Cases.* Lincoln: University of Nebraska Press, 1990.

Kopelman, L. and Moskop, J. (eds.) *Children and Health Care: Moral and Social Issues.* Dordrecht, Netherlands: Kluwer, 1989.

Resolving Differences:
Ethics in Internal Medicine
and Surgery

Internal medicine, often considered the heart of the profession, traces its conceptual roots to the publication of Sir William Osler's famous text, *The Principles and Practices of Medicine,* more than a century ago. Intended to inspire diagnosis and treatment in the most modern form, Osler's book was used and admired for generations. Now, the enormous growth of information and research results, as well as the world-wide expansion of medicine, has rendered the summarizing of internal medicine into a single, readable volume impossible. The discipline is organized around subject areas, each of which demands a thoroughness of understanding never imagined in Osler's time. The major realms of study and practice include cardiology, immunology and rheumatology, hematology and oncology, endocrinology, infectious disease, gastroenterology, and pulmonary and renal medicine. The list of what general internists need to know does not stop here. Neurology, usually deemed a separate field, interacts with internal medicine routinely. The newer field of geriatrics is in many medical centers a division of the department of internal medicine.

The role of the internist as primary care physician is well-established (see Chapter 4). Dealing with adults, internists may be spared some of the dilemmas encountered by pediatricians (e.g., when older children and parents come into conflict over treatment options). This is probably the *only* kind of problem not seen by internists. The full range of human difficulties, from deciding whether or not to insert a feeding tube in a patient with advanced dementia to helping patients with renal disease in their attempt to find a donor kidney, is everyday work for the physician who practices internal medicine. Questions involving patient lifestyle and other psychosocial and behavioral elements of health care are rarely absent.

The variety of cases seen by internists accounts for the large number of ethical dilemmas encountered. As generalists, internists see patients in many settings—the office, the clinic, the outpatient treatment center, the nursing home, the rehabilitation center, the hospital, even (though rarely) at home. Most medical training emphasizes acute care decision making. But internists know that the drama of an ethical decision about cardiopulmonary resuscitation occurs much less frequently than a routine discussion such as having to refuse a patient's request for a diazepam prescription. As gatekeepers, often within the confines of a managed care organizational structure, internists necessarily act as allocators of health care resources. Always, however, fidelity to the patient, which can take the form of advocacy, should claim the loyalty of the primary care internists.

Ethical problems are often inseparable from interpersonal and psychological difficulties. Getting the noncompliant patient to take her diabetes medicine can invite the physician to act in a threatening or even a coercive manner. Is this a violation of patient autonomy? Telling the fussy, difficult, nasty patient to find another doctor is the limiting act in dealing with what has been called the hateful person. Is it also a repudiation of the duty to benefit when a doctor realizes that he or she simply cannot stand the persistent and insulting phone calls and office visits of a patient who makes life miserable? Among the other psychological complications encountered by the general internist that may cause ethical problems are pressures on the primary care physician who treats more than a single family member, difficulties working with consultants (e.g., the psychiatrist or radiologist) in other medical specialities whose work may be in doubt, feelings of being trapped in the middle by loyalty to the patient and responsibility to the managed health care organization.

Few doctors are as consistently clinical as surgeons. The "blood and guts" of surgical procedures requires enormous fortitude and, especially in emergency situations, alacrity of mind in order to make decisions swiftly and clearly. Surgeons, whether in the operating suite, the trauma center, or at the bedside of a patient, have limited time to theorize. Their work must be active and decisive. General surgeons and those who specialize (e.g., in neuro-, cardiothoracic, ophthalmologic, gynecologic, orthopedic, maxillofacial, gastrointestinal, plastic, or transplant surgery) make use of the most sophisticated equipment available in the modern hospital. Dependent on both laboratory and clinical research, surgeons deal with every variety of medical problem: from breast reconstruction for the patient diagnosed with cancer to replacing a failed liver for the person who has irreversible hepatic disease. From the patient's perspective, the prospect of morbidity or mortality may not be as burdensome as the fear of disfigurement. Every surgical decision has a different and complicated ethical foundation.

One crucial decision faced by surgeons is whether or not to operate. The request of a patient, or even a referring primary care doctor, for surgical intervention should not mean surgery is automatically scheduled. No physician should perform a procedure when it can do little or no good. Because surgeons must often project a future based on uncertain results, they inevitably make judgments about the benefit-to-risk ratio of an operation. Predicting mortality or estimating morbidity is never done abstractly: The needs, lifestyle, family situation, and personal goals of the patient have to be taken into account. The fairness and justice of such assessments are always subject to scrutiny. For a surgeon to agree to perform cardiothoraic surgery for a patient with advanced renal disease, more than just a statistical assessment of survivability or rate of recovery is involved. The meaning of a limited recovery for such a patient naturally includes concerns about religious and moral sensibilities. For the cancer patient, issues about quantity versus quality of life must be faced. For the person with serious or borderline reconstructable cardiac processes, the nature of independence or dependence that might follow surgery is encountered.

Surgery has always been an exhausting task: "How long did the operation take," is a common inquiry. Fatigue, stress, and the pressure of having a patient's life literally in one's hands are truly burdensome, no matter how stoic the model presented to surgical residents during their training. Today danger for the surgeon arises as a result of the perceived life-threatening dangers of treating patients affected by the HIV virus. As the AIDS epidemic continues to grow, many patients who can infect the surgeon (no matter how careful the surgeon is, no matter what precautions are taken) are candidates for surgeries. Whether as a result of unprotected sexual activities, intravenous drug use, or transfusions taken when the blood supply was not satisfactorily screened—each patient, whether on an emergency or elective basis, will test the Hippocratic obligation to care for the sick in need. Protecting health care professionals while treating patients with HIV is the sort of challenge faced by doctors caring for plague victims in fifteenth century Europe and not very often since. Among surgeons, and out of the public eye, debates continue about safety and the moral responsibility of practitioners most vulnerable to cuts, punctures, and exposure to body fluids.

For patients with a terminal disease, the role of the surgeon can become crucial. The effort to rid the body of a tumor is not the sole occupation of the surgical oncologist, however. When curing is impossible, palliative surgery becomes an option. With the collaboration of other medical specialists, even the dying patient can exercise surgical options. Surgery, however, is often difficult and always risky, so decisions about an operation for a dying patient should be made in the most noncoercive and supportive climate possible. Ineffective or unwarranted treatments are not difficult to resist, but both tried and experimental therapies should be recommended only if they make medical sense. Removing an obstruction due to colon cancer is wise, but doing a liver resection in the face of diffuse adenocarcinoma is not. Surgeons have an enormous authority—their experience is the source of their power—and their recommendations necessarily reflect a desire to improve the quality of life of all, not just some, patients.

Internists and surgeons often meet in the ICU. This complex and highly technological environment represents, from the patient's perspective, all that is good and bad in modern medicine. Immediate and dramatic interventions such as CPR can save lives. But dehumanizing patients is also common. Both realistic and unrealistic fears inform the experience of ICU patients and their families, and such normally uncontroversial matters as explaining a procedure can become a source of anxiety resulting in the diminution of choice-making capacity for the patient. In the emergency room, another locus of collaboration between surgeons and internists, the swiftness of decision making can impede (and not always necessarily) the chance to reflect on ethical dilemmas.

■ FIVE ESSENTIAL CASES ■

Case 6-1

Fidelity to the patient is a clear and basic duty for the physician. But when *other* health care practitioners must take risks in the course of helping the patient, unlimited obligations may be resisted.

Mr. S.J. is a 44-year-old single male, a successful industrialist who was in good health until recently. During a long bicycle ride, Mr. S.J. experienced sustained chest pain. He visited his internist, Dr. V., a longtime personal physician whom he considers his friend. After the initial appointment, Dr. V. ordered an exercise stress test along with blood work. Mr. S.J. stayed on the treadmill for only a few minutes before he showed considerable ischemia. Two days later he underwent a coronary angiography that showed substantial blockage in at least four of the main arteries that could not be treated by angioplasty. Dr. V. advised his patient to see a cardiothoracic surgeon immediately, recommended a leading physician, and made an appointment for Mr. S.J.

The surgeon, Dr. B., examined Mr. S.J. the next morning and agreed that he should have a quadruple coronary artery bypass graft (CABG) procedure right away. Medical management, she told the patient, would be debilitating and potentiallly life threatening. The surgeon told Mr. S.J. that the chance for a successful operation was very good because of his good health, young age, and positive attitude. She also noted that the patient is lucky because the surgery would be performed prior to a heart attack. Mr. S.J. agreed with the recommendation and two mornings later was admitted to the hospital for the CABG procedure. The operation was scheduled for midafternoon. Dr. B. and the internist, Dr. V. lunched together, coincidentally, that noontime in the hospital cafeteria. Mentioning the upcoming surgery, Dr. V. said quite casually to his colleague, "I suppose Mr. S.J. told you that he is a homosexual?" Dr. B. said, "No, he didn't. Has he been tested for HIV?" A swift check of the patient's medical record revealed no evidence of HIV testing. Dr. B. knows that a blood test for HIV can be done immediately and that the results of the test can be available in as little as 2 hours. She says to the internist, "Will you ask this patient to have the test?"

■ ■ ■

The medical dimensions of this case seem clear. Mr. S.J. needs CABG surgery. Without it he will not die immediately—medical management will be provided, no matter what the decision about surgery, at least until the patient checks into the hospital for his operation. But for a patient of Mr. S.J.'s age, history, and general condition, CABG surgery is the treatment of choice. If successful (and here again the statistics are very encouraging), Mr. S.J. will survive to experience many years of vital health. He will be riding his bicycle again, probably in a matter of weeks. With careful follow-up (including monitored diet and exercise programs), Mr. S.J. can expect to live almost as long as a person who has not had a CABG operation.

Suppose, however, that this patient has been exposed to the HIV virus? This remains unknown. But assuming it *is* the case: What can Mr. S.J. anticipate. First, it could be many months before the antibodies develop that will show, on testing, that he is HIV positive. If such a test is confirmed (the first screenings can yield false positive readings; only a second test is confirmatory), Mr. S.J. may develop the first signs and symptoms of AIDS in a matter of months or years. He *will* develop AIDS, even though prophylactic use of drugs, inhalants for pulmonary infections, and other cautionary methods can be used to lengthen his period of relative well-being. During these months and years, Mr. S.J. will need, and want to have, a heart that is getting as much blood-flow as possible.

The real source of ethical anxiety in this case is as yet the property of the two physicians and not the patient. Dr. V.'s fidelity to Mr. S.J. has been demonstrated over the course of years. He has screened his patient carefully and made a sound recommendation for a surgical consultation. As a primary care giver he is ready to facilitate Mr. S.J.'s hospital experience with all that his experience allows. Yet some ambivalence, or at the very least tension, is evident in the quiet phrase spoken to his surgical colleague. In asking Dr. B. if she is aware of Mr. S.J.'s lifestyle, with its attendant risks of contracting the HIV virus, Dr. V. may be working from several, or mixed, motives.

As an advocate for his patient, the internist may be giving the surgeon information that can be useful to all parties. Because Dr. V. chose to mention his patient's homosexual lifestyle on the very day of the scheduled CABG surgery, he may presume that the patient has disclosed this fact to the surgeon already. On discovering that all of this is news to Dr. B., however, the request to solicit an HIV blood test from Mr. S.J. becomes a very serious matter. Assuming that the patient is anxious about the imminent surgery—and this is a virtual certainty—what justification for making this request can the surgeon have in mind? What reasons could the internist give the patient in soliciting consent to test?

Various states have legislated the conditions under which HIV testing of patients or prospective patients in hospitals can be secured. All press for confidentiality of data, usually limiting test results to a "need-to-know" basis. Does Dr. B. have such a need? As an experienced surgeon she undoubtedly practices universal precautions for blood and body fluids. Cardiothoracic surgery, however, is very invasive, requiring cutting bone, tissue, and blood vessels (including the major coronary arteries), and the careful suturing of venous and arterial grafts. It can be a long and laborious procedure, with much blood flowing and abundant opportunities for needle sticks, bone shard cuts, and fluid spurts. We can understand why Dr. B. would want to know the HIV status of her patient.

The assumption that Mr. S.J. is in a high-risk category is a statistical one. Homosexuals who practice anal or oral sex and IV drug abusers constitute the major population of male AIDS patients, but the concern of these two doctors must be for Mr. S.J., taken in a realistic context. Should he be asked, right away, to give consent for the test? Will the results tell enough to be useful? (Aside from the problem of false positives, HIV antibodies may not have appeared in his bloodstream.) It is fair to ask just who is being served by this request. Who, for that matter, should initiate it? Dr. V. is the primary internist, Dr. B. the surgeon who wants the results prior to surgery. Determining just who will assume responsibility is the next decision to be made in this case.

A search for an underlying principle that will resolve the case is no easy task, in part because every hospital requires universal precautions in surgery. In order for either physician to justify a full inquiry regarding this patient's HIV status, some plausible and consistent reason has to be found. Fear, anxiety, and ambivalence about nontraditional lifestyles are not reasons, although they may motivate the desire to test Mr. S.J. The principle of justice, on the other hand, demands equity of treatment for patients of varying backgrounds, classes, races, and economic status. To "go after" Mr. S.J.—as Dr. B. wants the internist, Dr. V., to do—places a colleague in a double bind, from which ethical escape seems unlikely.

Case 6-2

The acute-care emphasis of medical training—in surgery as well as in internal medicine—differs fundamentally from the chronic care/rehabilitation model applicable to professionals who care for patients with long-term disabilities. Conflicts between these two perspectives present questions of power and authority as well as ethical responsibility.

N.N. is a 34-year-old woman who has had cerebral palsy since birth. She has long been in the custody of the state. She has been labeled "mentally retarded" and, more recently, "developmentally delayed." She cannot speak and has a hearing disorder that requires an aid. N.N. had lived in a large state institution since early childhood and her level of functioning was not very high. Now, due to the state policy of deinstitutionalization, she has been transferred to a smaller, community-based facility. She has been receiving occupational and rehabilitative therapy, but only for the past 8 months. Presently she can dress herself, wash her face and hands, and go to the toilet. N.N. is also working on gross motor skills. She has recently learned to say a few difficult-to-comprehend words.

N.N. has never learned to walk. In the state hospital, she crawled on her knees and hands. Her feet are fixed in equinovarus deformities; both tibial plateaus show large callous formations from years of crawling. After being transferred, N.N. was taken by her physical therapist to an outpatient orthopedic clinic in the hope of having the physician prescribe a wheelchair for her use. The attending physician, a surgeon, took x-rays of her lower limbs and recommended surgery to reduce the deformities and to bring N.N.'s feet plantigrade so that she could stand. When the physical therapist asked the doctor for a wheelchair prescription, he stated that she would not need it, that the surgery would make her just fine.

The therapist told the surgeon that N.N. had the gross motor skills of a 5 month old and had been using primitive reflexes to achieve mobility. Repairing N.N.'s feet would not provide the motor control necessary for walking. The rehabilitation specialist felt that the surgery would be harmful because persons with mental retardation often regress after such an operation, becoming aggressive or self-destructive. The surgeon disagreed completely, feeling that repairing N.N.'s feet was the only feasible approach. He said that after the surgery the patient could continue rehabilitation therapy and would certainly be in a "condition to do more things better."

■ ■ ■

Questions about *who* makes medical decisions are often answered by the law (e.g., parents make health care determinations for their minor children) or by relying on principles ("I respect your treatment refusal because you are an autonomous adult."). If an appropriate decision maker can be found, only half the battle is won. An efficacious treatment option must still be selected. The case of N.N. is complicated in two ways: (1) Though decisions about treatment can ultimately be made by the appropriately designated guardian, there is no guarantee that such a person will make the "right" choice; and (2) reasonable caregivers differ significantly in their assessment of the patient and in their recommendation about care.

When professionals are in conflict in the medical center, matters of fact and opinion often overlap. Perspectives—based on specialized training and, just as important, on style of intervention—are very influential. Some doctors are conservative in their attitudes toward surgery or the use of new and recently proven drugs. Others are risk takers whose practices involve forthright intervention, even when there is a small chance of success. Is the surgeon in N.N.'s case such a practitioner?

When a struggle ensues, the decision may be based not on who is *right*, but on who *governs*. Just as physicians may have more clout than nurses and most allied health care professionals, surgeons are often seen as powerful and decisive due to the swiftness of their assessment and interventional skills. In the case of N.N., the surgeon seems to believe he knows what is best and will not be persuaded otherwise, but he is not, as yet, insisting on a surgical solution. The therapist, on the other hand, has the more sympathetic role of patient advocate. What if her clinical judgment is faulty? What if the surgeon *could* bring about a restoration of function that would grant N.N. an independence almost unprecedented in such cases?

The communication problem in this case is obvious and paramount. N.N.'s therapist has known many similar cases and has a vivid sense of the limitations of persons with such severe development disabilities. She knows that mental capacity influences physical capacity; she has tried to tell the surgeons about this dimension of the case. The surgeon knows about feet, and about how impossible it will ever be for N.N. to walk well without major repairs. That is his premise—and he seems unwilling to entertain another form of care. It seems a natural first step to try to encourage a dialogue between surgeon and therapist. The perspectives of the rehabilitation specialist and the surgeon have created a divergent set of foci on the case of

N.N. Both want the quality of the patient's life enhanced, but they are speaking incompatible languages; teaching them both to hear one another is a mandatory first step. The problem of *who governs* may, however, render such a discussion unlikely.

Many options remain. Another surgeon can be consulted. A physician, perhaps a primary care doctor connected to the community facility, can try to intervene on N.N.'s behalf. The ethical issue at stake in this case is masked, in part, by the social-psychological structure of the situation. N.N. is in the middle and is unaware of her status. The principle of beneficence will need a lot of support. To find the best and most ready way of helping N.N., all participants in the case must move toward a common ground of language and understanding. The search for a compromise in this case requires ethical sensitivity and political acumen. Bringing the patient "home" is an option. But will N.N.'s interests be saved by such a mode of conflict resolution?

Case 6-3

In the ER, time taken for reflection is often believed to be better spent on immediate patient care. But the intensity of moral dilemmas can be greater in the ER than in other medical locales.

Mrs. G.P., aged 88 and a long-time Alzheimer's disease patient, is brought into the ER of City Hospital from the nursing home in which she has resided for 12 years. She has not spoken or moved from her bed (spontaneously) for almost 1 year. The patient has only two living relatives, her daughters who take turns visiting her each day. She has been fed via nasogastric tube for a long time. She does react to some external stimuli and often seems comforted by soft music.

General sepsis due to pneumonia has resulted in respiratory insufficiency. When she arrives in the ER, Mrs. G.P. is still breathing spontaneously, but in a very labored fashion. Accompanying her in the ambulance is a nursing home LPN who has brought the patient's chart. It contains a statement by the patient's two children that, "If our mother stops breathing, do not put her on a respirator. Let her die if her time has come." There is no living will or durable power of attorney for health care document in the record. The LPN tells the ER resident, Dr. M., that "we couldn't let this lady die with us. You know how it is. We couldn't be really sure what was wrong with her. We had to send her here." The emergency medical technicians (EMTs) acted swiftly and now Mrs. G.P.

is in the hands of emergency medicine specialists. Dr. M. knows that intubating the patient is a clear and obvious first-step, but she wonders if doing this is right and necessary.

Emergency physicians have no real chance to know the patient. Intervention cannot wait and a detailed history is rarely evoked. There is no time to consider the factors that led the nursing home to send this patient to the hospital. (Reasons or rationales abound, including the fear of legal vulnerability, institutional policy, staffing problems, and difficulties in getting a physician to take responsibility within the long-term care facility.) Swift action is the mode of reaction. Medical records may be requested and friends or family members can provide information, but it is still difficult to find the time to get all the necessary data to make a determination *not to treat*.

ER doctors are skilled at risk-benefit analyses: Calculating the prospects for a very ill person remains a medical judgment in the absence of a sense of the values or prior lifestyle of the patient. So such doctors try to restore health and either save life or prolong it. They see Mrs. G.P. as a very sick person, and, almost instinctively, begin the assessment and treatment process, in the hope of keeping this patient going. Even if this goal is unattainable, the ER staff often feels impelled, perhaps due to legal fears, to relieve symptoms and to restore as much physical function as possible to the patient.

Such an approach to this case will probably yield the following results: By erring on the side of life Mrs. G.P. will be intubated and placed on a ventilator. She will then be given the very best of care by being transferred to the ICU where her sepsis and pneumonia will be treated aggressively. She will, perhaps, improve sufficiently to be removed from the mechanical breathing device and, after some time, may be taken to the general medical-surgical floor for a more complete recovery. Eventually (if we are "lucky") she will be returned to the nursing home. This is what happens to thousands of older patients—of the millions of persons with Alzheimer's disease—each week in major hospitals.

The ER team ignores financial cost when it initiates care for a patient. But more than one clinician in this case may ask, perhaps silently, "What kind of resources are we going to use on Mrs. G.P.?" There is no definitive answer (costs vary by region) but the answer, were we to follow the usual scenario, could be in the tens of thousands of dollars. But when a very sick patient presents in an emergency setting, to think of cost is deemed unprofessional. Yet the remarks in this patient's chart may have such a concern in mind. Many other notions can be entailed in that somewhat obscure annotation, "Let her die if her time has come."

The patient does not have the benefit either of a specific set of advance directives or of having appointed a person to act on her behalf if she is incompetent. Thus, the two *best* modes of pursuing the patient's interests are unavailable. Mrs. G.P.'s family, however, has conferred with the caregivers at the nursing home and convinced them that dramatic interventions should *not* be undertaken. But huge gaps exist—certainly between the legally secure (in most jurisdictions) living will or durable power-of-attorney procedure and the loose and informal sentences in her chart. More than just documentation is missing. What is the patient's resuscitation status? In the absence of a DNR order, Mrs. G.P. is a full code patient. Presumably, she has received good care—tube feeding has gone on for a long time, but planning for likely contingencies has not proceeded apace. Suppose Mrs. G.P. were to sustain a urinary tract infection, spike a high fever, and develop pneumonia? Would she get massive antibiotics in the nursing home? We do not know.

Such details are, at this moment, relatively unimportant. The ER physicians must decide what to do for this woman. Can they, and should they, wait before treating her? Should they give credence to the written statement and to the LPN's affirmation of it? Should they try to contact Mrs. G.P.'s children immediately? They do *not* need permission to intervene. The emergency exception to the doctrine of informed consent will cover their erring on the side of life (See Fig. 2-2). Will they be doing the patient any good (beneficence) if she is sent to the ICU? Will any restoration of function be accomplished? Will they be harming her if they treat her only to send her back to die of Alzheimer's disease?

Who is the patient whose fate is to be decided? She is unconscious and nonresponsive and certainly lacks communicative capacity. Is Mrs. G.P. still a person? This is a philosophical, not a medical, question and is dependent on our definition of personhood. For those who see life per se as an inherent good, Mrs. G.P. is worthy of continued care. For those who value self-awareness and the possibility of relationships as indispensable minimal characteristics of a person, the status of Mrs. G.P. is in doubt.

The decisions about to be made in the ER must be viewed not just as they relate to this case but to ethical considerations in general. Are *all* lives worth living? Are *all* lives worth saving? The only way in which ER doctors can deal with such questions is to raise such issues routinely. To provide an educational forum for all emergency personnel to air such concerns is an obvious first step. In some American cities, EMT organizations, in association with local and county medical societies, have suggested a portable DNR or limited treatment document. Some emergency rooms keep computer files with lists of patients who are not to be intubated. Advance planning is the best preparation. Of course, attention to the needs of the specific patient must transcend even the most sensible policy. In this case, much more than the life or death of Mrs. G.P. hangs in the balance.

Case 6-4

Advocating for the competent patient being treated by medical specialists in the large tertiary-care medical center is not easy for the internist. But when the patient's decision-making capacity fluctuates, and when physicians disagree about the nature and extent of treatment, there are forums for resolving conflicts and reconciling differences.

More than 3 years ago, Mrs. R. was diagnosed as suffering from terminal bone cancer. It was expected that she would die in less than 1 year. A widow aged 66, she told her doctor (an internist) that she knew that when she died she would go to heaven. She survived, in and out of hospitals, for an unexpectedly long period of time. A large and inoperable tumor at the base of her spine caused great pain. When the cancer caused bones in her left arm and hip to break, she was operated on and rods were inserted into the bones. She did not resist these treatments. But she did tell the internist, Dr. G., that she wanted to die and that "I would never want to be hooked up to a breathing machine. I would rather be with God."

Six days ago Mrs. R., who had been living at home with her brother, was admitted to the hospital due to difficulty breathing. Without her consent she was placed on a ventilator in the ICU. Her brother protested, but the physicians insisted, stating that this was an emergency. When Mrs. R. was stabilized, a pulmonary medicine resident approached her and asked, "Do you want the machine?" Mrs. R. replied, "Machine."

Dr. G. visited his patient later that day and she seemed coherent and alert but was incapable of speaking due to the respirator. She did write a note, in his presence, that said: "I am sick of being kept alive. My tumor is not going to go away. Can I just be allowed to die?" Mrs. R.'s primary nurse noted in the chart that the patient sighed a great deal and stated once: "I've had enough. When will they just let me go?"

Mrs. R.'s condition deteriorated rapidly. She was no longer communicative. Based on his earlier "conversation" with the patient, Dr. G. had a DNR order placed on her chart. It was signed by her brother as well. The next day, another intensive care resident performed a tracheotomy, noting in the chart that the DNR order did not prohibit other useful medical interventions. Two days later the director of the ICU told Dr. G. that his staff wanted to perform a gastrostomy so that the patient wouldn't starve to death. (Mrs. R., it should be noted, had no living will or durable power of attorney for health care document.) When Dr. G. stated that he and the patient's family knew that she would not want to be on the ventilator and certainly, if alert, would refuse the feeding tube, the ICU director conferred with the hospital's attorneys. The lawyers met with the intensive care specialists and told them about Mrs. R.'s earlier wishes and her brother's involvement, but the doctors continued to feel that failing to intervene would be medically and perhaps legally unwise. Because they thought it possible to get her through this crisis, the intensivists were reluctant to let her die. They agreed that they would not oppose the withdrawal of life-support if a court order were obtained first. The chief hospital attorney happened to be an ex-officio member of the institution's bioethics committee (BEC). He suggested to the parties that perhaps that body could help reconcile the differences.

What, exactly, are the presumed motives of the director of the ICU? Are they shared by the residents on the unit? Are they explicit or implicit? Are ethical realities being influenced by legal concerns? A reliance on patient autonomy — at least as expressed recently by Mrs. R. — would seem to lean in the direction of nonintervention. Are the intensive care physicians contemptuous of such prior expressions? More than likely, they are not. They are, rather, asking two very basic questions: (1) In the absence of concrete documentation, to what extent should a patient's "former" self govern decisions for her "present" self? and (2) should the views of patients regarding continuing care or the refusal of treatment be the preferred source of authority for medical conditions in situations like this? The intensivists, reared in a tradition of intervention and wanting to keep Mrs. R. alive, seek the wisdom of others. The hospital attorneys recommend a meeting with the institution's ethics committee.

In many acute care hospitals, the absence of a patient's competence to make a medical judgment is dealt with by having a close family member become the surrogate decision-maker. When there is no documentation or oral statement by the patient about treatment refusal, family members are presumed to share the patient's values and to know her way of thinking. But in the case of Mrs. R., the patient has made her views known several times. The intensivists are simply not satisfied with the content and the ostensible meaning of those expressions. Would it not be natural then to go to family members for clarification or confirmation? Were this tactic pursued, Mrs. R. would surely be allowed to die.

The ICU doctors, however, either mistrust the validity of the patient's and her brother's perspective or simply believe that some moral and perhaps legal authority compels them to continue to treat Mrs. R. with substantial aggressiveness. Given the litigious climate in which contemporary physicians practice, such a view is hardly idiosyncratic. Moving the question to the forum of the bioethics committee is also not an unusual procedure.

BECs, which date from the mid-1970s, do not make decisions. They are interdisciplinary groups based mostly in acute-care hospitals. Such committees reflect a growing awareness that technology can open up moral dilemmas while solving clinical problems. BECs — with membership from medicine, nursing, social work, pastoral care, and the larger community — can take a mediating role in advising caregivers about ways of approaching ethical conflicts. In addition to their policy and educational roles, BECs often provide a "safe space," a forum in which persons with seemingly irreconcilable differences about treatment options can speak in a nonthreatening and supportive environment (Fig. 6-1).

If the physicians from the ICU agree to bring this case before the BEC, a variety of process questions emerges immediately. Who should meet with the committee? The director of the ICU? The residents who care for Mrs. R? Should the internist be invited to attend? Is it appropriate for the patient's brother to participate?

1. Acting as an interdisciplinary clearing house for ethical dilemmas encountered by patients, staff, and administration, especially by bringing together accurate information from all available sources.
2. Advising physicians, nurses, and other health care professionals about dealing with ethical conflicts.
3. Consulting on hard-choice cases on an emergency basis.
4. Reviewing problematic cases retrospectively.
5. Educating staff and others about the ethical dimensions of medical care.
6. Developing policies and guidelines regarding issues of biomedical ethics (e.g., DNR orders, life-support withdrawal protocols).
7. Counseling practitioners who are troubled by decisions regarding treatment or nontreatment of patients.
8. Providing a safe forum for the discussion of problems within the medical/health care hierarchy.

Fig. 6-1. Functions of Bioethics Committees

Because the primary nurse has also noted the patient's earlier desire to cease treatment, should her views be solicited before the BEC?

What will result from having brought the case of Mrs. R. to the BEC is unpredictable. Most committees try to take a middle course by allowing case participants to hear one another. Given that this patient is quite clearly incompetent, the committee will likely raise several fundamental questions for the caregivers: (1) Will continued care or a potential intervention (e.g., insertion of the feeding tube) serve to prolong the patient's life or will it extend the course of her dying? (2) can the family and the primary care physician be trusted to speak for this now silent patient? (3) what would be the results of withholding or withdrawing care in this context? (4) what is the appropriate role for caregivers who (either due to matters of conscience or as a result of anxiety about legal consequences) cannot agree with surrogate decision makers who wish to cease treatment? A balanced and nuanced discussion of the case will not guarantee a middle-ground solution, but it will provide an opportunity for all parties to be heard. Identifying the interests in conflict and asserting the values (and principles) that have initially led to implacable concern can yield agreement.

Many BECs have lawyers as members, either officially or unofficially. Such committees, however, are not substitutes for courts of law. Their function is to help achieve consensus so that legal authorities need not be involved (Fig. 6-1). If the intensivists in the case of Mrs. R. can hear the views of many practitioners about the moral permissibility of removing life support systems from this patient, their ambivalence about the case may be assuaged. But no BEC can provide moral certainty.

Case 6-5

The patient is the center of concern in nearly all clinical situations. But the needs of other patients for scarce organs may complicate the ending of a person's life and can push medical personnel—internists, surgeons, and others—into awkward situations.

Mr. H., a 22-year-old man, was severely injured in a motorcycle accident. He suffered massive head trauma when thrown from his vehicle. In the ambulance he was resuscitated and as soon as got to the ER he was placed on a ventilator. Two hours later, his EEG was flat, indicating brain death. (Most hospital protocols mandate another such test in several hours.) The nurse who filled out the admission papers for Mr. H. noticed that on the back of his driver's license he had agreed to organ donation in the event of death. Initial efforts to contact Mr. H.'s family were unsuccessful. A trauma surgeon in the ER said to the nurse, "Well, give them another call and if we can't find anyone, we'll go from there."

The nurse phoned once again, this time reaching Mr. H.'s mother. The nurse explained the situation: "Your son has had a very bad accident. Please come here right away and bring a friend or family member if you can. We need to make some decisions and will want your help." When the nurse reported this to the trauma surgeon, he told her, "Let's get this guy's heart and kidneys before they go bad, O.K?" The ER is in a state with a required request statute that mandates asking family members for permission to harvest useful organs from patients in Mr. H.'s status.

The declaration of death by a physician is the most irreversible and, thus, the most profound act that a doctor can undertake. The diagnosis of brain death in both adults and children demands accuracy and sensitivity. With the advent of mechanical venitilators in the 1950s, the very definition of death changed. Although most state legislatures and hospitals have accepted variants on the definition of brain death origi-nally provided by the Harvard Ad Hoc Committee to Examine the Defi-nition of Brain Death, published in *JAMA* in 1968 and validated by the President's Commission for the Study of Ethical Problems in Medi-cine in 1981, many legal, ethical, and clinical issues remain unre-solved. In and out of ICUs, the utilization of CPR has become routine in most hospitals. But complicating discussion of brain death are (1) debates about the condition called persistent vegetative state (PVS) (see Chapter 8); (2) the right-to-die movement, a patient-centered effort to raise public concerns about both extending and lim-iting life; (3) changed secular and religious views on allowing patients to die; (4) innovations in organ and tissue transplantation and the scar-city of donor material that necessitate public faith in the credibility of physicians engaged in securing such vital material. The founda-tional Harvard criteria list four essential elements for assessing the patient in deep coma to determine if brain death has occurred:

1. Unreceptivity and unresponsivity
2. No movements or breathing
3. No reflexes
4. Flat electroencephalogram ("of great confirmatory value")

(The Ad Hoc Committee of the Harvard Medical School to Examine the Definition of Brain Death, Report, JAMA 205(6): 337–340, 1968.)

This official promulgation (and there are others) does not neces-sarily relieve the anxieties that professionals and members of the public have about the diagnosis of brain death and the use of donor material from patients such as Mr. H. Such concerns include:

1. The theoretic and practical reliability of the criteria
2. Discussion about the meaning of the term function as it applies to brain activity
3. Debates about determining the time of death
4. Problems encountered in dealing with complicating con-ditions such as drug intoxication, hypothermia and shock, and especially the reliability of criteria in dealing with very young children

Compounding the real, if limited, medical uncertainty in brain death cases are the facts of life and death. Mr. H. is dead by all clinical criteria. But, tethered to the ventilator, his chest rises and falls, his heart pumps, and his blood circulates. He is warm to the touch. Though there will inevitably be organ deterioration, at the moment he will not *appear* to a loved one to have died. Even if his family accepts the certainty of Mr. H.'s having died, they may be in no position to give considered or reasoned consent to the request for organ donation. The driver's license notation is a useful tool here—it will allow medical personnel to state, with honesty, that Mr. H. would have wanted to be a donor. But by law and custom such a prior statement is not compelling. All hospitals must ask immediate family (if they can be contacted) for permission.

Most American states have required requests laws that obligate physicians and other caregivers to ask for donor organs at appropriate moments. Most state regulations try to ensure that there is no conflict of interest; the ER doctor should not be the attending physician for a patient awaiting a new kidney. Assuming no such conflict, it is also apparent that all physicians know how much help a single set of body parts can be for a plethora of patients in need. Not only the obvious organs (i.e., heart, liver, kidneys) can be utilized, corneas, inner ear material, and all sorts of tissue can also be transplanted. Asking for such a donation is not a neutral task.

How should one approach Mr. H.'s family? As is common, they come to the hospital *not knowing* that Mr. H. is clinically dead. Time is truly essential in salvaging donor organs. How much of this precious commodity should be given to the family? What information do they need to make a truly informed consent to donate? Who should make the request? If Mr. H.'s mother gives a negative response, or simply seems reluctant, how far should the health care team go in trying to convince her of the benefits of donating her son's organs? Indeed, whose rights and responsibilities are at the center of the agenda in this case? Mr. H. is dead and no longer has the same interests he had earlier that evening. But do all his interests vanish when the EEG goes flat? Is there some kind of magical transfer of interests from the deceased person to his immediate family? Can we say that society, the state, or other persons in medical need now have an interest in Mr. H.'s remains? If there is doubt about such matters, who is best qualified to reconcile differences? Matters of life and death do not necessarily end with the death of the patient.

■ PRACTICE MODEL CASE ■

Mr. W.S. was a 53-year-old man awaiting discharge from an acute care hospital. Two days earlier he had undergone surgery that showed extensive and inoperable lung cancer. The surgeon opened and closed, and Mr. W.S. was taken to the recovery room. While Mr. W.S. was there, the surgeon told his wife that the patient had cancer, that it was likely widespread, and that though chemotherapy and radiation might extend her husband's life, they would not do so for very long. Mrs. W.S. told the surgeon, "I will tell him about this in my own way." She then spoke with her husband's primary care physician, an internist, who agreed that the person to give Mr. W.S. the news should be his spouse of 30 years.

The next day, Mrs. W.S. told her husband that he was "very sick and there is nothing more that can be done to help you here in the hospital." He told her that he was feeling very weak and nauseated and that he thought this was due to his recent weight loss. Mrs. W.S. made no response to this comment. Their adult son came to visit and told the internist, in the hall, that he hoped "there is something that can be done for my dad." The physician asked wife and son just how they wished to proceed. Mrs. W.S. said, "Well, we just don't know. I wish he could die here." The son responded, "It's a real tragedy, but I just can't bring myself to make a decision about what to do. What would you recommend, doctor?"

Patient

Mr. W.S. is in the dark, but not completely so. He is well aware of his illness. He is experiencing pain and pressure in his chest due to the lung involvement and has gastrointestinal symptoms as well. He is in the process of recovering from surgery and is certainly tired and in need of a great deal of care. His mental status has not been checked, but it is a fair guess that he is scared and, having heard that nothing more can be offered him in the hospital, may well suspect that his condition is terminal. Yet he has not heard the precise words, from the surgeon or the internist, to confirm a diagnosis.

If Mr. W.S. is to leave the hospital, a variety of decisions about his condition, prognosis, and welfare have to be settled. The facts indicate that his capacity to exercise his autonomy is in no way compromised. Yet without the information necessary to state a preference or make a decision, Mr. W.S. is no better off than an infant whose interests are protected by his parents. From Mr. W.S.'s perspective, being a patient (and one very ill and in need of much care) sums up his status at the moment.

It is also a medical fact that Mr. W.S. is in a terminal condition. While definitions of that status vary, most center around the notion of imminent death in a finite period. Mr. W.S. will not live, no matter what the intervention, for more than a few months. He could die within days. Does this labelling of the patient mean that decisions about his treatment should differ from determinations about a patient whose recovery is virtually certain. Does terminal status confer burdens or benefits on patients? Many physicians agree that when a patient is actively dying, she should be granted dignity and respect. Do such cliched certainties apply only to this select clientele?

Relationships

The person closest to the patient is his wife. It is not unusual for a spouse or close relative to hear the diagnosis or the treatment results for the patient. Mrs. W.S. undoubtedly sat in the surgical waiting room while her husband's exploratory operation transpired. A participant in the long-standing and common ritual of "waiting for the doctor to clean up after surgery," Mrs. W.S. was the first to hear the news about the inoperability of her spouse's tumor. She has become, in effect, the case manager and has secured the agreement of the other person with a primary relationship to the patient, his internist. They agree that information about the cancer and its care should be transmitted by Mrs. W.S.

As the matter presently stands, their adult son is also in possession of information about the patient's illness. Like his mother, he is in doubt about how to proceed. We can assume that both family members want to do what's right for Mr. W.S. Their concern, which seems paternalistic, originates in concern for the patient's vulnerability. Because they are doling out information in such small doses, however, Mr. W.S.'s relationship to them is unusually one-sided. The object of their concern is without much voice, and many important decisions need to be made.

At the fulcrum of the case is the internist. He has already served as the gatekeeper for his patient, having arranged for the surgery and having supervised the beginning stages of Mr. W.S.'s postoperative care. Though we know nothing about the internist's prior relationship to this patient, we can assume that the doctor has told Mr. W.S. that he will be hearing the results of the surgery very soon. All relationships in this difficult case are in a state of suspension as the internist tries to answer the son's challenging request for a recommendation.

Advocacy

In a rudimentary sense, we may portray Mrs. W.S. as an advocate for her very ill husband. She is asking questions on his behalf. If she is a minimally effective case manager, she is watching the nursing and medical care Mr. W.S. is getting and is, at the very least, making certain that he is treated well and carefully monitored. But the notion of advocacy is only minimally an observational function. It is a process through which a person (or persons) acts on behalf of a patient and with the patient's interests of primary importance. An advocate for Mr. W.S. will have to ask not only "what can we do to make him feel comfortable," but also "what will he need to know in order to regain the autonomy that can be permanently compromised by his physical condition?"

The internist, as a primary care doctor, is pledged to advocate for his patient. Realistically, however, he knows that he cannot speak for every one of his ill patients. He can never know enough, and possibly never even care enough, to be a surrogate family member at all times. Instead, he consults with Mrs. W.S. and her son. The collaboration between internist and family is beneficent. It is encountered routinely when a patient lacks decisional capacity. If Mr. W.S. were in a coma, no one would doubt the procedural wisdom of having the physicians consult with close family members. Mr. W.S., however, is only temporarily "out of it," a time during which effective advocacy is most indispensable.

Conflicts

The principle of veracity mandates that the truth be told to the patient and to all directly involved in a treatment decision. But truth is an evanescent commodity: It vanishes and reappears in strange guises. Mrs. W.S. has told her husband a version of the truth—that he is ill and that hospital care is not a viable option for him. In response to his self-report that his condition was "due to his recent weight loss," Mrs. W.S. has averted a discussion of the real reasons for her husband's physical weakness. Is she being fundamentally dishonest with Mr. W.S.? Does keeping quiet amount to the same thing as active duplicity?

The internist may also be experiencing conflict. His fidelity to Mr. W.S. entails a concern for both the patient's physical well-being and his psychological condition. The doctor's choice of decision-maker will have an enormous impact. If the internist says to Mrs. W.S., "We have no business even discussing this matter out of the earshot of your husband. It's his life, and his body," he will affirm patient autonomy as the supreme consideration. But if he recognizes the gravity of the situation and the necessity of working with this family as Mr. W.S. dies and says, "Well, I don't think radiation and chemo are going to do your husband and dad any good and will likely cause him much useless discomfort. Let's just try to get him home and have hospice take over this case," another entirely different set of maneuvers is set into action. The internist's internal conflict has important consequences for Mr. W.S. and the family.

Treatment or Nontreatment Options

This cancer patient—or the surrogate decision-makers if they maintain authority in the case—has many choices regarding future care. The most remote choice would be to find another surgeon who might be more of a risk-taker and who might try to cut out or reduce the original tumor. Beyond this unlikely option, Mr. W.S. can pursue radiation, chemotherapy, or a combination of those treatments in an effort to reduce the size and change the configuration of the primary tumor and to slow the spread of the metastases that will eventually cause both organ failure and pain. He might also consider some experimental cancer treatments, either by enrolling in a medical center-based drug trial or by consulting alternative health practitioners locally or in another country.

Mr. W.S. can also choose where he wants to die. The hospital is an unlikely place: After his recovery from surgery he does not need to be in an acute-care facility unless palliative surgery or other sophisticated treatment for the purpose of comfort is begun. He can go to a nursing home, for he is likely to require skilled care, or he can enroll in a hospice program, opting either for in-patient care or more likely home care while he dies. Presumably, his spouse and son would provide primary coverage for such home care and would be assisted by hospice staff (e.g., nurses, social workers) and volunteers. This list of options could be extended and depends on the patient's needs and desires. He might want to visit a favorite place before he dies. He might want to keep fighting no matter what. His religious views and his secular concerns surely figure into the decision.

Eventually, Mr. W.S. faces life-extending procedures. Does he want to be resuscitated via CPR? If he develops pneumonia (not unusual for patient with pulmonary problems) does he want a full course of antibiotics? If he becomes unconscious, does he want to be tube-fed? Is being placed on a ventilator a possibility? How vigorously should Mr. W.S.'s treatment be? Can he go so far as to choreograph his own death?

Interests

A strict autonomist approach to this case would ask a single question about interests: How can those of Mr. W.S. best be served? Such an absolutist approach is not without merit. The opportunities for health care professionals and family members to take over a sick patient's case are legion. Those who want to restore Mr. W.S. to the center of decision-making authority have an important axiom on their side: The patient is the presumed best judge of his or her own life choices. The merits of such an approach—that it affirms individualism, privacy, the very notion of selfhood—should not be denied.

For many patients in Mr. W.S.'s situation, there is a paradox to be faced. Can being honest with the patient also be an act of cruelty? Few would recommend bombarding Mr. W.S. with all the medical data about his condition and with all the financial, insurance, placement, and treatment-option data that revolve around his case. Yet anything short of providing this information necessarily limits the patient's central role of decision-maker. If there is a small justification for shortening the list of things that need be told Mr. W.S., then the same justification can be used to shade the patient from many other unpleasant and difficult matters. Sparing the patient necessarily results in a form of procedural weak paternalism.

Assuming that Mr. W.S. has certain basic interests that ought not to be compromised (an interest in remaining as pain-free as possible is an intuitively obvious one), what should be done if he determines to proceed without regard to those interests? Suppose that Mr. W.S. says, "I am walking out of here. Since nothing can be done to make me any better, I am just going to check into a hotel, get a bottle of whiskey, and watch television. I want to be alone." Does our respect for his own sense of his own best interests extend to behaviors we think silly, stupid, or irresponsible?

Consequences

A utilitarian calculation about best results in this case would have to take into account the needs of the patient and his family. The cost of care might also become a matter of interest. If Mr. W.S. gets maximal hospital-based care, his (or an insurance company's or the government's) costs could be more than $1000 each day. If he goes home to die, hospice care might cost less than a third that amount. Providing for the patient at home, however, would be very burdensome for Mrs. W.S. and her son; it is hard to keep a cancer patient comfortable and clean. How can one calculate such a burden, especially since the benefits of caring for him at home might include the joy of being with Mr. W.S. during his last days, the chance to "speak the truth" one last time, or simply witness the death of a loved one in peaceful surroundings?

For the internist, consequences in this case suggest problems and possibilities in others. If he defers to the family and keeps Mr. W.S. less than informed, this can work out for everyone's presumed benefit. But establishing family precedence in this case can make it easier to resist veracity in similar cases he may encounter in the future. If the physician takes a firm stand with the family and insists that Mr. W.S. be brought into the discussion, the doctor may be perceived as insensitive, cold, and unempathic with regard to family needs. How the internist acts will have long-term results for many other parties.

Ethical Principles

We have already spoken of our concerns about veracity and autonomy in this case. We have also assumed that everyone is trying to benefit the patient. But the principle of beneficence always surfaces when dependency is a result of severe or terminal illness. To want to help, to minimize pain, and to ease the suffering of others are admirable desires. To give Mr. W.S. some peace during his last days is by no means a malevolent notion. But beneficence seems to turn into paternalism with remarkable ease. Acting *for* Mr. W.S. converts into acting *as* Mr. W.S. when we allow his spouse to use information sparingly.

Strictly speaking, confidentiality has been broken in this case. As natural as it is for the surgeon to report the results to Mrs. W.S., we would be surprised to find that this doctor has asked the patient to waive his right to be the sole recipient of such news. The conversations between Mrs. W.S. and the doctors depend on her knowing a variety of details about her husband that even he is unaware of to date. This may be common procedure, but it also can be viewed as harmful to the patient's integrity. Whoever undertakes the task of restoring Mr. W.S.'s autonomy in this case will be working to bring an assortment of other fundamental ethical principles into balance.

As is often the case, an abstract commitment to doing the right thing cannot be put into action without effective communication among the parties in a case. Mr. and Mrs. W.S. needed a chance to set the parameters of decision-making with the internist long before the present hospitalization. Choices about treatment or nontreatment might have been discussed by this family years ago. The son should also have been an important participant in these negotiations. Just as there is certainty that Mr. W.S. will soon die, it is more than likely that the son may some day face a similar set of dilemmas when Mrs. W.S. is at the end of her life. It is never too early to begin the troubling task of talking about dying.

■ CASES FOR DISCUSSION ■

Case A

Mr. D. was a 62-year-old man admitted to the hospital with a history of shortness of breath and marked exercise intolerance. An angiogram showed coronary artery disease, aortic valve disease, and depressed ventricular function. Mr. D. also had a long history of hypertension and diabetes along with chronic obstructive lung disease. In the year prior to his admission he had two episodes that seemed to indicate small strokes; they cleared without residual neurologic effect.

The consulting surgeon discussed with Mr. D. his risk factors (which were multiple) and the significant operative risk. Mr. D., his wife, and the doctor agreed that an operation should take place. Accordingly, Mr. D. underwent replacement of his aortic valve and CABG surgery. A few days after surgery Mr. D. awoke, was able to follow commands, and gave no evidence of neurologic deficit. His pulmonary function was poor, however, and he remained intubated for 5 more days. In the step-down unit, Mr. D. appeared confused and often sleepy. He was taken back to the ICU for aggressive pulmonary care.

The next day Mr. D. became unresponsive with severe respiratory distress while sitting in a chair. He was reintubated and placed on the ventilator. His right side was flaccid; his left side could be moved spontaneously and responded to painful stimuli. He could neither communicate nor move on command. Mr. D. remained ventilator dependent and required a tracheostomy. Nutrition was supplied at first by hyperalimentation and later by tube feeding. Mr. D. spent 3 months in the ICU in this condition. The physicians approached his wife and asked her opinion about resuscitation should Mr. D. arrest and about continuing his intensive care.

Questions

1. Who should be making decisions about Mr. D's care?
2. What are the medical as well as ethical bases for deciding to withhold or withdraw life-sustaining respiratory and nutritional support?
3. If Mr. D. is transferred out of the ICU, what considerations should be discussed in determining an appropriate place for him?
4. Suppose that Mrs. D. tells the physician, "Well, doctor, I just don't know. What would you do if this were your father?" What would be your response?

Case B

Ms. E. is a 36-year-old unmarried accounting executive. She has never had any children and regards her success in financial circles as a very important aspect of her life. On inquiry, she states, "As a woman it's always been hard to compete with the guys." She also tells her physician that "how I look seems to count for a lot." Recently Ms. E. has met a man and is considering marriage. Three weeks ago while showering she discovered via self-examination a 2–3 cm lump in the upper right quadrant of her right breast. Her internist sent her immediately to a consulting surgeon who examined her and initially found no clinical sign of the cancer having spread. A mammogram shows no evidence of lymph node involvement, but the surgeon interprets the data as strongly suggestive of malignancy.

A needle biopsy confirms the cancer. The surgeon has no reason to believe that there has been any spread of the disease, but he does believe that immediate surgical intervention is appropriate. Aware of Ms. E.'s reluctance to have an operation, the surgeon ponders his next step.

Questions

1. Should the surgeon communicate his findings directly to Ms. E., or should he speak first with the internist?
2. If the surgeon and internist concur that a modified radical mastectomy with appropriate reconstruction is the best choice for Ms. E., how should they present this perspective to the patient?
3. If Ms. E. insists that radiation and chemotherapy will be enough for the time being, should the internist and surgeon go along with this conclusion?
4. If Ms. E., after time for reflections, tells the doctors, "I think I'm going to be just fine. I cannot have this surgery or any other treatment. Getting married is my first priority," what should the physicians' response be? Is there any justification for asking the patient for permission to bring in Ms. E.'s husband-to-be?

■ THINK PIECE: MEDICINE/SURGERY ■

The commitment of medicine to new ideas, techniques, and procedures is seemingly invulnerable, and for good reason: The development of antibiotics ushered in an era in which millions of lives that would have been lost have been saved. New surgical techniques and support services have made the replacement of vital organs possible with only *some* risk of rejection of the new heart, kidney, liver, or bone marrow. Suppose that the entire entity—all the elements that compose our makeup—could be charted and understood. Imagine that with enormous and costly effort the genetic basis of our very selves (and the roots of our diseases, disorders, even behaviors) could be mapped out for study and transformation.

The very notion is filled with promise *and* fear! We haul out some chemicals from the laboratory closet and, in no time, we synthesize a functioning gene that is alive. Creating genetic replicas is quite simple. But is it *right*? We know from earlier efforts that possibility often encourages action; *can do* is readily converted into *should do*. At present, the pregnant woman at high risk (due to family history, age, or exposure to toxic substances) of giving birth to a child with severe disorders is given a chance to see, via testing, the genetic material of her fetus and determine if it has Down Syndrome or spina bifida. Guidance for a woman's choice in such a situation is not a simple medical recommendation. Another illustration: Gender selection is now a possibility for every couple contemplating parenthood. Is it *right* to accept a pregnancy only if the potential offspring is the desired sex?

No one will deny the importance of genetic factors in human health. Some disorders, such as cystic fibrosis or Huntington's disease, are caused by a defect in a particular gene. Identifying the gene is a first step, after diagnosis comes the prospect of genetic manipulation and then a cure. Genetic analysis and its byproducts—the development of biotechnological interventions, which include new drug therapies—will surely provide a set of tools for studying the whole range of diseases. Our optimism is real. Should it be guarded?

There are two reasons to doubt the consequences of gene manipulation. One concerns policy. Should we undertake a given project? Does it make economic and human sense? The present effort at mapping the human genome, of identifying and studying the structure of the 100,000 or more genes that "make" us, is an international effort begun in 1987 and destined for completion at the beginning of the twenty-first century. It will cost about 3 billion dollars and use major laboratories across the world. Reasonable scientists have voiced doubt about the possibility of ever completing the work. Others have questioned the allocation of scarce dollars for this enterprise while babies die for lack of prenatal care. All of us can wonder if cancer can be "conquered" soon after we know the genetic structure completely. These kinds of worries are purely utilitarian: Will the consequences justify the effort?

The second reason for wondering is rooted in matters of principle. Many ask, "Are we playing God by acting with such arrogance in attempting to vary the very course of human life?" Others fret about interfering with nature. Human pride has made trouble in the past. Our memory of the eugenics movement is not limited to the Nazi experiments. Will our ability to use biotechnology race far ahead of our capacity to understand the ethical basis of what we are doing?

How far are we likely to go? Will the ability to cure sickle cell anemia and diabetes impel us to fix color blindness and left-handedness? Is the pursuit of genetic knowledge, and its achievement, likely to do harm or to help those who are most vulnerable?

No one can give a firm answer to questions of policy or principle. If a cure or an efficacious treatment for Alzheimer's disease results from the genome project, the applause will be deafening. If the prospect emerges of eliminating, before birth, a prospective off-spring with a just-below-average IQ or with the high probability of being a heavy drinker, responses will be more controversial. Scientists who claim that their research is value-neutral are either badly educated or irresponsibly evasive. Every discovery in genetics has within it the seeds of promise or tragedy. Every scientist in the laboratory, genetics counselor in the clinic, or administrator of biotechnological ventures is a moral agent. The time to ponder the basics, to ask hard questions about the kind of world we want, is now.

■ VOICES: PSYCHIATRIST-CONSULTANT TO ■ MEDICAL/SURGICAL TEAMS

Very frequently I am called on to help surgeons and internists when patients are afraid or are having difficulties making decisions. Surgery can be traumatic, but anticipating it can be overwhelming. I often see in these patients a high level of anxiety; some patients respond by becoming deeply depressed. There are often issues in the doctor-patient relationship: something has gone wrong. When I get called in, it's because some kind of problem exists. Surgeons, for example, rarely get to see the patient prior to hospitalization—this is a reflection of both the specialization of contemporary medicine *and* efforts at cost effectiveness (which give responsibility for preparing patients for surgery to their primary care doctors). The possibilities for miscommunication between surgeons and patients are enormous. If the patient is scared—placing yourself in the hands of another can be terrifying; being dependent often causes a psychological regression among sick people—it's hard to get through.

The fear of death is always there; I encourage patients and physicians to talk about this. Some studies suggest that the capacity of a patient to verbalize feelings about the fear of dying or of being dismembered can *help* patients gain a sense of control as they face surgery. Surgeons are not especially experienced at exploring these feelings. But it's a tradeoff: The ability of surgeons to distance themselves from their patients makes it possible for them to do their very difficult work. Surgeons are supreme technicians. We wouldn't want them to be preoccupied with feelings if that impeded their surgical task.

We see a lot of noncompliant, negative, oppositionist, even abusive patients. They may refuse surgical or medical treatment. A psychiatric consultation may be requested. Is this patient suffering from a major mental illness that is causing such behavior? Often this is the case, and we can treat the illness. Sometimes the patient is not only rational and well, but genuinely, ideologically resistant. That's a real problem. With the patient who is upset or indecisive, we can usually gain compliance by waiting and cajoling. Ambivalence is usually resolved in a short period of time. Surgeons are interested in results. Problem patients are those who do not go along with the system. I get called in when the normally smooth process is interrupted.

The principal ethical issue that arises in my consulting with surgeons and internists involves questions of patient autonomy. Assessing the patient's decision-making capacity—what courts call competence—is a technical challenge for me. I need to understand a great deal, but must make such a determination in a very brief amount of time. Experience certainly helps. Another difficulty arises in assessing a patient who wants to end treatment. For example, the patient who has long been on renal dialysis says "Stop." This patient will surely die if care ceases. Of course, I look for depression first. A profound sense of helplessness or hopelessness *can* be treated. I also believe that there can be a rational choice to end one's life. A person without mental illness who has *had enough* needs to be understood. The thoughtful patient who faces a very low quality of life has the right to die. Staff, however, especially in situations when something *can* be done to keep the patient alive in a modicum of comfort, are often upset by this kind of decision. This flies in the face of the health care professional's sense of omnipotence. These kinds of consultations usually come after the battle lines have been drawn on the ward.

I often ask myself, "Is medicine ageist?" We have come a long way in sensitizing our students and residents in this area, but we have only begun to accommodate the "graying of America." There's still a fair amount of negative attitude toward people at the end of their life cycle. We just don't hear such people. As medical educators we need to get doctors-in-training to the bedside of patients who are not in acute-care hospitals. Most older patients are at home or in a nursing home. We need to see them in their real-life contexts, not only when they have problems that bring them into the hospital for surgery or some other treatment.

RECOMMENDED READING

American College of Physicians, *Ethics Manual*. Philadelphia: American College of Physicians, 1989.

Beauchamp, T. and McCullough, L., *Medical Ethics: The Moral Responsibilities of Physicians*. Englewood Cliffs, NJ: Prentice-Hall, 1984.

Isserson, K., et. al., *Ethics in Emergency Medicine*. Baltimore: Williams and Wilkins, 1986.

Moskop, J. and Kopelman, L., (eds.) *Ethics and Critical Care Medicine*. Netherlands: Dordrecht, Reidel, 1985.

Robertson, J. *The Rights of the Critically Ill*. Cambridge, MA: Ballinger, 1983.

▪7▪
Mind Matters: Ethics and Justice in Psychiatry

Is psychiatry fundamentally different from other medical specialties? Does dealing with the mind, with mental illness, disease, and disorder, mean that this medical speciality is clinically and ethically more problematic? Philosophically, psychiatry has always held great interest. Separating mind from body, interpreting the "possession" of persons by alleged spirits, wondering about the alternative realities experienced by patients with schizophrenia, trying to locate emotions in sections of the brain—these are challenging conceptual issues.

From the perspective of clinical medical ethics, psychiatry presents a substantial set of challenges. No medical specialty has such power to limit the freedom of patients. No other group of practitioners is so closely intertwined with legal constraints and concerns. In addition, psychiatrists are routinely consulted to deal with ethical issues faced by other doctors: "Is this patient refusing treatment because he is depressed?" is a common inquiry for psychiatrists. Psychiatrists work in many settings including acute-care hospitals, community psychiatric facilities, and long-term care facilities, and in private practice. Even those who limit their practice to functional patients deal with issues of freedom and restraint every day.

As consultants, psychiatrists perform tasks that are immensely useful to other clinical specialists. Assessing a candidate for heart, kidney, or liver transplantation; helping family members and, often, hospital staffs deal with the death of a patient; providing a biopsychosocial perspective on the noncompliant patient; and helping nurses, doctors, and administrators evaluate the seriousness of a suicide threat are stimulating and difficult jobs encountered almost routinely by psychiatrists. Each entails value judgments, and all press the psychiatrist to remain a clear-thinking and objective adviser.

The power of psychiatrists is real and considerable. The following contrast is suggestive: When a seriously ill patient disagrees with a physician in deciding about an elective surgery, further discussion is initiated, but when a severely depressed patient disagrees with a psychiatrist who is recommending brief hospitalization for the purpose of diagnostic studies and the patient refuses, significant ethical and legal issues emerge immediately. After all, the "disagree-ing organ," say some psychiatrists, is the "impaired organ." A pa-tient's rejection of recommended treatment might even be evidence of the *need* for such care. The authority of psychiatrists to commit patients, voluntarily and involuntarily is substantial.

For example, when a trained member of a treatment team in the psychiatric emergency service (PES) approaches a potential patient for the first time, two questions emerge: (1) "What is happening with this person?" and (2) "What is the right thing to do for this person?" The answer to the second question is unlikely to be purely medical, for doing the right thing always entails judgments about moral, legal, and sociologic matters. Some of the kinds of judgments psychiatrists frequently make are illustrative:

Determining the "competence" of a patient can influence a claim the police have regarding the criminal responsibility of the person.

Assessing the dangerousness of the patient can determine the short- and long-term liberty of the person.

Evaluating the degree of rationality of the person can control future treatment choices for the patient.

Doing the right thing, often conditional on the availability of scarce resources (e.g., bed space), can be decisive for the patient's future as a client in the mental health and medical care systems. No judgment in a psychiatric emergency is merely medical. Because life and death can hang in the balance, bringing to light the ethical assumptions and moral and legal difficulties found in difficult psychiatric cases is indispensable.

Psychiatric care is controversial. Debates among professionals about how diagnoses are made (are they objective measurements or subjective impressions?) and about the biologic or psychological nature of mental illness itself continue. Clinical questions are often ethical: Should persons be free to entertain deluding ideas if others are not harmed? If services *can* be provided, *should* they? For instance, should homeless persons with histories of mental illness be coerced into treatment centers for their own good? Or should they be allowed to die on the street if that is their conscientious wish?

The powerful tools now used by psychiatrists in treating severely ill patients have had mixed results. Psychoactive drugs are seen as both a blessing, allowing the deinstitutionalization of chronic mental patients *and* by some as nothing more than "chemical straight-jackets." Psychiatrists can serve as surrogates for police authority (e.g., helping to determine who goes to jail and who goes to a mental hospital) as well as family authority (e.g., incarcerating teenagers who are uncooperative at home and in school). Simply dealing with the "insides" of patients (normal or pathologic) entails the examination of values and opens up questions of rights, duties, and, especially, the role of rationality in human interaction.

■ FIVE ESSENTIAL CASES ■

Case 7-1

If a patient announces a desire to take her or his own life, treatment choices must confront issues of autonomy, decisional capacity, and the beneficent, but sometimes paternalistic, desire to save a life.

J.R., a 44-year-old man, enters the PES and tells the second-year psychiatry resident that he has recently lost his job and his wife, and his life is no fun. He says that he has no history of psychiatric illness or care. He seems clearly upset; an examination shows him to be quite agitated. He does not seem to be clinically depressed or psychotic, but he says that he has lots of problems at home. The doctor suggests that J.R. talk briefly with the staff psychiatric social worker, but the patient refuses, saying, "It's you or no one, Doc!" The resident invites J.R. to elaborate his problems.

J.R. reveals that his wife of 20 years has been threatening to leave him and take their two teenage children with her. His appetite is down. He has no close relatives nearby. He has been thinking about suicide. When asked for a reason, he states, "It's either that or I kill her." The doctor recommends a temporary hospitalization to check things out, saying "Just let us get you upstairs for a while. Get some rest and then we can talk about this in more detail. I would hope to have you out of here in a few days." J.R. refuses: "Look," he states, "just give me something so I can get some sleep. I'm not staying here. If you won't help me, I'm getting out of this joint!"

■ ■ ■

There are several immediate dilemmas for the psychiatry resident. Professionals who deal with suicidal patients are potentially liable for all sorts of actions. If a doctor releases a patient who needs intervention, there could be a lawsuit. But restraining a patient and forcing hospitalization could also be the source of a charge against the doctor. Decisions about assessment, confinement, or release, and the involvement of third parties—complicated by legal requirements—are inherently ethical. They center around issues of justice, fairness, compassion, and honesty.

As J.R. heads for the ER door, a clinical-ethical question complements a medical dilemma: What is to be done? The resident in this treatment-refusal situation, an all too common one, might be taken aback at first. An effort might be made to get J.R. to wait. Additional staff would be called; hospital security might be called. The patient would be told that his depression is impairing his judgment, and he would be held, involuntarily, for observation. J.R. might yell about a lawsuit.

At a conference the next day, the case would be discussed. After a factual recapitulation, a series of questions would emerge about the actions taken. Had the resident let him go, remarks such as, "Well, we'll probably see him again over the weekend," or "I hope he has a therapist out there," might follow. Had the resident arranged for J.R. to be held, things would have sounded different. If J.R. had admitted, several hours later, that he had a gun at home, the hospitalization would have been validated. Had J.R., after taking some medication, expressed his gratitude for being held, the involuntary hospitalization would have been justified.

This follow-up discussion—a routine case conference for psychiatry residents—clearly involves underlying ethical questions. Why should a patient give up consent? Who determines his or her best interest? How are projected consequences of hospitalization or release assessed? What justifications can be given for the limitation of autonomy? When a psychiatric judgment must be made in an emergency setting, many ethical difficulties arise:

The patient has virtually no choice in accepting a physician in an emergency.

Sources of data about the patient are often self-reports, at least until confirming data are available.

Anxiety, pain, alcohol or substance use, and altered mental status can impede the accessibility of information.

The capacity of the patient to make informed decisions can be compromised.

The ER staff usually represents the policies and interests of the hospital administration; this can conflict with the interests of patients.

In a potential suicide case (Mr. J.R. has suggested that homicide is on his mind as well), psychiatrists face value questions. Medical values and psychiatric practice suggest that suicide presents one of the rare instances in which most practitioners are in agreement: Suicide is wrong, it must be prevented, it is the ultimate destructive act. Religious and secular commentators—from the Talmud and the Roman Catholic church to the writings of the deontologic thinker Immanuel Kant—sustain this impression. To be "for life" is to abhor self-destruction. Such virtual unanimity demands a careful analysis.

First, the ethical basis of intervention is quite logical: All medical personnel have a moral obligation to help those in pain. Suicide is closely linked to major psychiatric disorders such as depression. Successful suicides are irreversible. Thus, responsible medical personnel must prevent suicide. Second, even for those who do not state that all suicidal behavior is psychopathologic per se, good reasons remain for intervening. If suicide is not evidence of mental illness, it is either a cry for help or a demonstration of patient ambivalence. In any case, it calls for responsible intervention. Whatever the hidden agenda, we must not allow the patient to die. Still, agreement on the rudiments of an ethical response to threatened suicide does not close the discussion. Rather, it opens up other, equally grave, concerns. Suicidal ideation or behavior makes us ponder:

What sorts of promises should be made to suicidal patients?

What are the limits of protection that should be offered to suicidal patients?

Is paternalistic intervention always therapeutic, or does it support
the manipulative patient in unpredictable ways?
Can suicide ever be rational?

If we involuntarily institutionalize suicidal patients for what
is considered their best interests, we claim to help them regain
the freedom lost temporarily to psychiatric disorder, overwhelming stress, or difficult interpersonal relationships. In other words,
should we temporarily limit autonomy to try to establish future
autonomy?

Case 7-2
**The legal obligations of the treating psychiatrist can
complicate patient care. The medical perspective of the
psychiatrist can also have implications for the punishment or
treatment of patients who act violently.**

Louise E. is a 26-year-old woman who lives alone and works as a
salesperson at a large department store, and who has been seeing Dr.
K. for psychotherapy for 7 months on a weekly outpatient basis. She
originally reported feelings of depression. He has reviewed her history
and has evaluated her thoroughly and believes that she is suffering from
a bipolar disorder. With appropriate medications, however, she does
not require hospitalization. Ms. E. complies with the drug regimen and
has never missed an appointment for psychotherapy. Recently, however, she has told Dr. K. about a very disturbing problem. She started
dating a young man, Kevin M., about 5 weeks ago. They seemed to be
getting along just fine but he suddenly stopped calling her. She tried to
reach him, but he never returned messages on his answering machine.
Ms. E. wrote to Mr. M. but received no reply.

Two weeks ago Ms. E. told Dr. K. in a psychotherapy session that she
had been thinking about stabbing Mr. M. The doctor asked her if she
were serious and she replied, "No, not really; I just think about it once in a
while. I can't seem to get over him. It's more than rejection; he just won't
talk to me at all any more." The psychiatrist asked if she had a knife or
other weapon, and she replied in the negative. He then began exploring with her the feelings of anger and grief regarding the termination of
her relationship with Mr. M. Yesterday, Ms. E. was arrested and was
charged with first degree murder. She had allegedly waited for Mr. M.
outside his apartment house. When he approached the building she

ran up behind him and plunged a knife into his back, puncturing his lung. He died before the paramedics arrived. Ms. E. did not leave the scene and was subsequently arrested.

■ ■ ■

Dr. K. is flabbergasted! He faces at least two critical difficulties. First, should he have warned Mr. M. or someone who might have protected him that his patient was pondering murder? Second, if he is called on by the criminal justice system—either by the prosecutor or the defense—to provide information or assistance, what should he do? Dr. K. is involved, and the nature of that involvement remains to be seen.

Confidentiality is one of the oldest and most consistently held doctrines in medical ethics. Based on the safeguarding of privacy, confidentiality is the foundation on which people establish and maintain relationships of intimacy. Psychiatrists have access to personal and secret information about individuals, families, and relationships. Ms. E. told her psychiatrist the details of her life because she knew that he would tell no other person. Confidentiality is the basis of trust in the therapeutic relationship.

Patients expect privacy in health care, and institutions and professional organizations have policies designed to protect such information. Disclosure of clinical information requires informing patients and getting their consent. Third parties are given information only after patients have permitted such disclosure. But Dr. K. did not even ask his patient about warning Mr. M.

Patients routinely make statements in psychotherapy about killing people. Should every such threat be divulged? The exception to the general rule of confidentiality centers around the possibility of dangerousness to others. The unpredictability of such dangerousness, however, makes the premature revelation of private information a touchy ethical problem. In psychiatric circles the well-publicized Tarasoff case has instigated the radical rethinking of patient confidentiality as a moral absolute in psychiatry. That influential case involved the threat of murder spoken in confidence to a health center therapist by a young patient, Prosenjit Poddar, at the University of California, Berkeley. Mr. Poddar ultimately killed Ms. Tarasoff. Her parents sued, and the judgment stated that there is a *duty* on the part of psychotherapists to warn designated third parties if serious bodily harm appears to be imminent.

(Tarasoff v. Regents of the University of California, 188 Cal Rptr 129, 529 P2d 533, 1974).

As a result of this ruling, psychiatrists and other therapists must now concern themselves with threats to designated third parties and they must, on occasion, breach promises of secrecy. Psychiatrists clearly have moral obligations to nonpatients. Preserving life—a clear state interest and also a moral maxim in medicine—can require a Tarasoff warning. Courts have required psychiatrists to take "reasonably necessary" steps to protect nonpatients from serious violence. Does such a public policy demand that the privacy of an individual patient be sacrificed if a solid "hunch" makes it evident that some other designated person(s) may be in substantial danger? In the aftermath of the murder, Dr. K. surely wishes that he had made at least a gesture of warning the victim. But could he have known that there was going to be a murder? It is not easy to assess the magnitude of a potential harm or its imminence. Psychiatrists must balance the probability of an occurrence with potential damage to the threatening patient.

There are other complications. Should a psychiatrist tell a potential patient about her duty to warn? Should police authorities have advance warnings about possibly violent patients? Can psychotherapy proceed in an atmosphere of suspicion? The Tarasoff requirements are presumably based on social utility: We want fewer murders and we oblige psychiatrists to act, in effect, as surrogates for the police power of the state. But what principles can be violated as a result of this apparently positive social goal? Had Ms. E. made her revelations to Dr. K. and *not* gone on to kill the victim, would our view of the case be significantly different?

Still, the murder did take place. Ms. E. *may* be tried for homicide. If she is unable to understand the charges against her and cannot assist her attorney in preparing a defense, she may be found incompetent to stand trial (by a court). Let us assume that she is presently competent to be charged and tried. She will have several psychiatric examinations prior to appearing in court for the trial. Given her history, which is likely to be revealed by her attorney, both defense and prosecuting lawyers will want her examined. The records of Dr. K.

Table 7-1. Categorizing behavior as moral (bad) or medical (mad).

Bad	Mad
Moral evaluation	Medical evaluation
Legal attention	Psychiatric attention
Value-laden judgment	Value-neutral judgment
Opinion	Empirical observation
Punishment	Treatment
Retribution	Understanding
Perpetrator's choice	Patient's compulsion
Imprisonment	Hospitalization
Police supervision	Psychiatric care
Responsible	Not responsible

may be subpoenaed. Eventually, Dr. K. may be called as a witness. How this doctor conceptualizes the motives and behaviors of his former patient will entail matters of both clinical and moral judgment to decide whether Ms. E. is bad or mad. How we categorize a behavior, either in moral (bad) or in medical terminology (mad), has dramatic consequences for the ways in which we diagnose, assess, treat, or punish persons whose behavior has been aberrant (Table 7-1).

Only individuals who intend to commit criminal acts are held responsible by law for those acts. The insanity defense is rooted in the value of just deserts: Only people who deserve punishment should receive it. The measurement of mental illness and the degree of impairment of mental functioning necessary to demonstrate nonculpability are highly controversial. Expert witnesses usually appear on prosecution and defense sides in a trial where the insanity defense is evoked. What will the role of Dr. K. be if this case comes to trial? The conflict between fidelity to one's patient and devotion to the goals of societal safety is manifest. The normal premises—that humans are free and capable of rational choices—inherent in punishing socially unacceptable behaviors are not necessarily those of psychiatry. If Dr. K. has to publicly evaluate the disease process of his patient—and he will have to do so if confidentiality is waived when an insanity defense is raised—he will have to speak in a language unique to psychiatry. It is difficult to know if his words will be understood by a jury. But it is probable that the psychiatrist will feel torn by the conflicting obligations of trying to help his patient and attempting to see that justice is served.

Case 7-3

Getting the best results is a fundamental and utilitarian goal in clinical medicine. Psychiatrists can attempt to predict future behavior for patients who require a dramatic and expensive intervention such as a new heart or liver. In doing so elements of social and moral judgment inevitably arise.

Forty nine years old and the father of six children, Mr. A. is currently on welfare. He had his first heart attack 8 years ago and sustained another 3 years later. He has been unable to work since the first incident. Mr. A. claims to have lost his sexual function after the initial heart attack, but his wife says that this problem began earlier. Mr. A. has often been depressed during the past 8 years. He admits to having occasional suicidal thoughts. "What do I have to live for?" he has said. He was told to give up alcohol after the first heart attack, but he has continued to drink about a six-pack of beer each day.

Mr. A. has been married for 31 years. He has spoken of having hit his wife about four times during the marriage; on each occasion he was drunk. Mr. A.'s children live in the same small city as their parents. They visit frequently, in part because they do not know how long their father will live. When one of the daughters heard about a heart transplantation program at a major medical center 50 miles away, she convinced Mr. A. to try to get one. He asked his primary care doctor to contact the university-based hospital directly, and was scheduled for a thorough physical and psychological workup to see if he is a viable candidate for cardiac transplantation.

Mr. A.'s physical condition is quite suitable for transplant. He is neither too sick (his major organ systems other than his heart are working) nor too well (without the transplant he may die within 6 months or so). The psychiatrist-evaluator, however, reports to the transplant committee (an interdisciplinary group that will determine whether or not Mr. A. will make the list of potential recipients) that the patient is currently suffering from a major depression and anxiety disorder. The evaluation states that the patient has a long history of alcoholism, with frequent overdoses. His marital and family situation has not been very stable. He will likely have difficulty complying with postsurgical requirements of careful drug therapy, frequent clinic visits for examinations and biopsies, and gradual reintegration into vocational and social life. The committee takes the psychiatrist's findings under advisement.

■ ■ ■

Patients who wish to be candidates for transplantation are routinely assessed by a psychiatric team: Such evaluations include the patient's mental status, psychological and family history, and attitude toward surgery and recovery. Both informal interviews and the completion of projective instruments are utilized. A new heart is a rare commodity. Several thousand donor hearts become available each year — usually the result of the whole brain death of young males who sustain head trauma in auto and motorcycle accidents. About 20,000 persons between the ages of 10 and 54 are potential recipients, suffering conditions for which heart transplantation is indicated. Selecting the appropriate candidate is a challenging job. Is it a value-neutral task?

Mr. A. is an apt candidate, medically speaking: The usual criteria are age under 55 years and the absence of severe pulmonary hypertension, severe or irreversible liver or kidney dysfunction, systemic infection or unresolved pulmonary infarction, or diabetes mellitus. He has met these requirements. But psychiatric illness and the supposed absence of family support have clear medical consequences. If Mr. A. misses a follow-up appointment or fails, even for one day, to take his immunosuppressive drugs, he can die. On the other hand, faithful compliance after surviving the transplant surgery leads to a 1-year survival rate of more than 75 percent.

Many heart transplant teams exclude patients with mental and emotional problems. They reject active drug addicts (including alcohol), persons with mental retardation, schizophrenia, and severely hostile or uncooperative behavior. Common psychiatric diagnoses for rejected patients include depression, antisocial personality disorder, borderline intellect, and paranoid disorder manifested in noncompliance. Psychiatrists realize, of course, that patients can change. Were Mr. A. to "see the light" and abstain from alcohol, would the evaluation of his candidacy alter?

If Mr. A. does not make the list, one thing is certain: He will not survive for long. About 90 percent of such patients die within 3 months. Of course, placing Mr. A. on the list of possible recipients could mean death as well: Many persons enrolled in a transplant program die waiting for a compatible heart.

A variety of ethical and scientific questions can be asked of Mr. A.'s psychiatrist-evaluator. How valid are assessments of antisocial behavior and psychiatric illness or projections of future noncompliance? (It is very difficult to measure the behaviors of patients rejected from programs: They die too soon.) Are patients with a history of mental illness at greater risk for medical complications? If we eliminate Mr. A. from the list because of a mood disturbance (depression), should we do so prior to trying to treat that problem (e.g., with anti-depressant medications)? We do know that psychiatrists are not very good at predicting such future behaviors as violent activity, criminal behavior, or even regression into alcohol abuse.

We should also inquire why family and social support is so important for cardiac patients and should this be so. Certainly psychosocial stability and a supportive milieu can provide Mr. A. with some of the resources he will need to recover successfully. We also know that lifestyle problems such as alcohol abuse correlate with family instability. But are our assumptions clear or are they responses to a fundamentally white, middle-class value system? Is only the traditional, stable family morally acceptable? In the absence of a strong family structure, should we deny medical resources as a rule? The very words of the psychiatrist-evaluator suggest that the criterion of social worth has been smuggled into the process of determining the candidacy. Should we decry this evaluative perspective, or should we welcome it as a way of trying to provide hearts only to those persons who will profit from transplantation *and* who deserve a chance for a longer life?

Case 7-4

The psychiatrist who consults on medical cases involving the refusal of treatment faces ethical dilemmas in assessing the decisional capacity of patients. Fidelity to fundamental principles is always difficult in life or death determinations.

Mr. B., a 78-year-old married man, has had diabetes for many years. Kidney damage secondary to his diabetes has resulted in chronic renal failure. For the past 3 years he has been on hemodialysis; he has lived at home and has been transported by ambulance three times each week to an outpatient center. Three months ago he had a below-the-knee amputation caused by diabetic angiopathy. His experience with dialysis has been very unpleasant: He experiences severe nausea after dialysis and has had grand mal seizures. He has, in the past, said that he was "tired of all this" but persisted with the treatment for the sake of his two children and five grandchildren. Two weeks ago Mr. B. told his wife of 52 years that he had decided to discontinue dialysis. He had never been markedly depressed or despondent before, and his wife was unable to relate this change to any specific event or situation. Mrs. B. informed Dr. T. (Mr. B.'s internist, who had long managed the care of the patient) about the situation. He recommended that Mr. B. be hospitalized briefly in a geropsychiatric unit for the purpose of assessment. Mr. B. refused.

The family gathered with Mr. B. present to discuss his decision to stop dialysis. Mrs. B. and her children wondered if Mr. B. knew exactly what he was doing. With the support of Dr. T. the patient was admitted to a geropsychiatric unit involuntarily, on the grounds that he was a suicide risk. He did not receive dialysis for 2 days while being observed; his electrolytes and blood cell parameters were abnormal. When interviewed by the psychiatric resident he stated, "Why are you asking me these questions? It's already been decided." He did say, after being asked several times about his reasons for refusing kidney treatment, that he was weary of prolonged existence and, especially, of "depending on the machine." The attending psychiatrist, Dr. K., was called in to help determine whether Mr. B. had the decisional capacity to refuse life-saving treatment.

Hemodialysis keeps many patients with chronic renal failure alive. The quality of such a life varies substantially—some patients can lead almost full and active daily lives; others are forced into dependency with only limited autonomy. Mr. B. is in the latter condition. End-stage kidney patients are very ill: They suffer from weakness, nausea, and many other medical complications. They do not get better; rather, they are continuously sick. Spending 6 to 8 hours per treatment, three times each week (whether on an inpatient or outpatient basis) is burdensome at best. Mr. B. knows what dialysis entails. It is also evident that most dialysis patients also become depressed and despondent at times. Some demonstrate signs of delirium. Dr. K. has an enormous responsibility: Her consultation will, in effect, determine whether or not Mr. B. can stop the care that is keeping him alive.

Psychiatrists tend to treat patients, especially those who say that they want to die, with care and caution in the belief that a decision should be made for the good of that patient. To benefit a patient, especially one who is temporarily incapacitated, seems right in itself. It may well be, but this approach must be called by its proper name: paternalism. Mr. B.'s refusal of treatment will surely upset those who love him and, most likely, those who have provided kidney care for him for a long time. An almost instinctive impetus toward paternalism can result in resistance to the patient's expressed desires, limitations on patient liberty, if only temporarily, compromise of a potential therapeutic alliance, and potential legal complications.

At stake for the patient is his autonomy. To be autonomous is to be self legislating, at a minimum to be able to look at evidence, weigh it, and make a judgment. Is autonomy possible for a person like Mr. B. who is very sick, whose body is very weak, and who might be suffering from a compromised mental status? In the conflict between autonomy and paternalism, we see questions about the notion of mental disease and the ethical ambiguities that arise from it. If psychiatrists and other professionals could make completely reliable distinctions between so-called normal and allegedly psychotic people there would be little worry. The difficulties in differentiating potential mental patients from idiosyncratic "normal" people are substantial—predictions are inexact, and the liberty of coerced parties is at issue.

Whose needs are at stake in this controversy? Do the desires of the professionals, such as Dr. T., the internist, or of the hospital administration (which does not want a lawsuit if a patient is allowed to refuse treatment when incompetent) supersede the needs of the individual patient? Are institutional concerns paramount? Should they be tempered by fidelity to the rights of the patient and his or her claim to liberty? Placing Mr. B. in the geropsychiatric unit is itself controversial; it assumes (at least temporarily) that refusing kidney care is tantamount to suicide. Still, it does provide Dr. K. with an opportunity to assess the patient's decision-making capacity. Many issues need to be dealt with rapidly: Is Mr. K. certain or is he ambivalent? Is he acting sacrificially because he wishes to spare his family terrible suffering? Could he be clinically depressed—not in his "right mind?" Would it be useful to force him to continue dialysis treatment while receiving psychiatric treatment? Should we limit Mr. B.'s short-term autonomy in the name of some long-term goal? At a minimum Dr. K. has to find answers to the following questions:

Can the patient make a voluntary, deliberate choice?
Does the decision reflect the patient's past or present values?

Does the patient understand the consequences of either accepting or refusing recommended interventions?

A final complication could be added to this case, one found in many kidney dialysis refusal situations. Suppose Mr. B. suffers a seizure and does not recover cognitive functioning? His family, perhaps with the support of the consulting psychiatrist, will likely be the decision-makers: To cease or continue treatment will be the main concern. Mr. B.'s last expressions on the matter could be taken as his final word, but families often differ in judgments, especially in life or death situations. The psychiatrist—whose original task was a competency assessment—may be thrust into the role of mediator or negotiator in a family dispute about continuing or ceasing life-sustaining treatment.

Case 7-5

Patients may have to be coerced, presumably because they cannot act in their own best interests. Involuntary civil commitment, a legal construct, presents problems for psychiatrists, as does the occasional need to seclude and restrain hospitalized patients.

R.N. is 23 years old, mildly mentally retarded and capable of independent living, with a criminal record (three arrests, no convictions) for insulting verbal outbursts on the city's streets. His verbal skills are minimal. He can answer questions if they are posed slowly. He has been diagnosed as having schizophrenia, treated briefly, and given psychotropic medications. These drugs work: When R.N. takes his pills he does not behave violently. He is seen weekly at a community mental health center by a counselor. Monthly he meets with a psychiatrist there who regulates his medications and offers support. R.N. is supported by public funds (he is disabled and gets Social Security disability payments) and does not have a job.

On a Saturday evening, R.N. approached a teenaged woman on F Street. He asked her, "Do you want to go to a party with me?" She turned away and R.N. attempted to grab her by the hand so as to turn her face toward him. The young woman retreated (R.N. did not touch her) and screamed; the police came, and R.N. was handcuffed and taken away. The police officer noted the smell of alcohol on R.N.'s clothing. From a holding cell in the local station, he was taken to the court psychiatric clinic. An initial screening suggests that R.N. is hallucinating. The police agree that he should not be formally arrested at this time.

Instead, R.N. is brought to the L. Hospital's PES where he is evaluated by a psychiatry resident. He is screaming incoherently and struggling against his handcuffs. He is found to be decompensating and admits to having stopped taking his medications 3 days ago. R.N. is admitted involuntarily to the psychiatry ward for 3 days—the statutorily permitted time prior to a hearing on whether or not he should be committed for treatment. The grounds for this emergency hospitalization are that R.N. is dangerous to others. The psychiatrists also feel that he is in need of treatment and will recover his previous level of function. He is given a major tranquilizer by injection and taken to the psych unit.

The next morning, R.N. awakens in a somewhat drowsy manner. A doctor at his bedside asks him if he knows where he is. He says, "No!" When he sees a female nurse approach him in an effort to give him some medication, his hands flail forward. He strikes her on the cheek with his hand, his nails penetrate her skin, and she bleeds profusely. Hospital security is called and R.N., cowering in a corner, resists verbal efforts to calm him. He is maced, physically carried into a seclusion room, and put onto a hospital cot where he is tied down with leather restraints.

R.N. is hospitalized against his will. (He could have been sent to jail.) He is also restrained in the therapeutic setting and secluded from others. His freedom is manifestly diminished. The value bases for such actions are the need to protect society from antisocial behavior, the desire to help a man who seems unable to care for himself, and the necessity of guarding the therapeutic milieu—wherein many patients and staff reside—from severe disturbances. The assumption that R.N.'s dangerousness must, at least temporarily, be controlled is fundamental.

The empirical evaluation of dangerousness—itself a subject of methodologic conflict professionally—presumes predictive value. Holding a patient is more than a statistical activity, however, it symbolizes a moral claim: A patient involuntarily hospitalized in the mental health system is either nonautonomous or lacks significant decisional capacity. We are not worried about R.N.'s consenting to or refusing treatment. Other things are more important at the moment.

We can readily admit that the impediments to gaining consent from psychotic patients are considerable; those who can neither understand nor speak must have surrogates make their decisions. By law and practice, all patients being offered treatment, medication, or procedures must be told the nature of their condition, disease, disorder, or problem. The nature and purpose of the proposed treatment must be given in language that can be commonly under-stood. The risks and consequences of the proposed treatment, and any feasible alternatives to the treatment, must be stated. The patient's prognosis if the proposed treatment is not given must be described.

Can psychiatric patients in crisis grant a truly informed con-sent? Problems abound for those patients whose competence is in doubt. For patients demonstrably psychotic—deemed dangerous to others as R.N. is—the emergency exception to the requirement of informed consent applies. But for how long? R.N. has been in the hospital overnight. Ironically, he may have been given medication the night before that might impede his understanding of the clinical situation.

Decisions must be made swiftly in situations that entail violence or its threat; there is less time to establish the relationship necessary to discuss the content of proposed treatments, with time allowed for questions and responses, in the detail that might be possible in outpatient settings. R.N., restrained on the street by the police, might have been suffering debilitating delusions. Assuming that to be the case, who should be making decisions about his freedom? The ethical conflict in finding grounds for such a determination pits a desire to affirm autonomy against a need to act beneficently in the patient's interest. Society also demands justice.

Involuntary civil commitment, procedures for which vary from jurisdiction to jurisdiction, is always an alternative. Its rationale both medically and ethically is paternalistic: to protect the patient who cannot exercise decision-making power. Other grounds for such commitment also vary, but include demonstrable dangerousness to self or others, the inability to care for oneself (though care is not always defined concretely), dangerousness to property, and the controversial notion of "in need of treatment." There is considerable doubt about the consistency with which civil commitment stan-dards are applied in psychiatric emergencies. Because emergency settings prevent the fullest development of data and perspective, the likelihood of erring on the side of incarceration is considerable.

Several questions with ethical content should be posed during such situations:

Is the refusal of offered treatment seen as a major reason for attempting to commit the patient?

What weight should be placed on temporary factors (e.g., alcohol use, drug abuse) in the assessment that might lead to alternative discussions about the patient's capacity to be left at liberty?

What other interests (e.g., family, societal) are at stake in the commitment decision?

What are the likely effects of involuntary commitment (e.g., further psychotic decompensation)?

R.N.'s mental retardation is an apparent factor in this case. Does this label suggest that he will receive unfair treatment? Does his history of mental illness (he would be considered a dual diagnosis patient) and his use of psychotropic medications render him more vulnerable to a paternalistic or coercive response? For years, courts have held that mental patients do not automatically lose their rights when involuntarily committed: They may still refuse treatment, including drugs and electroconvulsive therapies. But when a patient like R.N. seems to be acting in a violent or threatening manner, courts and practitioners usually justify coercive intervention on grounds of safety and therapeutic efficacy for others.

R.N. is maced, secluded, and restrained. The medical justification for the seclusion is that an out-of-control patient needs to be contained and isolated; time out from external stimulation usually provides a calming effect. This beneficent argument states that the patient who is, or is potentially, assaultive needs temporary isolation for his or her best interest. Restraint is similarly justified on the grounds that preventing the patient from harming self or others to avoid subsequent arrest or punishment, or at least self-recrimination, is therapeutically necessary.

Neither seclusion nor restraint are to be meted out as punishments. That is the standard policy. It is often difficult, however, to distinguish disruptive from dangerous behavior. Staff members are often assaulted by patients, and a climate of fear is not unknown on units like R.N.'s. When patients are physically restrained in the name of aid and comfort, it is possible that other values are implicit, including the rights of staff members to work in an environment in which they are not harmed or even killed.

■ PRACTICE MODEL CASE ■

Lou G. is 37 years old. Eighteen months ago he was diagnosed as having amytrophic lateral sclerosis (ALS). He is not hospitalized. The disease has progressed to the point where he can no longer walk (he can sit and is mobile via wheelchair). He needs assistance with everyday activities such as feeding and personal hygiene. At the moment he has no serious respiratory problems: He can speak and swallow. Mr. G. lives at home with his wife of 6 years. They have no children or religious affiliation. No relatives live within 500 miles.

Prior to being stricken with ALS Mr. G., a college graduate, was a fashion model in this large midwestern city. He was also quite athletic and enjoyed competitive sports. He was self-employed for 3 years prior to becoming ill. Mrs. G. is also a successful fashion model; the couple met on a collaborative project. She is still modeling and is the sole source of their income. They pay for health insurance from their own funds.

Mr. G. has been the patient of Dr. I., an internist who has been managing the case. She has sent Mr. G. for a variety of tests, consulted with neurologists regarding the progress of the disease, and met with Mr. and Mrs. G. many times in her office. The G.'s are aware of the nature of ALS and know that few patients live more than 5 years after onset. They are also knowledgeable about the unpredictable, yet certain, degeneration during the course of the disease.

Recently, Mrs. G. has confided in her husband that she is scared and depressed. Her combined responsibilities as breadwinner and as principal physical and emotional support for Mr. G. are draining her. The G.s are suffering financially—their insurance premiums are very expensive and their income is falling rapidly—and they do not have any close friends. After a lengthy discussion with his wife, Mr. G. evaluates his life and future, and decides that he will commit suicide very soon. He states, "It's not crazy for me to end it while I still can." His wife supports his decision.

At their next meeting with the internist, they tell Dr. I. of their common resolve. The physician is taken aback. She suggests that the couple meet at least once with a psychiatrist, Dr. P., who is experienced in dealing with terminal illness. Mr. and Mrs. G. reluctantly agree to go to the conference. They remain firmly convinced that suicide is not only appropriate but the right thing to do.

Patient

Lou G. is suffering from a disease that is always fatal. ALS is a progressive, degenerative motor neuron disease that usually strikes males over the age of 40. The motor cells in the spinal cord, lower brainstem, and cortex degenerate and are replaced by a fibrous tissue. Surviving cells atrophy. There is no treatment for ALS and death occurs within 2 to 6 years of onset. The course of the disease is not predictable, but most often loss of dexterity and fine motor movement is followed by wasting of hand, forearm, and leg muscles. Lou G. is presently experiencing this level of impairment. Further progression is hard to predict, but eventually he will experience damage to the respiratory system. He will lose his ability to speak, though not to think, as a result of paralysis.

ALS is characterized by psychological as well as physical disability. Lou G. knows what his future entails. He also carries with him daily reminders of his past levels of functioning. We may assume that as a former fashion model appearance is important to Lou. Whether or not Lou is clinically depressed is a factor to be investigated. But beyond such a psychological response to his disease state, he has become almost totally dependent on his wife. Though Mrs. G. may not be the patient in this case, her involvement is integral and significant. Lou has told her about his desire to die, and she has agreed with his plan.

If Lou G. does not commit suicide, his next few years will be characterized by total physical immobility, loss of muscle tone and wasting, impaired circulation, and possible ventilator dependency. Among the complications found in patients with ALS are decubitus ulcers, edema, and congestive heart failure. Understanding the future that both Mr. and Mrs. G. face is a requirement for both the internist and the consulting psychiatrist in this case.

Relationships

One difficulty in this case derives from the paucity of relationships available to Lou G. With the sole and important exception of his wife, Lou has no close friends. He has no children and is not in contact with his family. Therefore, the nature of his relationship with Mrs. G. is significant. However bonded or distant they may be, their marriage is the principal focus of their social lives. The pressures on both of them need to be understood empathically. Mrs. G. certainly did not expect to be a caregiver for a husband with a short life expectancy. And Mr. G.'s dependency, which will increase, is central to his connection to his spouse. The psychiatrist they have agreed to consult needs to know a good deal; not just about the G.s' physical and mental status, feelings, and needs right now, but about their history together. Only 1½ years ago they were active, fully employed, and planning a life together. Now one faces certain death.

Also absent in this situation are institutional supports for the G.s. They do not belong to religious or secular organizations. Like many urban professionals they are not rooted in a neighborhood or an ethnic subculture. Mr. G. does not have an employer and colleagues. This is a family very much alone in the world. The recognition of this fact may play a role in their common determination to see Lou G.'s life end sooner rather than later. At the moment, Mr. and Mrs. G. have medical relationships with Drs. I. and P. It is fair to state that the content of those connections go beyond the norm of conventional health care issues.

Advocacy

Lou G.'s primary care physician has a moral obligation to care for his patient and to look out for his rights. This duty derives from the physician's fundamental obligation to prevent harm to a patient and, if possible, to do good as well. Does the imperative to pursue nonmaleficence and beneficence mean that Dr. I. is Lou's advocate? She is the gate-keeper: She sends Lou out for consultations, including the initial discussion planned with the psychiatrist. But is she obliged to do more? Should she be helping Lou to end his life or should she be informing appropriate authorities about such plans? Dr. I. is likely to defer such a decision until after Mr. and Mrs. G. see Dr. P.

The psychiatrist, Dr. P., is about to assume an extraordinary responsibility. Her involvement with Lou G. and his spouse will depend on her perception of the doctor's role as patient advocate. Advocacy has both neutral and value-laden connotations. An advocate who acts as a faithful spokesperson for a patient who temporarily lacks a voice behaves properly by accurately conveying the patient's perspective. The advocate works as a substitute autonomist. But a physician, in a dangerous situation involving suicidal ideation, might see advocacy as the adoption of a critical stance that, paradoxically, could result in the psychiatrist's advocating a position that opposes the patient's expressed wishes. Dr. P.—thinking that Lou G. is reacting emotionally though nonpsychotically to the fear of dying dependent and debilitated—might press the patient and his wife for a contract in which they promise to try several months of psychotherapy and counseling. In an effort to get to the "true self," Dr. P. may overtly or subtly cajole the patient in the name of advocacy.

Conflicts

There are both internal and external conflicts evident in this case. Lou G. *seems* to have resolved the problem of his future by announcing his intention to end his own life. We shouldn't take his words as definitive or final, however; instead they are invitations to further explore Lou's mind-set, his sense of potential pain and suffering, and his ethical principles. Externally, Lou has set out on an apparent course of suicide by immediately (and necessarily, given his condition) involving others. Mrs. G. states her support for his decision, but we must discover the process by which she has come to such an agreement. Are there unstated assumptions: Does Lou's fear of dependency result from the rejection of his wife? Or does her fatigue—rooted in concern and the anticipation of his loss—lead him to want to end things soon? How are they communicating now that the matter has been made public, at least to the physicians? Within the G. family, conflicts might be localized, but they still remain.

In the broader context, difficulties abound. It is not against the law in most jurisdictions to commit suicide (such decriminalization is a phenomenon of post-World War II American state legislation). But in virtually every state it *is* against the law, with severe penalties, to assist another person in committing suicide. Mrs. G. might be asked to help: Lou may be able to swallow, but he cannot reach the medications or pour the water needed to ingest the pills. Notice that Mr. G. is not asking that treatment cease or that treatment not be initiated later. He wants to take an active role in ending his life.

There might be an ethical conflict for the psychiatrist and the internist as well. Suppose Lou G. asks for assistance from these physicians. Such a request could take many forms; an inquiry about the lethality of certain drugs or drug interactions is possible. Lou can also press for physician-assisted suicide. To state that the Hippocratic Oath prohibits such activities is to beg the question (see Appendix A). Physicians around the world help patients die by active means; rarely are such acts brought to light.

Treatment or Nontreatment Options

First, we must examine the approach Dr. P. wants to take with the G.s. She should check for the presence of severe depression, including psychotic depression. But Lou's psychiatric symptoms—his feelings of helplessness and his loss of self-worth—are not rooted in hallucination or fantasy. He wants to die because he is in pain and anticipates more. Many psychiatrists conceptualize suicidal ideation as based on one or more of three things: (1) a cry for help or support; (2) a result of mental illness, usually depression; or (3) evidence of great ambivalence about one's life and prospects. Could Lou's desire to die originate outside these traditional realms? Could he be rational, autonomous, resolved, even justified in wanting to die prior to his total and likely painful physical dependency? Dr. P. will certainly want to rule out depression which is reactive to the diagnosis of ALS. She will want to contract with Lou G. for some further meetings so that the true issues can be discussed. If a reversible depression is diagnosed, the option to treat it will be offered (at first by pharmacologic means). If it is determined that Mr. G. is both psychologically well, mentally competent, and morally consistent, Dr. P. can still suggest supportive psychotherapy (a nonchemical intervention) for the couple. How long should such a contract last?

There is no medical treatment for ALS that can promise any significant results. It is true that physical therapy can, for a short time, halt the deterioration of muscle functioning. But Lou G.'s course is part of an irreversible trajectory. Interventions are possible. Placing Lou G. on a ventilator when he can no longer breathe himself will extend his corporeal life, but it will not restore any useful function to him; nor will he ever be weaned from the machine. If Lou G. has a living will or durable power of attorney designation, he can ensure that no such device is used against his will. But this is mere projection: Lou never wants to get near the time when such interventions are necessary.

Interests

Does Mr. G. have an interest in dying? To put the matter bluntly: Is he better off dead? This seems to be his point of view. If so, what are his present interests? Being free of pain is surely one. Being free of anxiety about total dependence might be another. The extent to which this interest is the result of a well thought out reflection on his disease is something Dr. P. needs to explore. She will want to ask Lou to separate—for the purposes of analysis—his long- and short-term needs.

Mrs. G. has interests as well. Though the cynical might think that her support for Lou's suicidal desires is illicit, we cannot make such a statement without evidence. On the contrary, she may have an interest in seeing her husband released from the bonds of disease. She might have a complementary interest in getting on with her life: She is surely grieving for Lou already.

The physicians have serious interests as well. One is in not being implicated in a suicide pact that could become a subject of public scrutiny. For a psychiatrist, the suicide of a patient almost always precipitates traumatic self-doubt about one's skills and one's values. Dr. P. has an interest in making sure that Lou G.'s desire to die is rational and that, if agreement that is appropriate and ethical can be reached, it be done without a physician's help.

Consequences

The notion of anticipating, or even measuring, the consequences of making a hard-choice clinical determination can seem almost value-neutral. If we ask what the best balance of good over bad is, or happiness over misery, we may want to try moral mathematics. But consequences for Lou G. are not cold or hypothetical matters. Suppose that Lou is cajoled or coerced into accepting the idea that suicide is a bad idea, because such an act would set an awful precedent for society. Even were Lou to agree, he will be the person ventilator dependent. Any balancing act has as its focus the body and mind of this patient.

In the short-run, Lou could stay alive in a dependent and increasingly vulnerable status. We can't know what this will mean for Mrs. G. But certainly Dr. P. will want to suggest a range of community resources—including volunteers who can sit with Mr. G. as well as provide respite care for his wife. Still, such strategies are only temporarily useful. Mr. G., if he does not die soon, will have to be taken to a long-term care facility or to a hospital for extended treatment.

From the psychiatrist's perspective, though the death of a patient by his own hand may seem a defeat, the long-term results could be otherwise. Helping a patient understand his plight and face the inevitable with a modicum of dignity and self-respect can strengthen the therapist and, indirectly, help other patients too. A final concern about consequences for the doctors is this: What aid should be offered to Mrs. G. in the days or months after the death of Lou? Is grief and bereavement a medical or psychological service that physicians know how to provide? Should they be there for the long haul with survivors of either suicide or death resulting from terminal illness?

Ethical Principles

If Lou G. has decision-making capacity, and if his determination to die soon is based on a rational conviction (and not on either a resolvable relational issue or a terror that can be assuaged through the help of others), then his autonomous choice will, perhaps reluctantly, have to be respected. Lou is an adult and his illness is surely fatal; he has seen its beginnings and has a firm understanding of its endings. There is a paradox, however: Lou G. gets to assert his autonomy by ending it forever.

The physicians' principles of beneficence and nonmaleficence (see section on Advocacy) suggest that the doctors in this case might have to act as Mr. G.'s advocate. But the duty to protect his interests could go a step further. Should Dr. P. and Dr. I., if they see Lou's ending his life right now as a good thing, encourage him to end his life? How far does the principle of veracity demand that a doctor speak words deemed controversial and certainly nontraditional by colleagues and the public. If the physicians think Lou is right and if they keep such sentiments to themselves, aren't they acting hypocritically and, perhaps worse, aren't they harming their patient by isolating him in a time of enormous need?

The principle of justice asks us to confront the allocation of scarce health care resources. Should all patients with ALS get every possible life-sustaining medical therapy? Should hospital beds, and eventually intensive care unit space, be dedicated to patients like Mr. G. who cannot benefit by their use for long? In this case, affirming Mr. G.'s autonomy will release us from having to worry about his utilization of money, professional time, and insurance reimbursements. But are we putting a price on Lou G.'s life when we say that his desire to die is a just decision?

■ CASES FOR DISCUSSION ■

Case A

D.J. is a 25-year-old man, employed as a salesperson, with manic-depressive illness that has reached psychotic proportions on occasion. He has never been hospitalized. The mania is characterized by pressured speech, expansive and euphoric mood, grandiosity, remarkable physical energy, and sleeplessness. This bipolar disorder, however, has lengthy periods of remission and during that time the patient has told his psychiatrist that, if there is a recurrence, she should do everything possible to treat him, even if at the time he refuses medications or hospitalization.

When, a few months later, Mr. J. moves from a normal state toward a manic, psychotic episode, he begins to spend large sums of money, curse loudly in public, and act inappropriately in his interpersonal relationships. He still goes to work every day. His family, discovering that he has stopped taking his maintenance medication, attempts to talk him into seeing the psychiatrist. Mr. J. says "Absolutely not! There's nothing wrong with me!" Mr. J.'s mother calls the psychiatrist. The doctor's impression, based on the telephone conversation, is that the patient does not represent a danger to himself or to others; nor is he unable to meet his basic needs. Thus he does not meet the legal standard for involuntary institutionalization.

Questions
1. What consideration should be given to Mr. J.'s initial statement to the psychiatrist regarding care if there is a recurrence of the mania?
2. What fundamental ethical principle could the psychiatrist cite were she to move toward intervening with this patient on the request of his family?
3. Does Mr. J.'s earlier statement to the doctor hold in this situation? If so, why?
4. If the psychiatrist tells the family to try to take Mr. J. to the emergency room's psychiatry service, has she exercised her duty to this patient in an ethically satisfactory manner?

Case B

Dr. C. has been in private practice as a psychiatrist for 12 years. He has specialized in family and marital problems. He sees individuals and couples on an outpatient basis. Last spring he attended an intensive week-long workshop on sex therapy. The course involved lectures and discussions, along with videotapes and films. Dr. C. found the entire area to be quite promising because several couples he had in therapy expressed concerns about sexuality and, particularly, about the quality of their intimate relationships.

During a therapy session with one of those couples, Dr. C. asked Mr. and Mrs. R. if he could watch them make love, at their home and in their own bedroom. The couple regarded the question as unusual but, when Dr. C. told them, "I need this data directly, not from reports you give me," they consented. Dr. C. did not ask them to sign any release form; he did not regard his observations as a medical experiment or treatment. He simply wanted to get a sense of their experience so that he could be of use to them as they tried to improve their relationship. He did tell Mr. and Mrs. R. that he hoped that direct observation would lead to interventions that might aid other couples with their problems. The following week, in accordance with a collaboratively designed schedule, Dr. C. watched the couple make love for about 45 minutes.

Questions

1. If you believe that Dr. C.'s behavior is unethical, state why.
2. Professional organizations, such as the American Psychiatric Association, forbid sexual activity between therapist and client. Should such groups also prohibit the kind of therapeutic "information seeking" Dr. C. has done?
3. Why should sexual activity be so controversial a behavior? Had Dr. C. asked a client to let him observe her vocational activity because the patient complained of incredible pressures on the job, would this request seem similarly questionable?
4. If you were a psychiatrist practicing in the same town as the practitioner in this case and Mr. and Mrs. R. told you, during a therapy session, that they were very uncomfortable about having agreed to let Dr. C. watch them during intercourse, what would be your response?

■ THINK PIECE: PSYCHIATRY ■

Psychiatrists, as physicians, are pledged to resist death. The state, however, executes criminals convicted of the most heinous crimes, notably aggravated murder. In more than 35 states the death penalty is utilized; it is estimated that more than 2000 prisoners await execution. Should psychiatrists or other mental health professionals participate in the capital punishment process? Such involvement can take place at many stages: Prior to arraignment forensic experts assess a prisoner's competence to stand trial; at the pretrial stage, psychiatrists are often asked by prosecuting authorities to evaluate prisoners who may face the death penalty; as expert witnesses mental health professionals influence juries who may, if the defendant is found guilty, ask for the death penalty as a sentence.

Even more controversially, a psychiatrist may be called on to *treat* a death-row prisoner. Courts have held that severely mentally ill felons who are deemed incompetent for execution must not be killed but, rather, must be restored to mental health if possible. Forensic clinicians share a dual, and sometimes internally divisive, professional commitment to the individual patient *and* to the administration of justice. When a defendant has received the death penalty, should a psychiatrist offer therapy, including psychotropic medications, knowing that the restoration of function may lead, rather swiftly, to the end of the patient's life?

What weight should be given to the clinician's own views on the death penalty? Those who oppose state executions might face the need to conscientiously refuse participation in any stage of a capital case. But if evaluations and treatment are left to those practitioners who *approve* of the death penalty, wouldn't some proexecution bias creep in, resulting in the killing of persons who might otherwise remain alive? In providing execution competency assessments, a psychiatrist is not directly involved in administering the death penalty. (Other physicians who have been asked to administer lethal doses of barbiturates—as a more humane method of execution than hanging, the gas chamber, or the electric chair—have refused to do so on the grounds of violation of the Hippocratic Oath.) Can the evaluator role of the psychiatrist be held analytically distinct from the clinician's traditional role as therapist?

Finally, if a psychiatrist is asked to *treat* a prisoner presently incompetent to stand execution, is it ethically valid to do so? If refusal is the appropriate response, what are the ethical grounds for saying "No," especially if the prisoner is in mental pain, with symptoms that might be readily relieved by prompt therapeutic intervention?

■ VOICES: CLINICAL PSYCHOLOGIST ■

I am a clinical psychologist, working in an acute care hospital with often very ill patients. Some are depressed; others suffer from schizophrenia. Many are poor and come from families with unbelievable problems. Drugs and alcohol complicate their lives. I've always been fascinated with the human mind. My colleagues, who are physicians and psychiatrists, also see all kinds of troubles. I act as a consultant to a team of care givers who are trying to assess and help persons who are often in great mental distress. As a psychologist I try to see the patient in depth. Of course, I have to do this in a concentrated period of time. I give patients a battery of tests, but I always try to delve further into the patient's psychological makeup. Psychiatrists are less apt to do this. They are not trained to interpret behavior and feelings as we are. Most psychiatrists are interested in psychology. I do try to train psychiatric residents in such skills, but we really have very different perspectives on the lives of our patients.

The psychotic patients I see are not crazy all the time. Many have had acute psychotic episodes, but they often recover swiftly, especially after hospitalization. I am always looking for the strengths of such "crazy people." Psychologists are often accused of looking for psychopathology; I prefer not to do so. I believe psychiatrists are looking for things to fix, often with medicine. My job is to pass on to the psychiatrists (residents most of the time) what I see as the patient's essential problem. We often disagree in our assessments. Then I am in a dilemma. How hard should I push my diagnosis? The doctors are literally liable for the well-being of the patient. But many times I am opposed to the psychiatrist's analysis. It's an ethical issue: How aggressively should I press my views? How responsible should I be to the patient? I certainly admit that we need both approaches—a medical and a psychological understanding of our patients. If a serious error has been made in assessing a patient, however, I worry about the patient being jerked around, being committed involuntarily. I've come to realize that if I can make *some* impact on the system, I am doing the best I can. If I were a psychiatrist my credibility would be much greater, of course.

It really disturbs me that psychiatric facilities are being closed down and patients deinstitutionalized. The promise of community mental health centers has not been met. Many patients need a structured environment. They need a hospital, if only for transitional support as they try to return to their homes and jobs. I think that poor people get different treatment from rich people in the mental health system. *Where* you are hospitalized matters as well as what insurance you have; that's a real tragedy, and I see it all the time. The kind of care you get depends on who, if anyone, pays. It also depends on majority or minority status. In some places blacks get a raw deal. Elsewhere, it's Hispanics who are discriminated against. In other locations, impoverished Appalachians don't get a fair hearing. We're not very good at understanding different cultures.

A major ethical issue in my practice as a clinical psychologist is easy to portray by example. A man came to the hospital, allegedly suicidal. We then found out that he was having an incestuous relationship with his 15-year-old stepdaughter. The mother had left this child with the man. He put a gun to his head. I think because he was about to be arrested. When he came to the hospital I tested him. I think he is clearly a sociopathic personality. He was not insane. If a person is truly suffering from a major mental illness, you cannot hold him or her legally or morally responsible for harming others. There are a great number of paranoid patients—those with a fixed delusional system—who do need treatment. If they act out violently they need care, not imprisonment.

However, the man I am discussing was not crazy. He was using the system to get away with a crime. A few months later when he went to court I was subpoenaed to testify at his trial. What was ethically correct? He came to the hospital for help, for treatment. The hospital didn't want me to say anything. On the witness stand I said that my conversations with the man were privileged, confidential. The judge said that I *had* to tell the court anything I knew about this man and child abuse; this was mandated by law. I felt pulled both ways. In my heart, I felt that this man was morally wrong in what he had done, that he had full knowledge of what he had done to this child. I also thought he was faking in making the suicidal gesture. But professionally I thought I should keep quiet. When the judge ordered me to testify, I did so, but it was not easy to sort out the internal moral conflict.

Many of my patients are actually suicidal. I have come to believe that, on rare occasions, wanting to take one's own life can be rational. A young woman with cancer overdosed on pills. I don't think that this was wrong. She was trying to avoid the horror of a slow and painful death. She was rational and deliberate and was trying to help her family. It was an altruistic suicide. Her earlier mental problems did not enter into this decision. (When she was psychotic, she was very psychotic; but when she wasn't, she was just fine.) When people are under the influence of a serious mental illness, suicide is not *right*, but it is *understandable*. If something could be done to relieve the depression, we should make it available. For some chronically depressed patients, the quality of life looks pretty bad, now and for the future. But I do believe that there is always something we can do. Some new medications or intervention might be effective. Maybe I'm just showing my own rescue fantasies.

I also work with adolescents. A 16- or 17-year-old might tell me things that I would like to keep from the parents. It's a hard choice — do I work with the kid or with the parents, or with all of them? There's a clear confidentiality problem, no matter what I choose. Legally the parents have a right to know what goes on between me and the child. I try to set up a contract and get the parents to agree to privacy between me and the adolescent. I ask them to waive their right to know. I also try to avoid talking with the parent behind the kid's back. If the child, however, tells me of a potentially dangerous situation (e.g., serious drug abuse or the threat of physical violence), I might be forced to spill the beans. But I will tell this to the child. Oddly enough, if the kid were 19 years old, I would never tell the parent.

Another ethical problem in my field is therapist-client sexual relationships. It's strictly taboo. There are sanctions, but it does happen. I have been on the state ethics committee, and we really are clamping down on this kind of behavior. Sexual relationships between therapist and patient are obviously detrimental. But there are some nuances. What if the therapist is attracted to a patient and then suggests that she stop being his patient and refers her to his colleague. Then, 3 weeks later he calls his former patient and asks for a date. This might be O.K. according to the rules. But I have real problems with the scenario. Why is it almost always men who are acting this way? Why do they need to have illicit relationships? I'm at a loss to explain why men take more liberties. But I think there should be a strong sanction: If you do this, you're out, you're not a therapist any more.

RECOMMENDED READING

Battin, M.P. *Ethical Issues in Suicide.* Englewood Cliffs, N.J.: Prentice-Hall, 1982.

Beck, J.C. *The Potentially Violent Patient and the* Tarasoff *Decision in Psychiatric Practice.* Washington, D.C.: American Psychiatric Press, 1985.

Block, S. and Chodoff, P. (eds.) *Psychiatric Ethics.* Oxford, England: Oxford University Press, 1991.

Gutheil, T.G. and Appelbaum, P.S. *Clinical Handbook of Psychiatry and the Law.* Baltimore: Williams & Wilkins, 1991.

Hillard, J.R., ed., *Manual of Clinical Emergency Psychiatry.* Washington, D.C.: American Psychiatric Press, 1990.

Macklin, R. *Man, Mind and Morality: The Ethics of Behavior Control.* Englewood Cliffs, N.J.: Prentice-Hall, 1982.

■8■

Final Judgments: Ethics at the End of Life

What does it mean to disconnect a ventilator that is essentially breathing for a dying or persistently vegetative patient? How does this act differ from a decision not to place the same patient on the machine in the first place? Courts and philosophers have held, almost uniformly, that there is no significant difference between the two acts. Withholding and withdrawing care are morally equivalent, the conventional wisdom states. But if you ask a nurse or a physician if there is any real difference, nearly all such personnel answer with a resounding "Yes!" Withholding care, most will state, is easier; when we withdraw care, we feel as if we are killing the patient. Contesting such views by pointing out that, perhaps, withholding care should be *more* problematic because it is based on a statistical assessment of the patient ("Most such persons with this condition do not survive, so let's not start him on the breathing machine") only serves to harden attitudes.

Practicing medicine ethically in the realm of death and dying requires insight and patience and above all the recognition that emotion, fantasy, and a strong dose of ambivalence inform the work of healthcare professionals when their patients are near death. Though death has been called the great equalizer, no two experiences of dying are the same. There are, however, common problems. Many nurses have observed that doctors visit patients near death infrequently and for increasingly shorter periods. Though most physicians believe that it is their prime obligation to control human disease—through accumulating knowledge and perfecting skills—

this pledge is not unconditional. Doctors know that there are patients in futile conditions. Though the content of medical education is changing—there are now courses on death and dying in many schools of medicine; more medical students are gaining clinical experience in nursing homes than ever before—the major ideological thrust of contemporary medicine is aimed toward curing patients and secondarily toward caring for the dying.

Hospices—at least 2000 of them across the United States and Canada—provide a place for terminal patients to die in relative freedom from pain and without being sustained on life-prolonging devices. Yet only a small proportion of dying patients (perhaps 10%) are cared for under hospice supervision. Nearly 80 percent of deaths take place in acute-care or long-term care facilities where the impersonality of dying is often an established fact. Dying patients challenge the physician's mandate to cure, or at least to help. The experience of dying is only beginning to be subject to medical inquiry. Our paucity of knowledge and experience in this realm has authentic impact on the ethical dilemmas that we confront at the end of life.

The areas of law and ethics are both most concerned about the issue of dying. Most of the significant court cases since the Karen Quinlan case (see Appendix H), have dealt with the rights of patients or their surrogate decision makers to refuse care that would sustain life. Recently the issue of physician-assisted suicide, and the related issue of active euthanasia, has received public attention. Important questions about advance directives, living wills, and durable power-of-attorney provisions have provoked discussion in medical societies and in state legislatures as well as among the larger public. The Patient Self-Determination Act of 1991 has stimulated further dialogue, for example: How specific and how prophetic must patients' wishes be when they ask for certain kinds of care to be withheld from them perhaps years after making a request? Central concerns about real and symbolic matters include whether or not removing tubes providing artificial hydration and nutrition is ever morally acceptable. Should the relief of pain and suffering enable physicians to accelerate the dying process? What status should be accorded to patients who are not actively dying but who completely lack, and will never have restored, cognitive function and interpersonal capacity? Should a physician *ever* assist a patient in taking her own life? The role of the interdisciplinary ethics committees in resolving conflicts about treatment or nontreatment decisions near the end of a patient's life is still evolving.

There is much misunderstanding, and some prejudice, in providing care for patients who are near death. Our general attitude toward aging and toward persons more than 85 years of age, a growing proportion of our population, is not a positive one, although public opinion polls suggest a modest improvement in the image of the elderly in recent years. Older patients, especially those who, as a result of stroke, coma, neocortical insult, or advanced dementia, cannot communicate, may present very frustrating cases to younger physicians or physicians-in-training. There is an omnipresent temptation to evaluate the quality of life of very old patients—especially those who are dependent in long-term care facilities or in ICUs—with prejudices rooted in ageism.

Many health care dollars are fruitlessly utilized in caring for persons who will not profit, for long, from this expenditure. Perhaps one-seventh of all health care dollars (the total amount of which will reach more than a trillion dollars by the year 2000) is expended in the last 6 months of patients' lives. About half of the patients in medical intensive care units (MICUs) are too sick to benefit from care. Yet the way in which we treat dying patients is only partially a consequence of our socioeconomic concerns. Arguments about setting limits to the kinds of interventions allowable for persons older than 80 open up the question of fairness among the generations. Few would argue that the mere existence of technological means of sustaining life is enough to require the use of ventilators in all patients no matter what their condition.

It is widely recognized that decisions regarding ventilation, hydration and nutrition, orders not to resuscitate, and use of pain medications for terminal patients are much more than medical determinations. Each entails a reflection of values: those of the patient, the physician and other health providers, and the institution as well. Conflicts emerge often. Nurses ask, "Why are we always first to know that the time to stop treating has been reached?" Family members argue with one another and with doctors about such decisions, often feeling as if they have been left out. For example, when spouses or siblings are included in judgments about DNR orders, they may feel confused or patronized. Doctors, especially those who have to care for dying patients, often lack awareness of the nuances of the terminal process. Doctors also feel time pressure ("Why spend a half-hour at the bed of a comatose stroke patient who won't live out the week when I can offer something more useful to another person?") as well as emotional stress.

Some emerging common wisdom can provide guidelines for dealing with patients who are dying or who are permanently nonresponsive. The American Medical Association Council on Ethical and Judicial Affairs (see Appendix D) has stated that withdrawing or withholding life-prolonging medical treatment may be appropriate when a terminal patient will only be burdened by continuing such treatment. The AMA prohibits physicians from intentionally causing death, but allowing patients to die by removing life-prolonging equipment (e.g., artificially or technologically supplied respiration, nutrition, or hydration) is not unethical. Opinions of the AMA, or of judges, lawyers, or politicians rarely assuage ethical anxieties when our own lives or those of friends or family are at stake.

Even if physicians and other health care workers could agree that life-sustaining treatments *may* be withdrawn under appropriate circumstances (for example, from the patient in a persistent vegetative state who has mandated it in an advanced directive), there is another side to the coin. Patients or their surrogates (often family members) sometimes request the continuation of life-support systems when such treatments are considered to be futile by doctors and nurses. If we are to respect patient autonomy in refusing to continue treatment such as ventilatory support, can we also respect a demand to provide such an expensive and elaborate mode of life sustenance when there is no chance of patient recovery or restoration of function?

To achieve a humanistic understanding of death requires much more than the capacity to interpret neurologic tests that demonstrate that a patient on a respirator shows signs of whole brain death. Though our clinical understanding of death and dying is remarkably well developed, a sense of what this process means both to those dying and to loved ones who may suffer with and survive the death of another requires empathy. To understand others, however, is not necessarily to agree with them or to validate their moral position. For example, we can appreciate the frustration and desperation of a patient who has not achieved a successful remission from cancer and who then asks a doctor to "help me die now." Seeing the agony in that patient's request, however, does not mandate accepting the plea. Our views on active euthanasia in this case must be set into concrete contexts; flexibility is always desirable. There is no requirement that a health-care professional abide by a patient's wishes at all times.

■ FIVE ESSENTIAL CASES ■

Case 8-1

Decisions made at the end of life are influenced by *who* makes those determinations. Even patients who appear to retain decisional-capacity do not always get to assert their views.

Mr. V. was a 51-year-old man transferred to the hospice in-patient unit from a nearby acute care hospital. Three weeks earlier he had undergone exploratory surgery that showed liver cancer and widespread abdominal metastases. Mr. V. became aware of the seriousness of his condition when Dr. F., the attending physician, told him he had a tumor. A surgeon opened and closed, inserting drainage tubes to relieve pain. Mr. V. had been healthy for most of his life; only in recent months had he begun to lose weight and to state "I have been feeling bad."

Dr. F. told Mr. V.'s family (his wife of 26 years and 23-year-old married son) that he thought Mr. V. had less than 2 months to live. He did not communicate this message directly to the patient. Mr. V.'s physical condition deteriorated quickly while he was still in the hospital; he had continual nausea and vomited often. The doctor recommended to the family, away from the patient's bedside, that he be transferred to the hospice. Mrs. V. toured the facility and was told about the hospice's policy: It would provide palliative care, but not medical interventions such as CPR, for her husband until he died. Mrs. V. returned to the hospital and told her husband that he was going to be transferred to a place where he could get some of his strength back.

Mr. V. was taken by ambulance to the hospice in-patient facility. He was weak and tired and extremely nauseated. He said little to the admissions nurse but indicated that he wanted an emesis basin. He was taken to a room where he pulled up his covers, closed his eyes, and turned on his side. The son stayed with Mr. V. In the hospice admissions office, the nurse asked Mrs. V. if her husband understood why he was being admitted. Did he know about their DNR policy? Mrs. V. replied that she believed he knew his cancer was inoperable and that he thought that in-patient hospice care might allow him the strength to go home and be with his family.

The admissions nurse asked Mrs. V. if her husband was still able to understand and if he could sign his own consent form. She replied: "Oh, yes, he was still writing checks yesterday to pay bills." The nurse and the family proceeded to the patient's room. The nurse asked Mr. V. to read and to sign the consent form. He waved his arms, as though he did not want to be bothered. The nurse read him the contents of the form; Mr. V. kept his eyes closed. After she finished reading, Mr. V. turned his head away and said, "I don't care. Kill me if you want."

Mr. V.'s son was visibly upset. He left the room and the nurse and his mother followed him. When Mrs. V. told him about the hospice's DNR policy, he exclaimed, "Do you mean to say that if my dad's heart stops you won't resuscitate him? What will happen then?" Mrs. V. and the nurse spoke with the son about trying to alleviate Mr. V.'s symptoms and to help him live comfortably and fully in his time remaining. Eventually, Mr. V.'s son told his mother that it was all right with him if *she* signed the consent form. Mrs. V. did so and Mr. V. was admitted to the hospice.

■ ■ ■

Hospice care is available in many large and medium-sized communities in the United States and Canada. This alternative institution is intended to provide for dying patients in a dignified, comfortable manner, with aid and assistance from family members, community volunteers, and health care professionals. Hospices are generally available for patients in the last 6 months of life and provide at-home care for most of their clients, with in-patient services on a respite basis or, occasionally, for patients who cannot be adequately cared for at home. Most hospice patients suffer from advanced cancer. Pain control is emphasized in hospice care, as is concern for the whole patient, addressing physical, emotional, psychosocial, and spiritual needs. Hospice teams are interdisciplinary—physicians, nurses, social workers, and counselors are typical members. Though Mr. V. is admitted to the in-patient unit in great discomfort, hospices are experienced at dealing with patients like him.

Mr. V.'s cancer is widespread, terminal, and inoperable, and his attending physician believes that no treatment can be offered him in the acute-care setting. But how, and with what specificity, has this been communicated to the patient? Apparently not very effectively because the physician has spoken with the family but not to the patient. Mr. V. does know that he has cancer, but the basic decisions about the setting and the kinds of care he is about to receive have been decided for him by Dr. F. and his family. Mr. V. is being kept partially in the dark.

Is this an atypical situation? Thirty years ago a majority of physicians, including oncologists, tended *not* to directly and concretely reveal a diagnosis of cancer to the patients. Believing that a positive mental attitude (rooted in ignorance of the diagnosis) might lead to a longer and better quality life, physicians used euphemisms such as "mass" or "growth" instead of utilizing language immediately understandable by the patient. All this has changed in recent decades. Most physicians reveal the cancer diagnosis. The attending physician in this case has not *quite* misled the patient. But in discussing options with the family outside the earshot of Mr. V., Dr. F. has behaved in a typical manner. "Sparing the patient" is quite common, as is allowing family members time to absorb the bad news and to secure an appropriate place for the patient to spend his remaining days. What *should* Dr. F. have done?

The role of the family in this case is crucial. Some would argue that Dr. F. has violated the rule of confidentiality by discussing both prognosis and care options with Mrs. V. and her son. But Mr. V. was very uncomfortable in the hospital, and though we may not condone this apparent violation, we can understand why a physician would consult with the family on such matters. If Mr. V. is to be a hospice patient, he must have a primary nonmedical care-giver, and Mrs. V. is the obvious candidate. Sending her ahead to evaluate the facility is not an outlandish idea. But is it fair to the patient?

During the admissions process a variety of problematic ethical issues develop. We may assume that the patient was placed in the private room initially so that his nausea could be cared for, or at least contained. Later, Mr. V. *is* asked to consent to admission and is informed at least minimally about hospice policy and procedures. This follows the nurse's sensible question to Mrs. V. about her husband's capacity to exercise rational judgment. But Mr. V.'s response to the nurse is surprising and upsetting. When he remarks, "Kill me if you want," there is a clear indication that the patient's oral consent to admission has not been achieved. Yet the consent form is signed by his spouse, after consultation with the son. Is this an example of the emergency exception to the doctrine of informed consent (see Fig. 2-5)? Mr. V.'s situation is not directly life-threatening, but his capacity to make an important decision is dubious. Can a spouse consent for her husband under such circumstances? Can consent be regarded as temporary and subject to patient affirmation later on? Is there a clear assault on Mr. V.'s autonomy and, in effect, dignity?

All patients are entitled to know the treatment plans being prepared for them. Mr. V.'s wishes, not only about CPR or pain medication, but about being sustained by artificial hydration and nutrition (a service sometimes offered by hospices), need to be elicited. One way of discovering any patient's views is to make available a living will (see Appendix E) as a basis for the discussion of end-of-life care. This kind of dialogue would have been most efficacious *before* Mr. V.'s cancer diagnosis. At the very least it should have been offered to him while in the acute care hospital.

Finally, provisions for who should become Mr. V.'s surrogate decision-maker when he loses decision-making capacity ought to begin. Using a durable power of attorney for health care document would allow such a designation, and the person who will have this authority might as likely be the son as it would Mrs. V. This decision needs to be made by Mr. V. as soon as possible. Knowing the patient's values, including his sense of what may happen after he dies, will help those who make decisions on his behalf. Simply getting a spouse to sign on the dotted line is never a substitute for a sustained and detailed evocation of the patient's wishes.

Case 8-2

The dying patient who has the capacity to accept or refuse treatment and who is fully aware of a terminal status may ask the physician to accelerate the dying process. Subtle differences between allowing death to occur and hastening its arrival present serious moral challenges.

William M., a 33-year-old gay man, was diagnosed as HIV positive 3 years ago. Counseling provided by the local AIDS clinic had been very useful to him; he voluntarily reported all of his prior sexual contacts to the local health department. He left his job as an attorney with a large corporate firm to pursue less lucrative work as an advocate for persons HIV positive or with AIDS who experience discrimintion on the job or elsewhere. He attempted to take the drug zidovudine (AZT) prophylactically, but the side effects were devastating for him, so the medication was discontinued. Mr. M. did make irregular and inconsistent use of aerosolized pentamidine to ward off lung infections. He became a peer counselor for people with AIDS. He continued to see a physician, Dr. S., at the AIDS clinic. Nine weeks ago Mr. M. was hospitalized with his first episode of *pneumocystis carinii* pneumonia (PCP). His presumptive diagnosis of AIDS was confirmed.

Dr. S. visited Mr. M. to discuss the insertion of a catheter into his pulmonary artery as part of his treatment and evaluation for PCP. Mr. M. was well aware of the likely course of his disease and refused to consent to the procedure. Dr. S. tried to convince him that this first bout of PCP would not necessarily prove fatal and that he might have many months or even years to live. Dr. S. told the patient, "I will stick with you and keep you comfortable." The patient was very knowledgeable: He knew, for example, that corticosteroids could increase his survival temporarily. But Mr. M. told her that he knew that his illness would get worse ("I have seen so many of my friends die, and die miserably") and that he did not want that future for himself. Mr. M. stated that he had seen a lawyer and had made both a will and a living will and had designated his best friend, via a durable power of attorney procedure, to make medical decisions were he to become incompetent.

Mr. M. had no history of psychiatric illness; on the contrary, he was regarded by caregivers and by the wider community as a pragmatic, rational, moderate man who helped others readily. He was refusing medical treatment, Mr. M. said, because he knew that his condition was fatal. He did not want to die *later* in unpredictable or painful circumstances. He asked Dr. S., in the privacy of his hospital room, if she would "help me to die. I know that you can prescribe enough medications, and tell me which combination will work, so that when I leave the hospital I can end my life in my own way."

The clinical course of HIV infection and AIDS is not completely predictable. The visible symptoms of the disease become manifest eventually and can be painful and disfiguring. It is almost always relentless in its course and even periods of improvement are rapidly followed by relapses. An AIDS patient can look in the mirror and see evidence of wasting and disability. Pulmonary problems, development of unusual and rare cancers, raging and intractable infections (often with high fevers and accompanying pain) may be common. Central nervous system disorders, which may be masked as psychological or adjustment problems, can produce thought disorders, clinical depression, delirium, psychotic hallucinations, or dementia. Mr. M. does *not* seem to have suffered this complication, but he will need to be checked frequently, for if his cognitive capacity becomes impaired, his autonomously stated prior expression may require reexamination. A consultant-liaison psychiatrist can be very useful. But were Mr. M. to lose decisional capacity, this does *not* mean that all earlier requests can be ignored.

Perhaps even more threatening psychological and social pressures and fears accompany the virus. For example, facing death through the aging process during a normal life cycle is a gradual, though never easy, progression. Most people have decades to prepare for their dying. AIDS patients rarely have 5 years; many have less than 1. Like Mr. M., many persons with AIDS are young men and women in their 30s and 40s, a time of potential achievement and personal growth for people who are well. Death, statistically, is for the old, not those who have only recently left youth behind. For Mr. M., the disease also represents a loss of his community, support system, and affective bonds. Many of his friends and acquaintances have died. Ironically, he is already a survivor and he has rearranged his life to benefit others who are dying or who are trying to live with the disease.

Pain and the fear of pain add to the feelings of dependency and discouragement for patients with AIDS. Mr. M. is *not* in grievous pain right now; however, he has seen it in others. The physician, aware that pain is more than a sensory event involving nerve pathways, will want to investigate the psyhological dimensions of Mr. M.'s concerns. The level of distress Mr. M. must tolerate will be conditioned by much more than his own anxiety or coping skills. It will be a function of his social support and the extent to which it can be mobilized. Physicians are not accustomed to stage-managing social networks. But given Mr. M.'s unusual and troubling request, how far should Dr. S. extend her energies in organizing psychosocial systems on her patient's behalf?

Two other factors make AIDS so disastrous for its sufferers. First, the majority culture, which already disapproves of "alternative" ways of life and judges the worth of persons by their private lifestyles, places gay males and male and female IV drug users in the "high risk" category without regard to their individual traits or behaviors. Mr. M. has had to struggle on behalf of people with AIDS to secure legislative and constitutionally guaranteed prerogatives for them. He has had to deal with unconscious sexism and most likely racism. Second, Mr. M. is immersed in a health care system that has been torn asunder by the AIDS epidemic. Not always publicly, physicians have been divided about providing AIDS care and about expressing their own fears of infection. That AIDS is perceived to be a growing threat to the health of caregivers is no secret. If Dr. S. is to accede to Mr. M.'s request for assistance in dying, she must be certain of her motives.

Before Dr. S. can entertain her patient's request, she must check several things. She must speak with the interdisciplinary team to get their assessment of Mr. M.'s mood and feelings. She must ask her patient for permission to talk (in his presence) with friends and loved ones. Involving others is a delicate task (preserving confidentiality is a prime necessity), but in order to assess Mr. M.'s psychosocial needs, and how they are being met, Dr. M. must speak with other people. It is not enough just to be sensitive to this patient's requirements. His self-perception is tied to his place in his community. Dying patients continue to care about others. Is Mr. M. seeking an earlier death because he fears abandonment? Or is his desire based on a rational evaluation of what the next few months will do to his body and mind?

Mr. M. is asking his physician to help him die. We know that persons with underlying medical illnesses have a higher risk of suicide than the general population (see chapter 7). AIDS patients are no different: Their rate of suicide is significantly higher than others in their age range. But such data do not confront the ethical dilemmas posed for Dr. S. *Is suicide a rational choice for Mr. M?* Doctors, psychiatrists in particular, are trained to view suicide as a product of either patient madness or physician failure. The possibility of its being a manifestation of a mental disorder must be ruled out by careful neuropsychiatric testing. But, assuming that Mr. M. is not in this category, what should Dr. S.'s response be?

Physicians must obey the law. To assist in a suicide is a punishable offense in almost every American jurisdiction. Strong professional, religious, and secular traditions argue against helping another to die. Dr. S. must look within for wisdom, but if she views Mr. M.'s suicide to be rational and ethically acceptable, why must she be unwilling to provide the minimal information (and thus the potential means) necessary to do this in a pain free and comforting manner? Dr. S. may tell Mr. M. that he is "on his own" in this time of ultimate need. But has she discharged her obligation—a particularly strong one as a physician caring for a patient with a terminal illness—to stand by a suffering and dying person?

Case 8-3

Orders not to resuscitate have real, and symbolic, authority. For patients who are no longer capable of refusing treatment, justifying a DNR order evokes a discussion of quality-of-life considerations.

After suffering a myocardial infarction (MI), Mrs. S. is brought into the emergency room by the life-squad. No medical records or traces of family or friends can be found for this woman, who seems to be in her late 60s and who has been "living on the streets for years," according to the police. Her only identification is a county welfare card; the social agency supervising her case tells the hospital that Mrs. S. picks up her monthly check and her food stamps promptly, but they know little else about her. After she is stabilized, the patient is taken to the coronary care unit.

The heart attack has been quite massive; a good deal of the heart muscle is irrevocably destroyed, and Mrs. S. has not awakened by day 3. A neurologist says that she is in a coma and cannot predict if or when she will regain consciousness. The patient is not on a ventilator and is receiving IV hydration and limited nutrition along with medications for her heart. Late that evening the patient sustains a witnessed cardiac arrest; the crash cart is summoned and she is "successfully" resuscitated after a few minutes. Her condition seems to worsen: No moaning is heard, and her eyes do not open even for a second.

The next day a social worker arrives with a young woman who is identified as Mrs. S's niece. She confirms that there are no other family members and that she has not been close to her aunt for many years. After 6 more days in the ICU, the physicians feel as if they can do very little for Mrs. S. When the medical resident suggests that Mrs. S. be made a DNR her primary nurse asks, "Shouldn't we consult with the niece on this one?"

Letting go is very difficult: The removal of life support equipment should never be done lightly or readily. For many physicians, allowing a patient to die seems contradictory to the central purposes of medicine: to sustain life and to relieve suffering. But sometimes pursuing one goal conflicts with the other, and often the conflict is less than apparent. It is perhaps possible to sustain Mrs. S.'s life, but we are unsure how much she will suffer. Because nothing is known of this patient's values or preferences, the staff must pursue a decision with no knowledge of the patient. The only possible help is the presence of Mrs. S.'s niece.

Must a physician wait until a patient (if competent) or a family member or other surrogate accedes to a DNR order? Acute care and many long-term care facilities have policies about this matter. The Patient Self Determination Act, a federal mandate that went into effect in December, 1991, states that all competent patients on admission into such facilities must be made aware of state law regarding advance directives and institutional policies about providing as well as withholding or withdrawing life-sustaining treatment. Policies, of course, appear on paper. The actual task of communicating with patients and their surrogate decision-makers, often families and friends, is a delicate and complex endeavor. Using the "D" word, telling a very ill person that he or she is dying, is never easy.

Critically ill patients are often categorized. (There is a tendency to label those categories by color or number—a residue of the days in which such decisions were made without patient or family input.) The determination of resuscitation status is based on an assessment, subject to revision, of present medical condition. In some systems, for example, category III patients are not alive: They have suffered *whole brain death* but may be sustained on a ventilator in anticipation of organ donation. The body still requires a dignified and respectful attitude by professionals.

Category I conventionally requires *total support* of the patients: all available means of preventing death and reducing morbidity are used. Unless specified otherwise, all patients are Category I. Patients in Category II receive *no resuscitation* and are designated only by written physician order. For several years the American Hospital Association has required each accredited institution to have a formal policy on DNR orders. Most specify that Category II assignment be done by the attending physician *with the consent of the competent patient or the surrogate decision-maker for the incompetent patient.* A cardiopulmonary resuscitation is a complex event, and can include cardiac compression, endotracheal intubation, defibrillation, and the use of cardiac medications. Some DNR policies provide subdivisions in which, for example, a patient who arrests will not be intubated but may elect to receive a "push" of stimulating medications. Physicians need to be encouraged to write orders that are as concrete as possible: "pressors for hypotension" means much more than "use appropriate meds."

Mrs. S. is certainly not dead. She continues to breath spontaneously. If her niece accedes to the team's recommendation that she be made DNR, clarity is most desirable. Unlike many Category II patients who have requested that a DNR order be placed in the chart, Mrs. S. is not suffering from a terminal malignancy. Nor is there complete vital or multiple organ failure. She is, however, unconscious. Finding an appropriate care plan for her will be difficult. Family members often use archaic terminology, asking that no heroics be provided or that no extraordinary measures be used. Phrases such as "utilize only natural and not artificial" methods of life support make no sense. Such labels lack content and substance. Is a breathing machine artificial and a gastrostomy tube natural? Being concrete and patient-specific means that Mrs. S.'s doctors have to make a clinical assessment of her prospects and from the ethics perspective must find *reasons* to recommend not resuscitating her or limiting treatment in any other fashion.

A primary reason for wanting to resuscitate Mrs. S. were she to arrest once more is that it would save her life. CPR is a wondrous maneuver, snatching a dying person from death, providing temporary respiratory and circulatory pressure to keep vital organs sufficiently oxygenated. It symbolizes contemporary medicine: a technological innovation that may defy the disease process or a traumatic accident. But for Mrs. S. it may also symbolize potency without sensitivity. The reluctance to admit the inevitability of death can make CPR a punishment for patients, their families, and even for caregivers. Whether using CPR on Mrs. S. will be beneficial or not is not immediately evident. She cannot utter a word. We do know, statistically, that some DNR patients survive. A small percentage (such factors as whether or not the arrest was witnessed are crucial) do live to leave the hospital. Patients who are resuscitated in coronary or intensive care units have a *very* small chance of living if they arrest more than once.

The general wisdom regarding DNR status has only limited utility in the case of Mrs. S. In the absence of a competently expressed choice by the patient, physicians look to legal guardians and persons designated by proxy instruments (Fig. 8-1). In their absence a flow chart approach prevails. Next of kin in the following order are consulted: spouse, parent, adult child, brother or sister, aunt, uncle, nephew or niece, first cousin. (Of course multiples in several of these categories can present difficulties: Adult children often quarrel about what their parent would have wanted.) In Mrs. S.'s case there is a niece, but if the purpose of consulting her is to reveal the patient's hidden wishes there is little chance of her doing so. Respecting patient values is another rule of thumb: Mrs. S. may have had a history of moral choice-making, but it will be nearly impossible to trace it.

One alternative, of course, is to seek a court-appointed *guardian ad litem*. A lawyer, even a hospital administrator or physician, can be appointed by a judge. But if this is the decision-maker, no subjective or empathic leap of imaginative power will lead to a sense of what Mrs. S. wanted. Instead, a rational, benefit-burden test is likely to be applied. Weighing the costs (especially in terms of pain and suffering) of continued care versus the potential good is also not easy in this case. Because we think that Mrs. S. is unable to perceive her condition, continuing to treat her (even to revive her via CPR, often a "violent" and aggressive intervention) may not be noticed by this patient. If the medical cliche, "If you err, do so on the side of life," is applicable, will it lead to the right choice for Mrs. S?

Concern 1: Patient Competence

  Competent patient: not necessary to find substitute

  Never competent patient: always necessary

  Formerly competent patient: problem area

Concern 2: Assessment of Prior Expressions (by formerly competent patients)

  Documented Statements: living will, durable power-of-attorney for health care, medical advance directive, patient values history, written designation of proxy

  Informal statements: letters, diaries, reports of conversations, religious convictions, narratives

Concern 3: Finding an Approach

  Subjective: What would this patient want under these circumstances that would be consistent with her expressed values?

  Objective: What would the reasonable (average) person want under these circumstances? (Calls for application of a best interest test: Calculating the benefits versus the burdens of treatment or nontreatment, with special concern for the pain and suffering of the patient.)

Fig. 8-1. Decision Making in Terminal Care: Basic Concerns

Case 8-4

When a patient is in great pain, those who watch and wait may be suffering. Managing death, especially for a person who has asked not to be allowed to linger, can strain all participants.

Mrs. L., married and age 81, was healthy and active and enjoyed a full range of family and social activities until a diagnosis of lung cancer 8 months ago. The primary tumor was resected, and Mrs. L. received chemotherapy on an outpatient basis. A spry and engaging patient, she often entertained her caregivers with lively stories of her many travels. Her primary care physician, Dr. A., has known the patient for more than a decade and regards her as "a little like my own mother." Their relationship has been characterized by a rare honesty. Mrs. L. knows that she will likely die from the cancer or from related complications. On her physician's advice, Mrs. L. completes a living will, which is binding in her state of residence.

This document, which she has filed with her attorney, pastor, and physician (with copies to family members), is supposed to carry the force of her decisional power if she becomes incompetent. It states, "If I am going to die within a short period, please do not let me linger." It also states, "I want to be kept as free of pain as possible." Mrs. L. knows that lung cancer, especially with bone metastases, can be a very painful experience. Because of the weakness she has experienced from the chemotherapy, Mrs. L. enters a nursing home. One evening she is short of breath and the life squad is called. Mrs. L. is transported to the hospital and is found to be dehydrated, somewhat confused, and to have pneumonia. She is taken to the ICU where she is placed on antibiotics and fluids. Her condition improves and when Dr. A. visits the next morning she says, "I know that the time is coming soon. I certainly don't want any more of that chemo. Just give me the painkillers. Promise me that you will see to it that this thing is no struggle. Nobody needs to see me thrashing around, begging for relief. I've said goodbye to everyone and I am ready to be on my way."

Dr. A. does not believe his patient to be depressed. On the contrary, her affect seems both peaceful and expectant. Dr. A. asks her permission to meet with Mr. L. and it is granted. The husband affirms his wife's wishes and tells Dr. A., "If you can just make it easier for this good woman to leave her body I will be eternally grateful." Dr. A. knows that decisions about pain management in this case will be his. But he asks himself: "What are my motives here?"

Mrs. L. is requesting a managed death. She has made her views known and has had them documented in a living will (see Appendix E). Now the ball is in Dr. A.'s court. Most physicians, if asked to list and prioritize the factors to be considered in providing terminal care for a competent patient, would note the following:

Medical condition: Is the patient going to die soon, and is there anything I can do to sustain her life or improve the quality of her remaining days?

Patient wishes: Has the patient reflected on the future course of events and presented a reasonable and responsible set of desires?

Legal obligations: Will withholding or withdrawing care violate the norms of medical practice or state interest?

External factors: What role should be played by family feelings, financial burdens, or considerations of scarce health care resources?

In Dr. A.'s mind the notion that such concerns can be separated is a naive one: He is likely to wonder about all at once. If Mrs. L. can be moved to a medical-surgical floor and "free up" a bed in the ICU, the physician may feel a bit less pressure. But her request for assistance in dying peacefully is not waived when she is out of intensive care. The primary obligation to render medical services to Mrs. L. is strong. Dr. A. recognizes the distinction between curing and caring. Mrs. L. will grow increasingly weak and vulnerable to infection. The longer she lives, ironically, the more pain she will experience. Medical organizations, from the AMA (see Appendix D) to a consensus conference of the American College of Chest Physicians and the Society for Critical Care Medicine have agreed that therapies that cannot benefit a patient should not be given. They also concur that merely sustaining the life of a patient without good reason makes no sense. But is it ever morally permissible to *accelerate* intentionally the dying process? Mrs. L. seems to be asking Dr. A. to give her a "push."

Caring for the dying is a medical art that requires empathy, humane values, and practice. Not enough of that experience is gained in medical schools. Medical residents who anticipate the first time "being with" a patient in her last days or hours speak of it with dread. Concepts such as a "good death" are rarely found in the clinical literature or around the case conference table. Nurses have more hands-on opportunities to spend time with terminal patients.

Physicians, accustomed to making rounds and leaving orders and prescriptions for nurses or support staff, must make time for terminal care. Dr. A. seems willing to do so. He must be aware that dying patients feel isolated and abandoned and fearful of intractable pain.

The patient has also given Dr. A. a powerful documentation of her last wishes, if not a legal guarantee. The phrase she has used, "do not let me linger," could have been phrased more aptly, but there is no mistaking her intention. The living will should be attached to her chart to avoid any further ambiguity. The decision, however, about appropriate pain medications for this patient will be Dr. A.'s. To keep Mrs. A. free from pain, he will have to increase narcotics to whatever dose renders her comfortable, which can depress her respirations and lower her blood pressure. The narcotics may dull her cognitive capacity, make her very sleepy, and gradually lead to unconsciousness. If Mrs. L. dies not in 3 weeks, but in 3 days due to the use of morphine prescribed by Dr. A., has he put her to death?

Let us note that we are *not*, in this instance, scrutinizing a decision to withhold or withdraw care. We are talking about providing drugs in doses that could be regarded as lethal in certain circumstances. Physician-assisted suicide is a complicated notion. If a doctor injects the patient with potassium chloride and she dies, the active dimension seems patent. But if the same doctor tells the same patient, "don't take more than twenty of these pills I am prescribing," is this also an active intervention? A corollary concept for those who usually oppose active euthanasia, yet who might be willing to allow the morphine injections anticipated in Mrs. L.'s case, is the doctrine of *double effect*. Based on Roman Catholic theology, but used more widely, the basic idea is that if the doctor intends only to relieve the patient's pain with the narcotic, the probability or even certainty that it will also kill the patient is a secondary, or double, effect. Because death was not intended it is not morally wrong. But could Dr. A. truly hide behind this veil and escape responsibility by stating, publicly, that he did *not* intend that death would result? An ethics of motives (Dr. A. wants to honor his covenant with this patient and to keep her pain-free) is complicated by an acknowledgment of consequences (most patients would not survive that dose of morphine). Which should, in conscience, prevail?

The Hippocratic Oath (see Appendix A) prohibited active euthanasia more than 2500 years ago. Though medical students often swear a version of that original oath when graduating from medical school, the debate about helping patients die has never been settled.

In recent years, public opinion polls in the United States have shown that a majority of voters would favor legislation that allows physician-assisted suicide when the request was made by a dying, competent patient. The fundamental medical obligation to relieve pain and suffering for the patient has limits. Dr. A. may legitimately be confused about what sort of step he might be taking in providing the requested pain medication. Prescribing analgesics is a common practice; but is administering an overdose the moral equivalent of giving Mrs. L. a lethal injection? No one doubts that this patient can require a physician *not* to initiate or continue all sorts of care (e.g., dialysis, CPR, mechanical ventilation). Does this right provide a moral foundation on which Dr. A. can, in conscience, sustain Mrs. L.'s desire to "be on her way?"

Case 8-5

Most physicians and the AMA regard providing artificial hydration and nutrition to be medical treatment. Issues concerning tube feeding are both real *and* symbolic. Withholding or withdrawing such treatment from patients who are very ill or unlikely to recover cognitive function continues to be controversial.

Mrs. F.T. is a 66-year-old woman, a long-time widow, with a history of severe diabetes, hypertension, obesity, cardiac problems, and cerebral thromboses. A resident of a nursing home for many years, she has been hospitalized three times during the past 4 years. Her physician has never discussed end-of-life decisions with her. She has never filled out a living will or other expression of her wishes regarding terminal care. Most recently, she has been hospitalized for a major stroke and was in a coma.

On admission, her two brothers (her only significant family members) told the attending physician that "everything should be done." Accordingly, she was placed in the ICU on a respirator and IVs and was given a NG tube for nutrition and hydration. The brothers stated with regard to continuing care: "When God wants her, God will take her. Meanwhile, she should stay alive." Over the next several days, three EEGs were administered; they showed some brain activity. Mrs. F.T. did not regain consciousness. Two neurologists stated that she was most likely permanently unconscious (i.e., neocortically dead).

The attending physician then met with the brothers, who agreed to the removal of the respirator while Mrs. F.T. was in the ICU. The doctor ordered withdrawal of the respirator, offering to do it himself, but an ICU nurse volunteered to remove it. Surprisingly, Mrs. F.T. breathed spontaneously. When the doctor reported this to her brothers, they were perplexed, for they had expected her to die. They inquired about the feeding tube that was sustaining Mrs. F.T. One brother said, "Is this feeding going to do her any good?" The physician said that he could not remove it because "as a doctor I cannot starve my patient to death."

■ ■ ■

Mrs. F.T. is alive but is unaware. The euphemism "neocortical death" is a rather cold and seemingly clinical description of her. The alternative, persistent vegetative state (PVS), is no more humane. It means that she is in a noncognitive state and has suffered an irreversible loss of consciousness. Such a status is often associated with trauma from an accident and brain damage due to anoxia (sometimes caused by a cardiac or respiratory arrest) from asphyxiation. It can also be caused by a stroke or series of strokes, as in Mrs. F.T.'s case. What such patients have in common is permanent brain deterioration. They do not give any sign of self-awareness and are unable to respond behaviorally in any major or appropriate way to the external environment. The brain stem may continue to function—it apparently is working for Mrs. F.T. because she continues to respirate spontaneously. We are not looking at patients in the advanced stages of Alzheimer's disease or those who suffer "locked-in syndrome" as a result of a stroke. Persons neocortically dead do not remain in that situation very long; many die within weeks or months. Some, especially younger patients in the PVS, may breathe on their own for many years (see Appendix I).

Caring for Mrs. F.T. cannot lead to the usual ethical goals of patient care (i.e., promoting patient autonomy, restoration of bodily functioning and interpersonal existence, and relief of pain and suffering). It is impossible for the attending physician to help this patient except in the tangential manner of showing respect for her by providing care that gives the appearance of dignity. But Mrs. F.T. is not the only subject of this case. Her brothers have a vital presence, and their views will be influential. The importance of continued existence via tube feeding may be tremendously important for her family.

Methods of feeding patients who require artificially supplied hydration and nutrition are well-established procedures in nursing homes. About 2,000,000 North Americans live in long-term care facilities—and that number may double in a few decades. In many cases a NG or gastrostomy tube or a hyperalimentation line is indispensable for survival. That such methods of feeding are medical therapies is doubted by only a few. But serious questions inform the debate about stopping tube feeding. First, what is it like to die from dehydration and malnutrition? Second, what risks attend tube feeding? Third, beyond the empirically verifiable questions posed by tube feeding, what is the impact of the *symbolic power* of feeding persons who are ill and dependent?

Mrs. F.T. passively accepts the nourishment and water she receives. The decision to provide a feeding tube for her was made, almost automatically, on her admission by the doctor in consultation with her family. This is where the problem began. A phrase such as "do everything" has no medical or ethical meaning. Instead of taking the time to talk about treatment options and about the meaning of dependency on both the ventilator and the NG tube, the physician plunged straight ahead. Now, the doctor feels stuck, fearing that the withdrawal of nutritional care will amount to starving the patient to death.

"Do everything" is not the only meaningless phrase heard at the bedside or in the hospital corridor at the end of life. "No extraordinary means" and "just use natural, not artificial methods of life support" are others. When feeding is at issue, such cliches are frustrating and confusing. Isn't eating the most natural, the most ordinary thing in the world? Certainly for the conscious patient, and for professional and familial caregivers, seeing a sick patient eat is a sign of life and, often, a reason for optimism. But this basic function has no *real* meaning for Mrs. F.T. She will never know of it. Withdrawing care must be considered in a more complex way. Saying that we are starving a patient to death demands analysis. (When we remove a patient from a ventilator, do we claim that we are suffocating the person?) Larger and smaller questions must be asked by this physician. What are the benefits and burdens of this care? Is this patient going to die soon, no matter what the treatment? Will the continuation of the NG feeding entail suffering? Will Mrs. F.T. die more comfortably with or without the tube? Does the symbolism of compassion expressed by the ideal of feeding the hungry make any real sense in this case? If a decision is made to remove the NG tube, what orders should be written in the patient's chart to ensure a dignified death?

■ PRACTICE MODEL CASE ■

Mrs. D. is very ill. Presently 87 years old, she weighs 77 pounds and has been a resident of a nursing home since a massive stroke 4 years ago. A nearly complete right hemiparesis with spasticity was diagnosed. A CT scan of the brain showed a low density, nonenhancing lesion in the left temperoparietal region. She is bedbound and lacks speech capacity. A long-standing scoliosis is evident. Mrs. D. has been tube fed for years and has an indwelling Foley catheter due to urinary incontinence. She often develops decubitus ulcers on her back, despite her nurses' efforts to prevent them. The patient has no family. No prior expression regarding health care decisions is evident in her chart. A guardian has been appointed by the court to handle her finances, but this person's involvement has been minimal. Mrs. D.'s medical costs are covered by Medicaid. The nursing home's attending physician, Dr. V., has been seeing Mrs. D. since her admission. Dr. V. is board certified as a family practitioner and has been practicing in the community, on her own, for 8 years.

Early one morning Dr. V. receives a phone call from a nurse at the nursing home. (Dr. V. knows this nurse well and trusts her judgment completely.) It seems that Mrs. D. is running a significant temperature (103.9°F), is sweating profusely, and seems in great discomfort. She is heard moaning in the night, which has alerted the nursing staff. Dr. V. goes to the facility and examines the patient. Rales in her lungs and her high fever are strongly suggestive of pneumonia. It is virtually impossible to x-ray Mrs. D. because of her scoliosis, but Dr. V. is quite certain that her patient has pneumonia.

Even though it is nearly sunrise and Dr. V. is very fatigued, she thinks about the options for this patient. It is possible to proceed aggressively. That will entail moving Mrs. D. to the community hospital, inserting IV lines for hydration and antibiotics, and ordering a variety of laboratory and other tests. It will also mean that Dr. V. will have to see her patient at least daily and perhaps more frequently, changing the drugs if necessary. If Mrs. D. seems to be doing poorly, she could be transferred to the tertiary care hospital, about 75 miles away. There she will be seen by a specialist, probably a pulmonologist, and, if necessary, be placed in the ICU. It is likely that she will be placed on a ventilator to help her breathe.

Dr. V. regards these options as "doing a full court press." She wonders if a less "powerful" approach would be more appropriate. Mrs. D., even if she recovers in the hospital, will be returned to the nursing home where she will eventually succumb, to another bout of pneumonia, to some other kind of infection, or to another, fatal stroke. Dr. V. is inclined to wait until the afternoon to see what occurs. It is quite possible that in the interim, Mrs. D. will die. The physician feels torn. With another patient, she might feel bound to take action, to write an order for liquid penicillin and encourage fluids, but with Mrs. D. she is simply unsure.

(Based on Hilfiker, D. Healing the Wounds: A Physician Looks at His Work. New York: Pantheon, 1985. Pp. 100–105.)

Patient

Is Mrs. D. dying? We can only offer a yes-and-no response. *Yes*, this patient's lungs are infected and will fill with fluid; this process is apt to lead to her death. The pneumonia may have several origins, but its likelihood is compounded by Mrs. D.'s bedfast status and by her generally poor medical condition. If the infection is not reversed, the patient will die in a short time. *No*, if aggressive intervention is used it has the capacity to reverse the infection and to restore Mrs. D. to about the level of functioning she has been at for several years. Earlier in the twentieth century pneumonia was labeled "the old man's friend," because it commonly claimed the life of an older person, at home, and during sleep. With the advent of antibiotic therapies, pneumonia can often, but not always, be successfully treated.

We cannot be certain about the patient's level of awareness, but her response to the fever has not been completely passive. Dr. V. can try to assess her cognitive capacity, but any attempt to solicit her views will surely be fruitless. We do know that the patient is dependent on a variety of interventions. Unable to ingest enough food and fluids, Mrs. D.'s survival has been prolonged by tube feeding and IV fluids. How we conceptualize this care is a function in part of what we call it. If, for example, we state that we are "feeding" the patient, our picture of the process will shift dramatically if we add a single word and say that we are "force feeding" Mrs. D. Medical treatments are a means to an end: If they provide no benefit to the patient, should they be continued? Is the care provided for Mrs. D. futile?

Does Mrs. D. *want* to die? We may assume that in entertaining the possibility of limiting treatment that Dr. V. is trying to figure out what her patient would have desired were she capable of thinking and speaking. The questions make sense only if we imagine both Ms. D.'s past and present selves lying in the hospital bed. Today, Mrs. D. is unlikely to want anything except for relief from the pain she may be experiencing. But her prior self, the entity that existed long before her stroke and admission to the nursing home, remains silent. Who will speak for this patient?

Relationships

For patients with chronic and perhaps progressive neurologic disease or damage, a satisfactory treatment plan based on prior patient expressions is optimal. An assessment of what's best for the patient can sometimes emerge by looking at his or her past relationships. Again, this is impossible for Mrs. D. No family members can be contacted; no living will or other advance directive is available. Efforts to ascertain Mrs. D.'s prior sentiments *can* be initiated. Did the patient attend a church, synagogue, or other religious institution? Could her pastor be located? Are friends from the past decade available?

Without knowing it, Mrs. D. has had a relationship with her court-appointed guardian. The responsibility of that person has been financial. Is it possible that the guardian has made an effort to contact others who knew Mrs. D. when she was competent? This avenue should be fully explored. But given the frequent isolation, not to say abandonment, of older incompetent patients, it is unlikely to yield significant information. Mrs. D., after all, has been in the nursing home for 4 years, and she has been noncommunicative all of that time. Interestingly, even though staff at the nursing home may never have spoken with or engaged this patient, they *will* have a sense of her as a person. They will have had one-sided conversations with Mrs. D. and they will recall her nonspecific utterances in response to painful stimuli as well as the occasions during which she seemed to be comforted. Much of this assessment, of course, will be speculative. Still, it will be nearly impossible to locate a spokesperson who could demonstrate this patient's values or views to health care professionals.

Advocacy

The absence of an obvious surrogate decision maker does not prohibit advocacy on Mrs. D.'s behalf. The nursing staff at the long-term care facility is pledged, professionally, to promote the patient's well-being and to argue forcefully if they believe her rights are being violated. Dr. V's dilemma—to pursue aggressive care or to allow this patient to die—stems from her sense of duty to Mrs. D. She is an advocate and more. That *more* is terribly problematic, for, in her role as a physician, she wants to find the right course of action on her patient's behalf. In the absence of any other obvious voice, Dr. V. must also act as the authoritative decision-maker. Can she separate her advocacy role from her role as health care authority?

A neutral way of helping to find a less engaged decision maker would involve going back to the probate court and requesting a hearing to appoint a guardian who will be empowered to make health care decisions. When Karen Quinlan needed a surrogate to order her removal from the ventilator the court appointed her father (see Appendix H). Two procedural requirements imposed on Mr. Quinlan were that he act through his daughter's physicians *and* that a hospital BEC confirm the patient's diagnosis. If Dr. V. proceeds this way, she will likely become the principal adviser to the court-appointed surrogate. The second suggestion—moving the case for reflection by the BEC (such groups can often be mobilized within hours)—should also be considered.

Conflicts

What is the essential moral difference between acting and failing to act? In terms of this case, what is the difference between sending Mrs. D. to the hospital for intensive care and letting her fever proceed without aggressive treatment in the nursing home? Does nontreatment by a physician suggest the repudiation of a primary duty—the obligation to help a patient in medical need? Or could such nonintervention be viewed as merciful and compassionate? Our answer to this dilemma rests on our view of the patient, which will control Mrs. D.'s situation because her views are unknown. Do we see her as a drowning swimmer to whom we can throw a life preserver? If so, the doctor's failure to act—given the special demands implicit in the patient-physician relationship—appears malevolent. If this drowning person is struggling to remain at the surface and, approaching the life preserver, has it yanked away, the act becomes one of commission rather than omission. If Dr. V., to pursue the analogy, intubates Mrs. D. but then fails to connect her to the ventilator, we might find such a decision reprehensible.

If we see such hypothetical distinctions and their attendant conflicts as unnecessarily formal and theoretical, it is for a good reason. Such traditional dichotomies may stimulate and amuse lawyers and philosophers, but plain and clear orders regarding Mrs. D.'s care must be given. The entire subject of withholding versus withdrawing care needs clarification. An older and quite simple-minded observation assumed withdrawal of treatment to be an act rather than an omission, while withholding care was presumed to be an omission and not an act. Today, courts and most ethicists regard the two phenomena as morally equivalent. But are they? For Dr. V. the determination to hospitalize and most likely intubate her patient could proceed almost automatically. But if no improvement is obvious after a stated time (e.g., several weeks), the physician will have to face a decision to withdraw care. Were Dr. V. to withhold intensive care *now*, she might assert as a prime reason for doing so her concern for the patient. Allowing the natural course of the pneumonia to proceed should relieve whatever pain and suffering Mrs. D. is experiencing. It will, perhaps only symbolically, preserve her dignity by forestalling any further, futile interventions. But is this choice simply a physician's rationale, because it seems psychologically more difficult to withdraw rather than to withhold care? Is Dr. V. looking for a way to avoid a decision later in the course of Mrs. D.'s illness?

Treatment or Nontreatment Options

Dr. V. must devise a plan for this very sick woman. It will not be limited to a simple choice between treating at the hospital or waiting the night to see if Mrs. D. dies. Treating the infection at the nursing home is an option that the physician is already considering. Other options might include calling in a pulmonary specialist, administering lots of fluids, taking the patient to the community hospital for x rays and observation, and treating the pneumonia but withdrawing the artificial nutrition. The basis of such specific determinations must be Dr. V.'s sense of her patient's right to refuse treatment, a right now completely impeded by her impaired condition.

Prior to the development of contemporary medical technology, serious illness almost always meant certain death. Palliative care was the physician's job and death usually came swiftly. The modern capacity to cure communicable and other diseases—and the ability to reverse the cessation of heartbeat and respiration—means that deaths now result from chronic, degenerative diseases. An illustration: Mrs. D. has lived for years in a nursing home without the ability to swallow. For the alert and competent patient, balancing the presumed benefits of treatment against the burdens of further care is a given. Because Mrs. D. has left no hint of her desires, and is permanently without decision-making capacity, has she lost her right to refuse treatment?

While no one would say that an incompetent patient who is terminally ill must continue to receive all forms of care that would benefit her (e.g., palliative chemotherapy, radiation, or even surgery for a cancer patient; hemodialysis for a profoundly demented patient with end-stage kidney disease), finding the grounds for treatment refusal in this case remains hard. Mrs. D. probably will not die very soon if she gets some relatively basic treatment. Nursing homes are filled with patients like Mrs. D. They lie for years in bed, often in a fetal position, fed by machines via tubes, and are only remotely, if at all, aware of the existence of others.

Interests

Most state courts and, recently, the U.S. Supreme Court, have ruled or implied that incompetent persons retain a right to die that emerges from the right to refuse treatment (see Appendix I). Medical care that produces results thought to be either unbearable (usually codified in terms of pain and suffering) or an affront to human dignity have been ordered stopped by courts on behalf of patients who can no longer communicate or who have left no advance directive. The notion of *substituted judgment* may in fact be a masquerade for patient choice. Usually someone tries to assess what the patient's best interest is, right now. If Dr. V. is to take a principled position regarding any of her treatment or nontreatment options, she must say just how the treatment serves the interests of Mrs. D. She must state what those interests are and present them in the context of her patient's current condition, degree of pain, loss of dignity, the risks and side effects as well as possible benefits of each treatment option, and note the prognosis with each potential treatment.

Some have argued that the assessment of pain is the only objective way of determining patients' best interests in cases like this. But doesn't this detract from other ideals about dying (e.g., the notion that continued and fruitless bodily interventions rob the patient, even if unaware, of elemental human dignity)? Individuals and the larger society may disagree about which ideals should count, or count most. But must the absence of a firm social consensus mean that only *pain* matters? If Mrs. D. is oblivious to her existence, must any determination of her best interests be suspended?

Dr. V. has more than a professional interest in this case. She seems to be using this particular episode as a way of reconsidering the normal physician impetus to treat first and think later. Such reflection may have a value, but the doctor also has an interest in testing her capacity as both medical authority and patient advocate. Is it possible to simultaneously think with clarity and feel with compassion? In what ways is this physician identifying with the patient? In what ways may she be projecting her own fears of death and disability onto this case? Sorting out such questions is an often-ignored physician interest.

We cannot neglect the position of the nursing home. Though physician orders are usually compelling, policies and procedures of the long-term care facility must be followed. Any decision must be thoroughly documented and must specify plans and goals for Mrs. D. The nursing home will likely have its charts reviewed by a state licensing authority, and it must be prepared to offer a reasoned explanation of the course of treatment and nontreatment decisions made on behalf of this incompetent patient. Dr. V. must coordinate her efforts with the responsible caregivers in the institution.

Consequences

Consequences have *macro* as well as *micro* elements. One facet of this case that remains uninvestigated concerns the allocation of scarce health care resources. If an aggressive approach to her critical illness is pursued and Mrs. D. ends up in the ICU, the economic costs will be high. This consequence is normally ignored by physicians, particularly those who resent the efforts of quality assurance managers who are in permanent pursuit of cost reductions. Most doctors also acknowledge, however, the fundamental notion that fairness requires that physicians not waste limited resources in situations that are futile. Mrs. D. is a Medicaid patient. This state-administered federal program has suffered budget constraints in recent years. It is fair to say that one anticipated consequence of placing this patient in the ICU could be the limitation of primary medical care for several young children.

Even if we can find a convenient or simple way of paying for Mrs. D.'s care, the problem of scarce resources does not vanish. Budget cuts in hospitals, the shortage of nurses and other professionals nationwide, and the widespread use of ERs as segues to ICUs has meant beds in that unit can be hard to find. Should the patient with severe chest pain awaiting laboratory confirmation or disconfirmation of a MI wait for an ICU bed on a medical/surgical floor while Mrs. D. lies intubated? Conversely, should Dr. V. accelerate a decision to remove her from a ventilator in the ICU, a decision she would rather postpone, because that same patient's survival from the MI *might* hinge on placement in the unit?

Assessing results is always a problematic endeavor. If Mrs. D.'s problems remain untreated it is *likely* that she will die by this afternoon or certainly within a few days. But, as nurses will recall, nursing home patients have been known to linger for remarkably long periods. Physicians who treat patients with the dementia and the pulmonary problems experienced by Mrs. D. often say, "Well, let's just give it some time and we'll see where we are." But on whose side does time reside? What is the purpose of a temporary plan to watch and wait?

Ethical Principles

This patient's autonomy has long ago vanished. Efforts to recreate her autonomy by appointing an informed surrogate decision-maker who might speak with her prior voice will not work. Dr. V.'s conflict resides in a tension between her duty of beneficence, her devotion to benefitting her patient by sustaining life and treating reversible illness, and nonmaleficence, the need to avoid harming Mrs. D. by forcing treatment on her, even though her awareness of such care may be limited. Keeping Mrs. D. in the nursing home means that decision-making authority will reside with this primary care physician. Transferring her, especially to the tertiary care institution, may result in sharing responsibility with critical care specialists and hospital administrators. Mrs. D. may spend many days in an ICU cared for by residents and attending physicians who neither know her nor in the humanistic sense care for her.

The conflict between beneficence and nonmaleficence would be much more apparent if recommended technologies were to cause grievous pain to Mrs. D. Hurting a patient in order to keep her alive is not unusual in medicine. That is the bottom line justification for many surgical procedures. Still, the confrontation between these related, some might say reciprocal, duties remains. Can we help Mrs. D. by speeding up her dying? Proponents of a beneficence model have argued that for advanced dementia patients a hospice approach is the most caring and ethical way of dying. Others assert that we will harm her if we fail to send her to the hospital. Will we do this fragile woman an even *greater* harm by sustaining her breathing for several more weeks in the ICU, only to return her to the revolving door of nursing home residence followed by acute care treatment?

■ CASES FOR ANALYSIS ■

Case A

Ms. V.F. is a 77-year-old woman with a history of dementia and renal failure, who was admitted to the hospital from a nursing home with a necrotic foot ulcer and an extensive sacral decubitus ulcer. Her long-standing kidney insufficiency had required dialysis in the past several months. This treatment did not improve her mental status, as had been hoped. In fact, it worsened, and by the time she was admitted to the hospital she required tube feedings and total nursing care. Her dementia was found to be profound and irreversible. On admission, Ms. V.F. was awake but completely noncommunicative. She showed no signs of pain and her vital signs were stable. Only the grossly necrotic left foot and massive bedsore were remarkable. The internal medicine resident thought that Ms. V.F. would require an above-knee amputation of the leg, debridement of her ulcers, and prolonged antibiotic therapy. Her dialysis would have to continue. Several of the other physicians, including the vascular surgeons, were reluctant to undertake such measures. The patient's daughter, who worked at the nursing home where her mother usually resided, stated that Ms. V.F. had told her many times, "do everything you can for me, honey." The daughter agreed with this plan.

Questions

1. What plausible reasons are there to support the position of the surgeons and other doctors who do *not* want to continue active intervention in Ms. V.F.'s case?
2. What weight should be given to the daughter's claim about her mother's desires for treatment?
3. Must *all* of the treatments suggested by the resident be tried? Considering the best interests of this patient, which might be postponed or rejected? Why?
4. Ms. V.F. cannot speak for herself due to advanced dementia. But suppose that she were a stroke patient with a significant probability for recovery of cognitive function (but presently incompetent). Would this make a difference in your recommendation regarding appropriate care?

Case B

Mrs. O. is a previously healthy and active 82-year-old widow who has enjoyed a full range of family and social activities and has lived independently all of her life. She is diagnosed with lung cancer. The tumor is resected and she is given chemotherapy on an outpatient basis, but this is complicated by pneumonia that requires readmission. The patient presents as dehydrated and somewhat confused; this is thought to be secondary to hypoxia. She is placed on antibiotics and IV fluids. Mrs. O.'s mental status improves rapidly. After regaining alertness she states to the nurse that she does not want to continue with chemotherapy. When the doctor visits she says, "Why can't I just go home and die?" She shows no signs of depression or suicidal ideation, but she does question the cost of care relative to her prognosis. She is told that completion of the chemotherapy will give her a better than 50 percent probability of significant extension of survival. It is likely that she will be able to resume many of her normal activities. (Finances and insurance coverage are not problems.) But her children (two sons and a daughter) tell the staff that, "Mom has always been a fighter. She wouldn't be talking like this if she were herself." They want to have a guardian appointed who will order the treatment that will most likely extend the life of Mrs. O.

Questions

1. Which basic principles can be used in sustaining the desire of this patient to cease chemotherapeutic treatment?

2. Which principles can be utilized to argue for treating her, even though she says she wants to go home and die?
3. The argument that this patient is not herself suggests that her present wishes are clouded, if not by serious mental illness then at least by the dual trauma of having cancer and of being treated for it. Is there a way to hear the voice of Mrs. O.'s ostensible true self, the fighter her children know or remember?
4. As the treating physician in this case, under what circumstances, if any, would you assist the family in guardianship proceedings on behalf of Mrs. O?

■ THINK PIECE: END-OF-LIFE ■

Early in the morning of January 11, 1983 Nancy Cruzan, a woman in her midtwenties, had an auto accident on a country road in rural Missouri. The state trooper who found her, face down, thought she was dead. He did not initiate emergency procedures but did call for aid. When emergency personnel arrived they began CPR and other advanced life support. They did achieve the restoration of Ms. Cruzan's breathing and heartbeat, but her brain was without oxygen for a lengthy period of time and she never regained consciousness. After a brief stay in an acute care hospital, she was transferred to the Missouri Rehabilitation Center, a state hospital. Medical testimony states that she was permanently unconscious without any chance of recovering cognitive or sapient function. In a PVS, Ms. Cruzan was *not* dependent on a mechanical ventilator to help her breathe. She was, however, incapable of feeding herself and was being fed through a gastrostomy tube in order to maintain adequate levels of nutrition and hydration. Her parents petitioned a Missouri court to have her feeding tube removed, recognizing fully that this withdrawal would lead to the patient's death.

Care givers differed in their interpretations of Ms. Cruzan's organic status. All agreed that she had never spoken or given any sign of recognition either verbal or symbolically demonstrable (e.g., no code or system of eye blinking had been established). All agreed that she could not ambulate independently. PVS is a result of overwhelming damage to the cerebral hemispheres. The body retains the capacity to sustain vegetative functions such as respiration and temperature maintenance but the loss of consciousness is regarded as permanent. PVS may follow a variety of insults, including stroke, infections, degenerative disease, poisoning, or as in the case of Ms. Cruzan, head trauma caused by direct physical injury. Approximately 10,000 such patients exist at present in the United States. Recovery is possible in the first few days or weeks following the insult. Many patients also survive unchanged in PVS for months and even years if provided with nutritional and other supportive measures.

PVS is distinguished by chronic wakefulness without awareness and is often accompanied by spontaneous eye opening, unintelligible utterances, instinctive grunts or even smiles, as well as sporadic movements of facial muscles and nonparalyzed limbs. The demeanor of the patient may appear to be alert, though examination and observation show total failure to demonstrate coherent speech, comprehension, or capacity to initiate or make purposeful movements. Reflexes such as withdrawal from noxious or other external stimuli may remain intact. PVS patients do not track with their eyes, though they do demonstrate startle responses to loud noises. These and similar motions are often interpreted as evidence that the patient is aware of the environment. Neurologists and other specialists believe—based on experience with such patients from brain imaging studies—that persons such as Nancy Cruzan are, and always will be, unaware of themselves and their surroundings and have no chance of recovering any measure of cerebral function.

In requesting judicial authorization for the removal of Ms. Cruzan's life-supporting nutritional care, her parents, Joe and Joyce Cruzan, were seeking two kinds of permission. First, they believed that they were the appropriate decision-makers in this medical dilemma. Second, they asserted that they spoke with Nancy Cruzan's voice: They had heard her previously expressed views and her prior statements, witnessed her life and seen the expressions of her values, and participated in her relationships. Therefore they believed that they should be allowed to make health care decisions for her.

The trial court in Missouri affirmed these arguments, but the Missouri Supreme Court in November 1988 held that Ms. Cruzan's guardian's could not exercise her right to refuse treatment for her. The court expressed its concern for "the anguish of these parents," regarding them as "loving parents" condemned to an "indeterminable bedside vigil." But, holding that the debate was not between life and death, but rather between "quality of life and death," the

Missouri Supreme Court balanced patient's rights against the state's interest in preserving life. They ruled that family surrogate decision makers, in the absence of clear and convincing evidence (demonstrated by specific statements that would have anticipated the precise situation in which Ms. Cruzan resides), could not "choose the death of their ward."

During the summer of 1990, the United States Supreme Court ruled that Nancy Cruzan had to stay tethered to the feeding tube that sustained her. The Court held that a state can require "clear and convincing evidence" of an incompetent person's wishes regarding the withdrawal of life-sustaining treatment. In a split decision, the Justices did find a constitutional basis for the "right-to-die" and made no distinctions between feeding and other forms of medical care. But in the case of Ms. Cruzan, a majority held that the state of Missouri may hold those who wish to terminate treatment on behalf of another to a rigorous standard, because (said the Court) erring on the side of life is always preferable. Ms. Cruzan never gave concrete statements about the sorts of care she would accept or reject; she never signed a living will or other advance directive. So she seemed destined to remain in the rehabilitation center.

Later that year, however, her parents returned to the court of origin in Missouri. In a closed hearing the judge heard testimony from witnesses not identified earlier. They testified that Ms. Cruzan had quite specifically given her views and that she would *not* want to be kept alive via tube feeding. The Missouri Attorney General—who earlier had contested the Cruzan family's effort to stop the treatment Ms. Cruzan was receiving—decided that, this time, the state would not resist the petition. The judge then ordered the gastrostomy tube to be removed. Ms. Cruzan died about 10 days later, in December 1990.

Courts, of course, make legal and sometimes constitutional judgments. Rarely do they assuage excruciating personal and familial suffering. The larger question, which could never be answered in legal briefs or determinations, is Who is Nancy Cruzan? Biologically we can describe her situation in clinically useful ways. She was not dead in a medical or legal sense, nor terminally ill. We may add psychosocial elements to our portrait. She was, at the time of her death, a woman more than 30 years old who had been married at the time of her accident (her husband left her and filed for divorce after the accident). Ms. Cruzan was, for many years, in the custody of her parents (as guardians) and was dependent on the state of Missouri for the payment of her medical expenses. Her history could be embellished with many details: She was by all accounts a lively, vivacious, engaging, fun-seeking young woman who expected to live a long life.

Such a portrait only hints at the essence of the Cruzan story. It leaves out the years of family visits, the efforts to talk to Nancy, the gradual recognition by her young nieces that their aunt would never "come back." Beyond the specifics of this landmark Supreme Court case, the questions raised by the *Cruzan* case speak to the essence of ethical dilemmas: How do we know what we do is right, or just? Do we err, as a matter of policy and practice, on the side of life? What does the phrase "quality of life" mean, both for the competent adult and the formerly competent person in the last stages of Alzheimer's disease? If certainty in such matters is a vain hope, how do we muster the courage in less-than-certain decisions? Whose advice and support—not just authority—should we seek in resolving such hard choice dilemmas?

■ VOICES: HOSPICE COUNSELOR/SOCIAL WORKER ■

I see death almost every day. Patients are referred to hospice when all else has failed. They've tried chemo and radiation and surgery. Most of our patients have cancer. The exceptions are a few patients with ALS or end stage heart disease; we've also had several persons with AIDS. Most of them know that they will die very soon, and many of patients are initially quite terrified. I've literally seen many of them shaking. But we do have something unique to offer them. We give them a chance to *choose* the manner in which they will spend their final days. Most patients with a terminal illness lose their autonomy. We try as much as possible to preserve it.

Our team consists of nurses, social workers, home health aides, and, of course, volunteers. Strictly speaking, the decision to enter a hospice program is made by the patient, if he or she is aware. But practically speaking the determination is made by the physician. After the doctor can do no more, the cancer patient is sent to us. Our job is to provide palliative care, and we're quite good at it. We know a lot about pain medication. We're even beginning to teach doctors about the subject.

I do think that in the past 20 years, Americans have become a *little bit* better at discussing death. Cancer is not the fear word it once was.

Perhaps this is due to the reported cures that have come through research or the use of new technology. We don't see that same shudder when what used to be called the "C word" is mentioned. Of course, our patients have reasons to be scared. They know that death is imminent. They are sometimes in great pain. A great deal of this fear is culturally conditioned. Many of our clients come from an Appalachian background. These folks have known death—dying in the mines, for example—and also have a lot of religious faith. For them, it's probably not as scary as it is for our upper middle class patients.

Hospice, as a movement, has certainly grown. There are thousands of them, in big and small cities, across the country. But it's not a program for everyone. Most people think they will never die. It's unimaginable! So they try everything to prolong life. We don't provide any high tech treatment. A hospice patient knows in advance that he or she will not be resuscitated. We don't use IVs very much, and we don't feed patients artificially. Our experience tells us that providing nutrition by IV only causes more pain. And, as I said, we have become quite expert at giving pain medication.

Pain and suffering are complicated. Aside from literal, physical pain, there's much more. There's economic pain: Many of our patients are nearly bankrupt. They've spent a great deal on their cancer treatment. Even those who have insurance have had to pay about 20 percent of the bill. Over the course of years of treatment, that comes to a lot of money. So they are suffering economically. There's also psychological pain—the feelings of dependence and of isolation. We try to treat this kind of pain. That's why having volunteers who really care is an integral part of the hospice program.

I think our greatest strength comes from restoring a sense of control and autonomy to the patient and the family. When you have a cancer patient at home, and he or she and the primary caregiver (who is likely to be a spouse or an adult child) make the decisions about *when* and *how much* medication is going to be given, it is certainly very different from the experience anyone gets in a nursing home or an acute care hospital. The care given by family members, and volunteers, is of a very high quality. The hospice does, of course, have a medical director (actually we have two), but that job involves reviewing patient charts and helping to devise a care plan. The direct, bedside work is done by nonprofessionals with the help of nurses. Hospice is a viable alternative.

Even though I said that the subject of death and dying is a little more public and a bit more honestly discussed these days, I still believe that we have a way to go. Americans believe in the quick fix. We still have fantasies about living forever. All this transplant business is an example. We want to think of ourselves as replaceable parts. Well, it doesn't work that way. Not in the long run. Hospice is really a dose of reality, and a return to an earlier way of life. We believe that death is a natural thing, a part of the life cycle. We want people who are dying to know that they will not be isolated or abandoned.

RECOMMENDED READING

Beauchamp, T. and Perlin, S. (eds.) *Ethical Issues in Death and Dying.* Englewood Cliffs, NJ: Prentice-Hall, 1978.

Cantor, N., *Legal Frontiers of Death and Dying.* Bloomington, IN: Indiana University Press, 1987.

Hastings Center, *Guidelines on the Termination of Life-Sustaining Treatment and the Care of the Dying.* Bloomington, IN: Indiana University Press, 1987.

Lynn, J. (ed.) *By No Extraordinary Means: The Choice to Forgo Food and Water.* Bloomington, IN: Indiana University Press, 1986.

Meisel, A., *The Right to Die.* New York: John Wiley, 1989.

Rachels, J., *The End of Life: The Morality of Euthanasia.* New York: Oxford University Press, 1986.

Weir, R.F. (ed.) *Ethical Issues in Death and Dying,* (2nd ed). New York: Columbia University Press, 1986.

▪9▪

Physicians and Society: Ethics and Professional Responsibility

A baseball player bets against his own team. A stockbroker engages in insider trading. An attorney strikes a plea bargain with a prosecutor without consulting her client. Each illustration seems, intuitively, morally dubious. Why is this so? Though sports figures or even stockbrokers may not be seen as professionals per se, the conflict between role expectation and overt or covert behavior in each situation is obvious. Some sort of standard, explicit or implicit, has been violated. In addition, laws might have been broken. Physicians have obligations that go beyond those of ball players, brokers, and, arguably, lawyers. To be a doctor is to be a professional of a unique sort.

The term *professional* denotes exclusivity, specialized skill or knowledge, and many prerogatives. Professionals are adopted into communities and integrated into roles that are demanding, sometimes rigid, and often exhausting. Becoming a doctor entails education, licensing requirements, and eventually the securing of institutional privileges. It is no easy task. It is fair to ask what professional responsibility demands of physicians.

At a minimum, professionals are assumed to have a formal and specialized body of knowledge and the capacity to use it. Professionals pledge themselves, often formally through oaths (see Appendixes A and B), to social purposes that define a common good. To be a professional is to enjoy prestige and above-average social status. Professionals have traditionally regulated themselves. Teachers are scrutinized by administrators. Physicians are usually evaluated by peers. The authority granted by society for peer review obliges doctors to look carefully at the behaviors and practices of colleagues. Must a doctor who sees a questionable practice by another physician (e.g., driving while intoxicated) become a whistle-blower? Reasonable persons differ on this question.

Physicians are commited to a way of life that is more demanding than most: Doctors work long and hard and must constantly reeducate themselves. Most are available at all hours of the day or night. As servants of the public, they are also evaluated constantly. In a complex era—one in which doctors may have several offices and operate in four or five hospitals—the opportunities for evaluation multiply. The modes of assessment of physicians' professional conduct range from formal mechanisms (e.g., licensure, petitions for hospital privileges, or certification in specialities or subspecialities) to informal assessments (which include reputation among peers and other health care workers, referrals by patients, and invitations by medical societies or professional organizations to seek elected office). When doctors get into trouble, an array of procedures is available to censure them, most of them private and therefore not subject to due process rights, but some of them quite public.

Malpractice lawsuits must be included among the latter. Though many are frivolous and most are unsuccessful, attorneys argue that without the capacity to sue a physician for negligently inflicted damages, patients would suffer unduly (Fig. 9-1). Quasipublic investigations by professional societies or state boards of licensure exist but are rare. For example, the New York State Health Department's Board of Professional Medical Conduct, a three-member panel whose task is physician discipline, investigated the role of a doctor who

---

Liability for malpractice occurs when all of the following four elements of negligence have transpired in a medical/clinical setting:

DUTY: The clinician has a legal duty to the patient or client as a consequence of an established relationship.

BREACH: The clinician has breached (broken or violated) that legal duty.

DAMAGES: The patient or client has sustained legally recoverable damages.

CAUSATION: The breach of legal duty has directly caused the damages.

Fig. 9-1. Medical Malpractice: Basic Elements

admitted helping a suffering leukemia patient commit suicide. The panel concluded unanimously that no misconduct had taken place.

Most assessments are private, at least at first, and are peer-based. For example, if a practitioner feels that a colleague is advertising unfairly, a complaint can be filed with the local academy of medicine's or medical society's judicial or ethics committee. Were a physician to be suspected of practicing in an impaired condition— substance abuse is the most common charge—peers within the institution or a local professional group would likely investigate initially.

Some physician duties are mandated by law. A doctor who treats a gunshot wound in the ER is obliged to notify the police. Child abuse statutes in all 50 states require physicians to report suspected violations to the state, county, or municipal child protective service agency. Failure to report can result in misdemeanor charges being brought against the doctor. In recent years, the doctor who sees a patient who threatens the life of another may be obliged, even while violating confidentiality, to warn the potential victim and to notify the police (see Chapter 7).

While rules and regulations are important, physician responsibility is assumed to be more than a legalistic obedience to government authority. Doctors are *supposed* to be ethical, fair, honest, just, and consistent. Practitioners who are sexist, racist, or who express contempt for the beliefs of others are morally suspect. In addition, doctors are *expected* to contribute to public needs. Just as attorneys are supposed to provide (sometimes involuntarily) a certain amount of free labor for those who cannot afford a lawyer (i.e., pro bono work), doctors are usually called on to give some time to those in need. Such expectations are not mandated by legal or professional requirements, though some officials have asked that a minimal number of hours be designated as appropriate for voluntary contributions of time by doctors.

Finally, the manner in which physicians make money is a subject of debate and discussion in the area of professional responsibility. Entrepreneurship (e.g., physician investment in diagnostic and therapeutic facilities to which patients are routinely referred) has grown dramatically in recent years. Thus, conflict of interest concerns have emerged, stimulated in part by critics outside the field of medicine, but faced quite conscientiously by official bodies of practitioners, such as the American Medical Association. While no one has argued that doctors ought to be poor, the fact that medical professionals as a group are among the wealthiest in our society (there are significant variations between primary care doctors and specialists) has made physicians a target, fairly or not, when matters of personal finance are under scrutiny.

■ FIVE ESSENTIAL CASES ■

Case 9-1

In the medical profession there are practitioners who behave outside of the mainstream of practice. What is the obligation of a peer when he or she sees "eccentric" intervention that may be dangerous to patients? Is whistle-blowing the answer?

Dr. D. is a young family physician, in practice with a somewhat older and more experienced partner, Dr. G. Their office practice treats a wide age range and they pride themselves on paying personal attention to patient needs; both have admitting and treating privileges in R. Hospital, a suburban institution with 310 beds. Dr. D. cares for pregnant women unless apparent complications require consultation or referral and delivers three or four babies each month. She enjoys the obstetric and gynecologic elements of her practice, in part because as a family physician she can often see the wider context of individual patient needs.

Twice in recent months new patients have come for examinations with unusual gynecologic complaints. Both had children delivered at R. Hospital by Dr. J., an obstetrician-gynecologist with a large local practice. Each is now suffering considerable vaginal pain. On examination Dr. D. notes evidence of extraordinary surgical procedures. Both women seem to have had their sexual organs modified—the wall between vagina and rectum is notably thickened, the lower part of the outer lips of the vulva is sewn together. The women say that Dr. J. told them that he had "reconstructed a bit" during the course of the episiotomy and that "they would find that during sex their response would be much better than before." Dr. D. discovered that neither patient had given advance consent to the surgical procedures. Both say that they are now physicially uncomfortable much of the time. They ask Dr. D. for a recommendation.

When Dr. D. mentions the problems to her partner, Dr. G., he notes that Dr. J. has "been in business a long time. He thinks these operations will enhance the sex lives of his patients. A few of us at the hospital have told him we think it's a bit strange, but there's not much we can do about it. After all, surgeries don't require F.D.A. approval."

■ ■ ■

The extent of obligation to get involved needs clarification. The law, particularly in criminal courts, often makes a distinction between *commission and omission*. If you strangle an innocent person you are guilty of murder (i.e., commission). But if you notice a stranger drowning and fail to rescue him or her, you are unlikely to be convicted (i.e., omission). In medical practice, perpetrating a dangerous or heinous act (e.g., injecting potassium chloride into the veins of nursing home patients with the intention of killing them) will be legally and morally prohibited. But specific requirements of discovering, confronting, or reporting questionable practices are hard to codify, and the politics of everyday practice is complicating.

Dr. D. is clearly innocent of any wrong-doing in her own practice, but she is clearly perturbed by Dr. J.'s treatment of patients and her partner is certainly not encouraging her to pursue the matter. Suspicion of serious wrongdoing, which Dr. D. infers through her patients' presentations and statements, is worrisome: Does it require action? If Dr. D. stops to ponder, she may recognize two related things: (1) Her two patients are surely not the only women harmed by Dr. J.; (2) to press forward with an investigation and report may place *her* in a vulnerable position. Physicians charged with providing controversial therapies have been known to sue whistle-blowers. Both keeping quiet *and* going forward carry risks.

From the patient-care viewpoint, Dr. D. has many options. *Beneficence* requires her to help these women and to try to relieve their pain. Does this demand a strict accounting of past medical practices? Or should Dr. D. refer them to a surgeon who might try to correct Dr. J.'s "work"? Is *autonomy* retrospectively applicable? It seems that Dr. J. has ignored all the requirements of voluntary informed consent. But does Dr. D. have to compensate for that past failure? From a medical-scientific perspective, Dr. J.'s reasons for performing these "eccentric" surgeries *do* have a rationale: To provide increased sexual pleasure.

The principle of *veracity* is crucial here. Dr. J. may have hidden or shaded the truth about his obstetric and gynecologic practices. Can

Dr. D. look the other way; can she avoid any effort to pursue this other doctor? If she remains silent and other practitioners bring charges, what will her position be? The professional in medicine, law, and accounting often relies on peer review to monitor performance. In hospitals this is routinely done by committees with the power to sanction, suspend, or retract privileges. Within the community, the medical society (a voluntary association without legal authority) can bring pressure on nonconforming practitioners. The state medical board can revoke or, less punitively, restrict a doctor's license. If Dr. D. says nothing, it cannot be for lack of a suitable forum for further action.

The precedent value of a decision to blow the whistle is also important. If in a given city or county every doctor aware of Dr. J.'s practices "sat on" the case, a culture of silence would be maintained. But if it became more common, though certainly not routine, for doctors to report on one another, a culture of suspiciousness and conspiracy might develop. Finding a truthful, supportive, and secure environment for dealing with such cases is the obvious goal. For though doctors make errors, in this instance we are not talking about "mere" negligence. Dr. J. is acting intentionally and repeatedly.

Numerous cases of physicians, including psychiatrists, having sexual relationships with their current patients have come to light. Often there were multiple cases with the same doctor. Doctors who abuse their prescribing privileges have been found guilty of providing illicit drugs for patients. Supposing that colleagues had been aware of these practices—would we urge them to come forward then? It would certainly be hard to find an argument for ignoring such practices.

What might it take for a physician in Dr. D.'s position to take on Dr. J.? Certainly it would require a belief in values, a capacity to reflect, and a sense of responsibility to the community as a whole. These phrases need substance in order to motivate action. Dr. D. will have to have courage. Should she decide to act, there are many ways to proceed. Should she confront Dr. J. directly? Should she consult with other doctors, with the group of OB/GYNs at her hospital, with the institution's department of risk management? Each strategy carries with it risks and possibilities. From a utilitarian viewpoint, Dr. D. can weigh the possible benefits and costs. Deontologically, she cannot avoid confronting the professional duty to ask "Can I look away when obvious harm is being perpetrated by a peer?" If her answer is "No," then this physician has a necessary, though very burdensome job before her.

Case 9-2

The law in some jurisdictions makes a physician's duty to report activity once deemed private mandatory. Investigating behaviors within families and outside the literal purview of the doctor may place the physician in a difficult role.

Dr. V., a pediatrician at a children's hospital, has been caring for Cara M. since her birth 7 years ago. Cara was born with meningomyelocele. The lesion was not terribly high, but Cara will never walk without assistance and is presently using a wheelchair; she requires assistance with many of her activities in daily living. There were no other complications (e.g., no hydrocephalus requiring a shunt), and Cara's mental capacity seems age-appropriate. She is a demanding child, however, and her frequent frustration has been noted by family members and school personnel. She has been mainstreamed and is presently in the first grade.

The M. family consists of the mother, N. M. (age 27) and 3-year-old Sean. N. M. has a live-in boyfriend, R. F., who works in a nearby paint factory. He has been in the home for 2 years and is the parent of neither child. Dr. V. has never seen this man, though she has heard from the mother that he is a "good guy who contributes half of his pay check every week." The family lives in a trailer in a rural area about 30 miles from the hospital where Cara was born. Dr. V. sees Cara at the outpatient clinic about every 2 months.

On a recent visit, Dr. V. noticed that Cara had a small cut and some bruising on her left cheek. When Cara was asked, in the examining room with her mother present, what had happened, she remained silent. N. M. said that Cara had fallen while being helped from the wheelchair to the couch. Dr. V., in previous visits, had thought Cara to be quite an engaging and conversational child. Today, however, she seems subdued and withdrawn. When the physician asks the mother if Cara's mood is unusual, N. M. says "No! She's like that a lot." Inquiring about life at home, Dr. V. asks about the boyfriend, R. F. "He's doing all right," N. M. says. "Sometimes he gets a little rowdy on Friday nights after being out with the guys." Dr. V. wonders how to pursue the possibility that Cara has been physically abused.

Child abuse has a broad range of definitions and descriptions. At one end of the spectrum is nonaccidental physical assault and injury; at the other is verbal insult. The term *battered child*—sometimes used as euphemism for child abuse—was coined to portray children who, for example, had been burned by cigarettes by their adult caregivers. Child abuse occurs millions of times each year if we include *neglect*—situations in which there are deprivations of basic needs and denial of opportunities for physical and psychological development—in this category. Abuse should not be minimized: It is estimated that more than 1000 children die each year due to maltreatment. Causes proferred include adult substance abuse; burn-out and stress of parenting; the culture of poverty; sexual depravity; and psychological maladjustment. Some have gone further and argue that an abusing adult is suffering from a distinctive *disease* that is multigenerational, though treatable.

Just who is Dr. V's patient? The clear focus of attention by this physician is naturally on Cara. Concern for Cara's mother and sibling also is not unusual. Children with disabilities who live at home present unusual challenges, and inquiry about family matters is routine. R.F.'s role is somewhat problematic, but not unique. Can Dr. V. intervene in this case because of an authentic concern for family coherence? At the surface, perhaps so. But how hard and how far she digs *and* what the law and sound pediatric practice require of her will likely be a product of worrying about the child.

Physicians are mandated to notify a state social service agency when *any* case of suspected child abuse or neglect is found. Doctors are expected to do so on the basis of a physical examination and diagnosis. In situations in which sexual abuse is suspected, clinical signs may be apparent. But in cases like Cara's, the physical manifestations are historical and "explained." Diagnosis is much more difficult and there is no present treatment required: The abrasions are healing. If Dr. V. looks into the family dynamic more deeply, value assumptions may either clarify or impede her findings. The fact that the family does not fit the image of middle-class stability may lead the physician to be *unduly* suspicious. In fact, children of all races, sexes, religions, and economic classes can be victims of abuse and neglect. Poverty is no guarantor of guilt. Dr. V. must stay objective about family status.

If Dr. V. does report suspicion of child abuse, she can expect dramatic and swift consequences. An investigation by a child protective services agency will begin. The child may be removed, at least temporarily, from the household and placed into foster care, itself often a problematic course. If there is evidence of parental substance abuse, other enforcement agencies may be brought in. Initiating a report—which is required under varying circumstances of doctors, nurses, social workers, teachers, child care workers, and others—is a very serious act.

Dr. V.'s next step is crucial. Can she form an alliance with Cara's mother? Can she create a climate of trust and inquire discreetly about the child's "accident" and other possible occurrences? If she wants to see Cara again, how long is an appropriate interval? Should a home visit be offered? Clearly the right to privacy of the mother and her boyfriend requires some weight. Does the community's interest in protecting children always trump suspicious parental behaviors? In a few communities, teams of social service workers, police authorities, prosecuting attorneys, mental health specialists, and forensic examiners are available for consultation. Still, Dr. V. must take the first step if the process of investigation is to commence.

The fact that Cara is a chronic patient who has survived a serious and debilitating birth defect adds a paradoxical dimension to this case. During the past several decades, new interventions and technologies have allowed children with such conditions to survive into their adult years and beyond. The stresses placed on families in caring for such children are not relieved by a comprehensive system of financial, psychological, and social support, though there are agencies and clinics that can help. Dysfunctions such as alcoholism, drug abuse, and child abuse are found more and more in families in which "medical miracles" at birth have yielded children with chronic needs.

Case 9-3

Relationships between physicians and other health care professionals can involve controversies about fairness and justice as well as prejudice. Issues of race, gender, class, and belief-systems might be the focus of conflict.

A prominent surgeon working at C. Hospital, Dr. I. is well-known for his decisiveness, his surgical skill, and his temper. He admits, "I do not suffer fools gladly!" Many medical students and nurses have been brought to tears by his insults in the operating room. Dr. I.'s language is quite "colorful." When questioned about such remarks or behavior, Dr. I. usually states, "It's really not personal; it's a tension reliever. Besides, my criticism is fair. How are these incompetents going to learn unless I give them immediate feedback?" Dr. I. brings a great deal of business into the hospital. He has never been sued successfully for negligence or malpractice. He is regarded as a leading researcher into new surgical techniques and is widely published.

During a recent cancer surgery, Dr. I. referred to the patient, an African-American male aged 44 who was under anaesthesia, as a "monkey." His actual words were, "Does anyone know if this monkey was a smoker?" Ms. R., an African-American surgical nurse, took issue. "You shouldn't refer to a patient that way," she stated. Dr. I., never looking up from the operating table but clearly aware of the identity of the nurse, said, "What the hell's the matter with you colored girls? Can't you take a joke? I'm not going to put up with your crap!" Ms. R. was embarrassed but remained in the operating room. After Dr. I. left—allowing the surgical resident to close and clean up—the nurse stated, "That man is a racist and I don't intend to hear any more of that stuff!"

Is the scene portrayed in this case business as usual or an incident involving racial and sexual discrimination? Our response varies with our understanding of the hierarchic nature of the health care system. In particular, the changing relationship between nurses and physicians influences our assessment. While *words* alone are important— and Dr. I.'s expressions were directed to a patient and an operating room worker—milieu is also significant, not to explain *away* but to set the problem into a realistic context.

Tension relief in surgery is part of a long-standing "cultural" tradition—it includes the playing of music; "horsing around"; teasing and name calling; and, occasionally, statements about patients that they would not want to hear. This kind of conduct, while not epitomizing standards of professional decorum, is quasiprivate (it is meant for a select, invited audience). Are there limits to the rhetoric and behavior normally encountered in the OR? A *clear* violation of cultural norms would be, for example, physical assault on a nurse, resident, or medical student. Are words and phrases "protected speech"?

Two or three decades ago, doctor-nurse relationships were based on an unwritten covenant: Open expressions of disagreement were almost unheard of. Nurses who had complaints—unless they were terribly serious—remained silent. Nearly all physicians were men;

virtually every nurse was a woman. In an era in which women in general were socialized to behave in a subservient manner, nurses learned in nursing school and on the job to avoid even the appearance of questioning or defying physician authority. Had Dr. I. made his comments at that time, we can be sure that Ms. R. would *not* have spoken out and vowed to take action.

In the present era, the rules of the game have changed. As female professionals, Ms. R.'s colleagues work in a milieu of increasing wages, greater responsibility, and stronger group solidarity. Nurses are regarded as a "valuable" resource (perhaps because there is a nursing shortage); doctors are often female; federal, state, and local laws and institutional policies prohibit, with varying sanctions, racial and sexual discrimination; and procedures generally exist for pursuing job-related conflicts. The physician as deity is a distant memory (or at least a fading image). Nurses are regarded as fully qualified professionals, often highly educated, with specialized training, and part of the health-care team. Today, Ms. R. has the opportunity to go forward with her complaint. Should she? How should her coworkers respond? What, in fact, is Dr. I.'s responsibility in this case and how should his behavior and remarks be handled?

Part of the context of the case is also racial. African-Americans of all income levels lack access to the finest aspects of the health care system. They are sicker, die younger, receive fewer preventive services, and in specific kinds of interventions (e.g., kidney transplant) may suffer racial discrimination in the allocation of scarce resources. Surveys show that African-Americans are less satisfied than other groups with the care they get when in the hospital and feel that physicians treat them less respectfully than they treat others. While we cannot ascribe these specific concerns to Ms. R., we can assume that her reaction to Dr. I.'s nasty remarks about the patient was to take them personally.

Does Dr. I. deserve to be confronted and, if necessary, reported for his statements? His own earlier explanation—that he sees it as his job to be a critic in the OR—has a certain rationale. Does it justify this kind of discourse? Were his words clearly racist and sexist? Did his comment about the patient issue from personal contempt or a vain effort at humor? Did his reference to Ms. R. demonstrate insensitivity, harassment, or just the assertion of the surgeon's prerogative to run the show in the OR? One thing is certain, we will not learn the answers to any of these quite complex questions *unless* Ms. R., or a witness to the incident, takes conscientious action.

Let us speculate that one or more of the OR staff offered support to the nurse. Ms. R. would be likely to speak with her own supervisor. A decision would be entertained: Should the offended nurse speak directly to the surgeon? Or should the nurse-manager ask for a meeting with Dr. I. or should she, instead, speak to the chair of the department of surgery or even to the chief of staff? Should the hospital's offices of affirmative action or personnel be notified? Does a lawyer need to be consulted? Suddenly, the prospects of a serious confrontation seem increased. What will Dr. I.'s response be?

If nurses have an obligation to speak out on issues of racism, sexism, or class, what are the responsibilities of doctors? Not much attention is given in medical education to concerns about cultural and gender difference. Can one be a competently educated medical professional without mastering a body of knowledge about such differences? In the realm of patient care, understanding the psycho-social elements of a case is given lip service at least. Can a doctor know a patient solely through a symptoms list? Is it too much to ask that doctors confront their own values on issues of race, class, and gender? No matter what Dr. I.'s response, is there a useful method of helping the next generation of surgeons and other physicians learn to speak of patients and team members with respect and dignity?

Case 9-4

Physician impairment denotes the inability to provide medical care with skill, safety, and efficiency due to mental or physical incapacity. When a doctor appears to be incompetent due to such causes, the obligations of professional colleagues to report are not easy to fulfill.

A psychiatrist in private practice with admitting privileges to a general hospital, Dr. S. has admitted to his colleagues that he is overworked and fatigued. "I feel like I have six jobs," he says, "and I have no choice. I've got two kids in Ivy League schools and the tuition alone is stupendous." A friend and colleague, Dr. K., has observed that at parties Dr. S. drinks excessively and often must be driven home by his spouse. On hospital rounds Dr. S. seems competent enough, though lately he has been forgetting details about patient medication levels; a swift check of the chart has usually been enough to refresh his memory. A unit nurse mentions these lapses to Dr. K.

One morning, while sitting in the physician lounge, Dr. K. is joined by Dr. S. She notes the clear aroma of alcohol. "Were you out late last night?" she asks Dr. S. "No," he says, "actually I fell asleep in front of the T.V. at about 10:30. I'm really tired these days." Dr. K. is certain that her colleague has been using alcohol this morning: When he arises, she observes an uneven gait. As. Dr. S. starts to leave the lounge he looks back at Dr. K. and whispers, "I can see you're worried about me. Don't be! I can handle it. This is surely no worse than med school. I'll rest this afternoon. I have five patients in a row in the office. I can nap a little then!" He walks away, laughing softly.

■ ■ ■

The cause of a physician's impairment influences the responses by colleagues. If a neurosurgeon is losing his eyesight due to inoperable or untreatable cataracts, gentle persuasion and supportive counseling with the goal of retirement from tasks that require visual acuity are in order. But if the doctor is drug dependent or a heavy drinker who denies substance abuse, steps to be taken by an aware colleague are not so easy to pursue. What we call a physician in Dr. S.'s situation (and let us *assume* for the purposes of this case analysis that he *is* abusing alcohol but that Dr. K. is unsure of this) is relevant. Is he a disabled physician, a distressed or burned out doctor, a substance abuser or a functioning alcoholic?

If Dr. S. is suffering from a disease (both the American Medical Association and the American Psychiatric Association regard regular and recurrent use of psychoactive substances, including alcohol, as a disease or disorder) then treatment and a cure must be the goal. But just how physicians are to identify impaired colleagues and help them remains less than clear. The problem has wide scope: The AMA estimates that as many as ten percent of all practicing doctors are impaired. (It should be noted that levels of impairment and alcoholism are probably no different among lawyers, pharmacists, and clinical psychologists.) Still, detection remains difficult, because impairment from alcohol usually has a gradual onset, can be concealed from colleagues, and is a problem often denied; treatment is frequently resisted by physicians.

For Dr. K., it will be psychologically difficult to follow up on her concerns. She will not want to appear tactless; she will need to search hard for the exact words to use in this patent invasion of Dr. S.'s privacy. Dr. K. may be afraid that if she mentions her observations to others, she will appear malicious. Still, most hospitals have a well-publicized policy that imposes a duty on staff to report another's suspected impairment. Peer review is a powerful symbol of professional authority; it also carries an obligation to maintain high standards, particularly if the quality of patient care is in jeopardy. (Sometimes, such peer review responsibilities carry immunity from civil suits, an added incentive for colleagues to report.)

Doctors do talk with one another about colleagues' problems. ("Dr. X. is really falling apart," one may hear. "He needs a rest. I hope he can handle his practice. Let's hope he gets some help.") Taking action in a case like Dr. S.'s requires courage and support. Remaining quiet has the effect of *enabling* or covering up Dr. S.'s behavior. The common excuses—"How can I rat on him"; or "There but for the grace of God go I"; or "This will ruin his practice and his family"—are often stated. There are sometimes answers—physicians who are reported do not always have their licenses removed or restricted. A colleague who cannot confront an impaired colleague directly may be able to report indirectly to a committee or a medical staff official. But the goal remains the same: trying to help a physician in trouble.

Dr. K. can take a variety of steps. Underlying her determination must be a concern for the profession. If doctors are seen as looking away when other physicians practice medicine inadequately, the profession as a whole is legitimately vulnerable. Not only patient care is at issue in this case. No matter what Dr. S.'s response to further inquiry—and he is as likely to be receptive to advice as he is to be hostile to offers of assistance—the obligation of a colleague is tripartite: to patients, to the physician needing aid, and to the public as a whole.

Case 9-5

The physician as advocate is a real, though not always acknowledged, role. At times the desire to be there for an ill person may conflict with the legal and ethical obligation to conform to social and institutional rules and regulations.

Dr. L., a primary care physician with a large geriatric clientele, has been caring for an elderly patient, Mrs. U., for 3 years. She is a Medicare recipient and has no supplemental insurance or other significant means for paying medical bills. She suffers from diabetes and has high blood pressure. She has fainted twice in the past week. Though her heart seems quite normal, her breath sounds are a bit unusual. Dr. L. has her admitted to the hospital. He knows that if his grounds for admitting her are listed correctly, per the diagnosis related group (DRG) stipulations, she will have only a few days reimbursable by Medicare. He believes that this patient needs some time to rest, to be away from the demands of her large and still-dependent family, and to "get on her feet again."

The physician also knows, from long experience, that listing heart failure as an admitting diagnosis instead of clinical investigations of hypertension and diabetes, will allow Mrs. U. to remain with reimbursement for a significantly longer period of time. His notes in her chart (he intends to visit her daily) can easily reflect this tentative diagnosis. He knows that the utilization review people will not bother him. Dr. L. examines his own conscience and feels O.K. He says to himself that he will not profit from this slight alteration of the DRG; he will not send a bill to the patient for any of his own services; her best interest is his motivation.

Serving several masters is burdensome. Doctors rarely bring to the surface the role conflicts that caring for patients and serving the wider community engender. Some role separations are handled routinely, aided by legal authority and conventional practice: Reporting to the health department that a patient has a sexually transmitted disease (STD) speaks to the balancing act between concern for private interests and public order. In the STD situation, at least doctors can feel they are doing some good by preventing the spread of a virulent disease.

More patently conflictual are cases in which physicians feel they must *violate* an ethical standard in order to sustain another. If routine screening mammograms are not reimbursed by an insurance company, and the doctor feels that the patient cannot pay for the investigation on her own, the physician can write suspected cyst/tumor in order to secure third-party payment. Strict veracity can be sacrificed for beneficence. This is the short-run story. "It all worked out," the doctor may say, "She had the mammogram; the results were negative. Nobody was harmed."

In an era of cost control, do physicians have a greater responsibility to act honestly, even if patients may suffer consequently? Dr. L. faces this in a spirit of reflection, not overt defiance. In exaggerating Mrs. U.'s tentative diagnosis so that she can spend needed time in the hospital, Dr. L. is indeed being faithful to his patient. If he were asked about the diagnosis, could Dr. L. say in conscience that her pulmonary status was suggestive of heart failure? If he made this claim, would other physicians back him up? Probably not. He hopes, in fact, that he will not be challenged. This is an overt indicator not of a guilty conscience but of a desire to move Mrs. U. through the system with a minimum of obstacles.

Underpinning this situation is a rule-bound, highly bureaucratized, and very restrictive health care system. The use of technology obliges physicians to be aware not only of scientific data and clinical developments but also of cost-effectiveness and the risks and benefits of ever more sophisticated procedures. In the gatekeeper role it is a doctor's duty to do what is best for a patient; this includes not only accurate diagnosis but, for the primary care doctor, careful recommendations for specialized treatment and detailed follow-up. Does it also mean that Dr. L. must find a way to "slip" Mrs. U. through the regulations in order to do what he feels is best for her health?

The fact that this is a Medicare patient is of some significance. Providing a limited hospital stay and then allowing her to rest in a nursing home is not usually reimbursable. In another country's system, all such services would be guaranteed; no money would change hands. But in a system in which millions of people lack even basic coverage and the elderly pay higher and higher premiums for their health care benefits, Dr. L. seems to be in the position of medical economics decision-maker. DRG rules do not take into account individual differences and most often ignore the psychological or social needs of the patient. Doctors have little time to examine insurance coverages when seeing a patient in the office. Business managers are expected to help make appropriate arrangements. This goal is not always achieved.

In Mrs. U.'s situation, Dr. L. sees only gain and little harm coming from his efforts. This is true unless a much wider horizon is analyzed. If what Dr. L. is doing is indeed lying, then more general questions about physician veracity must be discussed. If Dr. L. is willing to lie for the patient, will this lead to other duplicitous acts less noble in their motivation? If hospital space and staff time are precious commodities, is Dr. L. not wasting resources in keeping Mrs. U.

days longer than others might want? And if physicians in general see themselves as "secret agents" working within the system but pledged to fidelity to patients alone, what does this say about their integrity?

Dr. L.'s solution to the problem appears pragmatic. Oddly enough, if it works all the time, health care costs will rise even faster and the next generation may find their access more restricted. Can busy practicing physicians always keep in mind such issues that are, by and large, beyond their control and still feel as if they are practicing medicine in the traditional mode? Must economics deteriorate the historically sacrosanct doctor-patient relationship? Where does the border between beneficence for Mrs. U. end and the territory of justice for all persons in need begin?

■ PRACTICE MODEL CASE ■

Dr. Foster is a board-certified ER physician in a tertiary care hospital's trauma center with 5 years of postresidency experience. He is also HIV positive. Dr. Foster believes that he was infected about 1 year ago by a needle stick. He admits to anger about this on-the-job exposure. He has known his HIV status for 8 months and has told his wife (and has pledged her to absolute secrecy) but not his two preteen children. His physician has put him on AZT prophylactically. Dr. Foster remains completely physically asymptomatic, but he is very worried, particularly because recent policy shifts from the Centers for Disease Control, the American Medical Association, and his own hospital (others may be legislated soon) have said that he must make his AIDS-infected status public. Dr. Foster believes that the mandate to reveal is unwarranted because the risk of his infecting a patient is insignificant. He also feels that to come forward, either by restricting his practice or by notifying potential patients, would end his career.

The guidelines state that infected physicians or other health care workers should cease performing invasive procedures *or* inform their patients. Dr. Foster feels that the scientific literature does not yield what he considers a political conclusion. There are virtually no documented cases of health care workers who have taken careful precautions infecting their patients. The few sensationalized illustrations have created a panic Dr. Foster believes. He does not want to sacrifice his professional life to a climate of panic and antagonism.

Dr. Foster has heard of other physicians who have conformed to the recommendations. Their patients have been panicked or outraged; the doctors have been barred from hospital practice or employment or have been shifted to meaningless busy work. He also fears a lawsuit if a patient who is now HIV positive or has AIDS ascribes the infection to his prior treatment by Dr. Foster. Adding to Dr. Foster's grievance is his supposition that *he* was infected *by* an ER patient. He realizes that there are many thousands of health care workers who are HIV positive, from a variety of possible causes. But he also knows that the greater danger comes not *from* doctors but *to* them (and nurses). He has heard murmurs about policies and procedures being developed to protect persons in his situation, but he has seen no action taken.

Dr. Foster is proceeding cautiously. He is certainly attentive to precautions in the ER, but he is still performing invasive procedures; that is part of his job. He has never refused to provide care to patients in high-risk categories (in his ER many drug abusers who share needles are seen); nor does he feel that his own reluctance to make his condition known is irrational. "I am not going to be a scapegoat," he tells his spouse. "I know that I am not going to live a normal lifespan. But I am going to keep going as long as possible."

Patient

We know very little about Dr. Foster except for our sense that he is isolated, angry, and seemingly definitive in his attitudes. Assuming that he was infected during the course of his ER duties and that he is exercising precautions not only at work but in his sexual relationship(s), we would still like to know much more. What did he know as he entered his residency program in emergency medicine about the risks of infection from the AIDS virus? What have been his attitudes toward patients and colleagues who have turned out to be infected? What kind of continuing medical education did Dr. Foster receive regarding AIDS? These questions matter for a single reason. The issue Dr. Foster is raising is singular: Does a physician have the right of what we might call conscientious objection when it comes to standards of care and behavior mandated by medical and legal authorities? Dr. Foster's information and, more important, his value base regarding AIDS will figure in our assessment of this question.

Without regard to Dr. Foster's specific situation, we can project a difficult future for him. He will become symptomatic, certainly within a few years. He will probably die prior to his natural lifespan. Dr. Foster can hide his situation for a limited period of time. When his status *is* revealed (and it could be posthumously), many will ask: "Why are we only finding this out now?" At the moment, Dr. Foster is acting with reason. But among the virulent symptoms he faces is AIDS encephalopathy. Will dementia have an impact on the kinds of questions he is introspectively raising right now? Psychosocially, one can only wish for a chance to hear Mrs. Foster's perspective. For she will be a part of this unfolding saga as well.

Relationships

Were we able to confer with the spouse—and we must remind ourselves that Dr. Foster has made her promise to remain silent—we would have access to hidden concerns. What are her fears? Has she been tested? Will she initiate testing? What are the couple's concerns about their children? Mrs. Foster might be able to elaborate on Dr. Foster's anxieties about social abandonment. She might also be able to confirm Dr. Foster's sense of his own injury and pain.

Other questions abound. What kind of relationship does Dr. Foster have with his physician; what kind of advice, if any, if he receiving? Does he have any person who could provide a confidential hearing? Dr. Foster knows that the risks of even a casual and seemingly innocuous conversation could be great. Though the AMA has told its members for several years that seropositive physicians or those with AIDS should consult colleagues or committees specially appointed for the task about finding risk-minimal activities, Dr. Foster has defied this admonition. His relationships, including ones that could be helpful, are almost nonexistent.

Advocacy

The definition of this situation *seems* to preclude finding someone or some group who can advocate for Dr. Foster. Such organizations do exist—in San Francisco there is a Medical Expertise Retention Program; in other cities medical societies are also acting on behalf of infected physicians—but Dr. Foster is not pursuing them. Dr. Foster can be fairly certain that other practitioners are similarly troubled, but he feels he cannot openly know them, or contact them. A lawyer (who would be pledged to confidentiality) might be useful for Dr. Foster. The attorney could acquaint the physician with the status of antidiscrimination legislation and court rulings, but only Dr. Foster can decide whether or not to reveal his HIV status.

It is the tension between private needs and public responsibility that makes this case so agonizing. We cannot, therefore, forget the public's perspective, even if such a thing is an agglomeration of real and perceived views. Bluntly put, does the next wave of Dr. Foster's patients have a right to know his HIV status? What details, if any, are patients entitled to know? Do we inform patients that their doctors are enrolled in impaired physician programs due to alcohol abuse? (See Case 9-4 above.) The most literal reading of the doctrine of informed consent would seem to say "Yes." Risks and benefits must be described to patients before procedures are initiated, but Dr. Foster's case departs from the norm for two reasons: (1) in emergencies informed consent is almost always suspended; (2) minimal risks need not be disclosed to a patient if they are routine. Dr. Foster thinks his risk of infecting another person is about zero.

Is there a moral obligation to reveal his HIV status? If so, who will advocate it? The professional societies who have asked their members to either limit their practices or tell their patients are not investigative bodies. Will hospitals make privileges conditional on frequent testing? How far will the balance of privacy versus public responsibility tip in the name of advocating for the potential patient's right to know a physician's physical condition?

Conflicts

There is an internal and external conflict in this case. Dr. Foster must wrestle with self-interest, conscience, and professional identity as he confronts his choices. This separation of concerns into three realms is somewhat artificial because all overlap. For example, as a professional Dr. Foster might see his determination to maintain secrecy as *affirming* the medical profession's true needs: to keep conscientious doctors working in ERs and to resist pandering to public outcries. To assume that Dr. Foster's internal dialogue is some sort of rational Platonic discourse is also naive; there is a deep emotional underlayer to this conflict. That this physician has to face this psychological burden almost alone is tragic, no matter what the outcome.

The external conflict at this stage pits Dr. Foster's need for career survival against a social justification for providing very private information to the public. The widespread nature of such a revelation must be emphasized. Even if Dr. Foster were to obey guidelines and tell patients about his status, such information would immediately become public knowledge. Media attention would be considerable and possibly flamboyant. Lest this conflict sound like a David and Goliath battle, we should recall that there are forces in the community who would aid Dr. Foster (e.g., civil liberties attorneys). But most of the armaments in any battle would remain in the hands of the authorities.

Treatment or Nontreatment Options

The issue of health care for Dr. Foster has been minimized thus far. The larger issue of physician responsibility versus individual conscience should not obscure the fact that this doctor will need comprehensive medical care. By comprehensive we include psychosocial and possibly economic care. Dr. Foster remains a competent, fully functional physician, but down the road he will become, if not impaired, at least ill.

Obligations need to be mutual. What does the hospital owe an employee such as Dr. Foster? When his status becomes known should the hospital do more than just transfer him to nonpatient care duties? Will it provide counseling? If he must resign for health reasons will it continue his health care insurance? Will the hospital treat Dr. Foster in its own clinics, for free if necessary? Beyond providing material benefits, what sort of atmosphere will Dr. Foster face? Will it be suspicious or contemptuous? When full-blown AIDS is developed, will Dr. Foster be a typical or atypical patient?

Interests

While we may have emphasized that Dr. Foster's integrity is in conflict with the public's alleged need to know, this is *not* a clear-cut case of self-interest versus public interest. Medicine as a whole has a stake in this case because it involves the examination of some central professional values. Doctors are supposed to be compassionate, loyal, and fair. The virtual monopoly they enjoy as professionals enjoins them to serve the sick in a nondiscriminatory fashion. Physicians are also obliged to guide their actions through reference to scientific and epidemiologic data and interpretation. Dr. Foster's silent stand flies in the face of the profession's definitive guidelines.

Does medicine have an interest in supporting or at least tolerating the idiosyncratic physician who is acting in conscience? Is there a role for the gadfly? These questions are eminently political, but so is the structure of power in contemporary health care. Must Dr. Foster, were he to decide to confront the authorities, become a martyr? Or is there room in the debate for dialogue about unexamined premises? Does Dr. Foster's view that the scientific data about physician transmission to patients is so lacking in foundation that it cannot form the basis for a policy deserve respect? Does his anecdotal but still real claim that telling patients he is HIV positive can harm them by raising their anxiety needlessly make any sense? The opportunity to look at premises usually accepted without reflection may be an unstated interest in the case.

Consequences

It is possible that Dr. Foster's HIV status will be revealed without his permission. Medical authorities have recommended that physicians who know that a seropositive patient is engaging in behaviors that endanger third parties should try to persuade the patient to cease the endangerment and, if persuasion is unsuccessful, should notify appropriate authorities. If no action is taken, notification of the endangered party is appropriate. Dr. Foster's own physician could do this, on fairly firm legal and ethical grounds.

If Dr. Foster's HIV status is made public, especially if his efforts at keeping it secret are discovered, then the consequences are serious. What will happen to his family is hard to say. He might lose his job. He could appeal, be transferred, or try to secure employment elsewhere. The upsetting of career and economic prospects he predicted earlier will come true. Who will or will not rally to his aid is impossible to know. AIDS support groups exist in every American city: Will they help a doctor who kept silent? We will not know the realities until Dr. Foster's situation is no longer his own.

The consequences more generally if Dr. Foster stays quiet are unlikely to be great. Will a patient in the ER become infected? Oddly enough, the fact that Dr. Foster knows his status may make him a safer practitioner than others who are unaware of their infectious capacities and who may be less thorough in utilizing precautions. The greatest danger from HIV is from those who are ignorant, not those who are knowledgeable. If Dr. Foster changes his mind and reveals his HIV status soon, he may be able to salvage the rudiments of a medical practice or a teaching position. Either way, he will soon develop symptoms and his vocational assignments will need to be reevaluated.

Ethical Principles

Dr. Foster prizes autonomy. He values it above the nonmaleficence claims that the profession uses to gain conformity to its rules and regulations. In many other cases in medical ethics, when a crunch appears between these two basic principles, autonomy has been seen to trump nonmaleficence, especially where clearly stated patient preferences are available. Should things be so different when a doctor is the subject of our case?

Complicating our consideration is the issue of veracity. Is Dr. Foster lying in not coming forward either by ceasing certain procedures or telling patients directly? Errors of commission and omission differ (see Case 9-2 above). Suppose that a patient, for whatever reason, asks Dr. Foster about his HIV status. (This is not a far-fetched notion in a climate of doubt and concern.) Were he then to either speak an untruth or finesse the question we could certainly say that the veracity principle has been traduced. But being quiet now may be another, subtle story.

Justice asks us to treat like cases alike. There is a notable imbalance between the personal and policy setting of this case. Though doctors are admonished to step forward, patients, including those who are knowingly infected, are not similarly enjoined. This asymmetry may be unjust, but it is the price paid by medical professionals. Being held to a higher standard of expectation and behavior than the public at large is what helps define a profession. In the realm of medicine, physicians like Dr. Foster have to suffer innocently so that the profession as a whole can enjoy the esteem it so desires from a skeptical public.

■ CASES FOR DISCUSSION ■

Case A

Andrea Newton is a medical student rotating on a geriatrics service. The chief resident, Dr. Maxwell, takes her to see Mrs. Reynolds, a patient with a variety of serious medical problems, including a heart problem and high blood pressure. He introduces the student by saying, "Good morning, Mrs. Reynolds; this is a junior colleague of mine, Andrea Newton. She'll be drawing blood from you today." After a brief physical examination the chief resident indicates to Ms. Newton that she should take blood from the patient. Observing routine precautions, the student makes four attempts before successfully drawing blood. The patient expresses significant discomfort, saying "Doctor, is everything O.K.?" Dr. Maxwell reassures her by stating "Yes, yes, this happens all the time."

Outside the room, the chief resident glowers at Ms. Newton. "What the hell is the matter with you?" he says. "Can't you do anything right?" The medical student begins to speak, saying "I felt uncomfortable from the beginning, when you implied to her that I was a physician...." Dr. Maxwell cuts off the student, shouting "I don't get you women. You can't follow orders and you complain day and night. If you can't stand the heat, maybe you should find another, easier career." Dr. Maxwell storms off, leaving Ms. Newton in the hall.

Questions

1. What is the appropriate way for a physician, whether an attending or a medical resident, to introduce a medical student to patients in a teaching institution?
2. How would you describe, in terms of physician responsibility, Dr. Maxwell's discussion of the forthcoming procedure with the patient in this case?
3. Is Dr. Maxwell's rebuke of Ms. Newton an illustration of medical student abuse?
4. Given the nature of the health care hierarchy, what is the proper response by the student to this episode?

Case B

Wilson Simms is a 54-year-old man with colon cancer that has spread to his liver. He has not responded to standard chemotherapy and is considering his other options. His primary physician, an internist, has been quite blunt, telling Mr. Simms that his disease is fatal and that his time is limited. He has recommended that the patient get in touch with the local hospice. Mr. Simms, however, says, "I know I can lick this thing. I've read about this new individual treatment they give over at the X Research Center. I'm going to try that." The doctor was unsure how to reply.

After reading a brief brochure about the research center given to him by Mr. Simms, the doctor reluctantly agrees to forward Mr. Simms' relevant records; the patient agrees to keep in touch with the internist. On a return visit, Mr. Simms tells the primary care doctor, "They got some of the cancer from me and they're going to process it and make an immune treatment so I can get well." The patient tells the physician that the cost of this experimental intervention is $55,000. "That sounds like a lot," says Mr. Simms, "but I think my life is worth it." After some preliminary inquiry the doctor discovers that the research center is owned by two local physicians, that their research is not federally or university funded, and that they, therefore, have not had to go through a "human subjects" review of their protocol. The primary doctor also learns that of the 83 patients seen at the research center in the past year, 77 have died. There have been no recorded complaints about the center at the local medical society.

Questions

1. When Mr. Simms originally proposed seeking alternative therapies for the cancer, what was an appropriate response by the physician?
2. Are there economic grounds that would allow the physician to condemn Mr. Simms' expenditure of such a large amount of money on an unproven treatment?
3. Does the primary care physician have an obligation to investigate this matter further?
4. If a different alternative therapy were being offered by, say, a clinical nutritionist, would your response be different?

■ THINK PIECE: PROFESSIONAL RESPONSIBILITY ■

The facts are in. Tobacco smoking is responsible for about 350,000 deaths in the United States each year. Most are a result of cancers (particularly those of the lung and respiratory tract, but also pancreatic and bladder cancers), cardiovascular diseases (coronary heart disease and peripheral vascular disease), and chronic obstructive lung disease. Smoking behaviors begin early, often at the outset of adolescence and some studies show that about one quarter of the young people who smoke more than a pack of cigarettes daily lose about 10 to 15 years of life. Another statistic is equally frightening: At any age, smokers are 68 percent more likely to die over the course of the next year than nonsmokers. Knowledge about the dangers of smoking is growing.

Warnings on cigarette packages (e.g., "Smoking by pregnant women may result in fetal injury, premature birth, and low birth weight.") are ubiquitous. The proportion of the population as a whole using cigarettes has declined but there are growth areas, especially among teenaged women. Smoking also has a class base in America: The tendency to smoke falls as persons get more education and rise in social class standing. Most smokers want to stop but cannot. The Surgeon General states that cigarettes and other forms of tobacco are physically addicting. In addition to the dangers to the smoker, passive smoking may harm family members, coworkers, and members of the general public who do not use cigarettes themselves.

What should be done about doctors who smoke cigarettes? Raising the issue, even with a group of physicians who do not smoke, often elicits a mixed response, partly autonomist and partly paternalistic. For example, many argue that if a doctor wants to smoke in the privacy of his own home, that's just fine. Doctors who smoke in front of patients, however, should change their habits. Should physicians be held to a higher standard of responsibility than others, even other professionals? Should doctors who smoke away from the health care setting *tell* their patients about such behavior?

The leading medical associations condemn cigarette smoking, recognize the duty of the practicing physician to prevent disease by encouraging smoking cessation among patients, and fight publicly for antismoking measures (e.g., research on addiction; imposition of bans on advertising, especially in settings impacting on minority populations; and encouragement of public, educational programming that might encourage people to quit smoking). Yet doctors do smoke—perhaps one out of ten does so. (Nurses are more apt to smoke than physicians.) Should they be made to stop?

Arguments for mandating nonsmoking for physicians, or at the very least, letting patients know that their doctors use cigarettes, are various. A consumer-based and clearly utilitarian demand says that the patient has the right to know about physician behavior that might impact the patient's well-being. Would a doctor who smokes neglect evidence of a spot on the patient's lung? Addictive behaviors might reinforce one another—smoking and heavy drinking are correlated. Should a doctor who smokes post a notice in her waiting room stating the fact? Would that not let the buyer beware?

A more principalist claim suggests that doctors who smoke are violating their oath to do no harm. They are, with full knowledge, hurting themselves and perhaps, given the dangers of ambient smoking, others. At the very least many doctors who smoke are acting in either a hypocritical or self-deceiving manner. Because they are pledged to keep patients from smoking via preventative means, or to aid those who want to quit, doctors who use cigarettes themselves are phonies, the argument goes. They are violating the principle of veracity and they should at least be held accountable for the deception.

There are programs and procedures for so-called impaired physicians, those doctors who are addicted to such harmful substances as alcohol and prescription and nonprescription drugs. No one wants to be operated on by a surgeon under the influence of such substances. Even in a less perilous setting such as the outpatient clinic the judgment of a doctor who abuses drugs is always dubious. Such physicians are scrutinized by their professional colleagues and if warranted must participate in drug or alcohol cessation programs. If they fail to change their behaviors, they may lose hospital privileges and, as an ultimate sanction, may lose their licenses to practice medicine. Is smoking at all like alcoholism among doctors? How, if at all, does it differ?

If we deem it important to stop doctors from smoking, how should we implement programs to achieve this goal? Will voluntary programs be good enough? In forcing doctors to stop smoking, are we going too far in trying to gain professional ethical consistency? Does a doctor lose some rights on entering the health profession? Should physicians be not only technicians and humane caregivers, but moral pillars as well?

■ VOICES: PHYSICIAN/MANAGER ■

There is a tendency to hold doctors to a higher standard of behavior than other people that I don't think is fair. Doctors are human. For them to act responsibly, with propriety and fairness toward others is enough. Unfortunately, not all doctors meet this general standard. Doctors' training and experience lead them to act independently. The fact that doctors are so important, so widely esteemed, places them on a pedestal so they get away with a lot. Sometimes I regret the fact that doctors are not trained to be managed.

For example, we know that physicians often break appointments with their patients, many of whom are willing to wait for hours. When there is a genuine emergency, I have no problem with a postponement. But sometimes doctors will just not show up. You could not run a conventional business that way. When doctors act unprofessionally, however, it is rare for a staff member or patient to call them on it. It doesn't take much for physicians to do better: They just need to be compassionate and understanding of others. But there are many in the profession who aren't. This kind of doctor just doesn't apologize.

Not much time is spent training medical professionals in matters of responsibility. It's not an aspect of physician identity, as is diagnostic ability or a good memory. Maybe it's part of the selection process. Medical schools seem to want smart people who can learn fast and learn a great deal. Communication skills, which are just as important in being a good and responsible practitioner, are emphasized less.

There are few great mentors, few wonderful role models in medical education or practice. Maybe the idea, which I have read and heard about, of having young residents spend some time as "pretend" patients will help humanize them. I know that my own experience in a hospital bed completely changed the way in which I speak with patients and consider their worries and fears. Understanding the patient's perspective is indispensable to practicing in a way that considers a person's feelings as well as symptoms. Maybe this view stems from my family practice orientation, but I really believe it.

Not many of the doctors I have encountered in both public and private settings are incompetent. Finding a colleague who is technically inadequate, poorly trained, or simply unaware of how to find data is rare; hardly any are completely incompetent. But many doctors I know are not clear thinkers and as a result make poor decisions (such as unnecessary surgeries) from the data they assemble. One approach, certainly not a cure-all, is to base a decision not only on the objective facts but also on what patients really want and need. Staying on a ventilator is not only a matter of pulmonary function; how the patient sees herself and what she wants with the rest of her life is equally important.

I welcome peer review and the ongoing evaluation process of, and by, colleagues. I also think we have an obligation to help other doctors in trouble. I've seen too many physicians impaired by alcohol and drug abuse. You try to get them into counseling, but very often that doesn't work. Many rehabilitation programs are ineffective. It's hard to know what to do next when seeing a colleague who is impaired. You want to intervene, but you don't know what will be effective. It's very difficult, in general, to be the boss of other physicians, and many managers are themselves undertrained in the art of management.

Do physicians have an obligation to serve society as a whole? Should they be required, for example, to help the homeless or treat the poor? I don't think such service should be mandatory. I may do it out of conviction or conscience or other motives, but I don't want to make others serve involuntarily. (If they occasionally work with those who need them the most, they will find out that it can be more rewarding than their routine practices.)

These days society seems to be making more and more demands on doctors. The public fear of getting AIDS from your own physician is irrational. This kind of public accountability puts doctors in an untenable position. Are we supposed to tell every patient about each of our habits? Should every provider in an alcohol treatment program tell this to the patient as part of the informed consent talk? This would be ridiculous; it would make no sense. But sometimes I feel that there is public pressure making all of us overly accountable.

In general, just as we cannot hold doctors to a higher standard of behavior than the norm, we need to learn, as practitioners, that we cannot be everything to everyone. We need to structure the system by which we provide services in ways that allow shared, though not diffused, responsibility. We need to help each other help others.

RECOMMENDED READING

Bok, S. *Lying: Moral Choice in Public and Private Life.* New York: Vintage Books, 1987.

Cassel, E. *The Healer's Art: A New Approach to the Physician-Patient Relationship.* Philadelphia: Lippincott, 1976.

Gorovitz, S. *Doctors' Dilemmas: Moral Conflict and Medical Care.* New York: Oxford University, 1982.

Jonsen, A., Siegler, M., and Winslade, W. *Clinical Ethics,* (2d ed.). Riverside, NJ: Pergamon, 1986.

Starr, P. *The Social Transformation of American Medicine.* New York: Basic Books, 1982.

▪10▪

The Pursuit of Fairness: Ethics in the Allocation of Scarce Health Care Resources

Health care is expensive (Fig. 10-1)! The percentage of the U.S. gross national product used for medically related expenditures has doubled in recent decades. Soon $1 trillion each year will be spent on health care in the United States. Medicine is very much a business. The balance of power and authority has shifted in recent decades from physicians working alone or in small groups to organizations such as HMOs, institutions such as hospitals or long-term care facilities, government agencies, and third-party payers. Some individual states, such as Oregon and Hawaii, have initiated plans to assess and prioritize specific medical interventions deserving of public funding. Nearly all participants in the debate about allocating health care resources agree on one thing: The American system of medical care, often derided as a nonsystem, is fiscally out of control.

A climate of blame has entered the debate about creating or recreating a health care system that is both rational and fair. Few parties to the discussion escape indictment. Physicians are criticized for inefficient management, greedy attitudes, and performing procedures and ordering medications with limited efficacy. For example, some estimate that more than $30 billion per year could be saved if unnecessary, redundant, and useless diagnostic tests were eliminated. Yet doctors claim that they must practice defensive medicine because of the fear of being sued for malpractice. Greedy plaintiff's attorneys are accused of initiating illicit lawsuits. Nasty comments by physicians extend beyond lawyer jokes. Hospital administrators who care more about the bottom line than about

---

About 12 percent of the United States' gross national product is spent on health care, a higher percentage than in any other industrialized nation.

Approximately 35 million persons, many of them children, lack access to medical treatment because they cannot afford it.

Medicare is the federal program that pays for health care for persons who are either over 65 years of age or who are younger and are eligible for Supplemental Security Income. Medicare also provides all costs for end-stage kidney disease treatment. In 1990 Medicare cost more than $105 billion.

Medicaid, through matching funds and grants-in-aid to the states, provides government support for health care for persons who are impoverished.

The federal government provides health care benefits to veterans of the U.S. military; such benefits amounted to more than $12 billion in 1991.

The U.S. Public Health Service provides some maternal and child health care services, focusing on the control of infectious diseases, especially via sanitation programs and immunization.

Fig. 10-1. The cost of health care in the United States.

patient care; quality assurance staff members who question procedures that do not go strictly by the book; insurance company and managed-care bureaucrats who press to have patients discharged from the hospital prematurely—all are routinely blamed for putting the economic squeeze on practitioners who prize independence.

Three strong currents influence present concerns about allocating scarce health care resources. First, earlier efforts at cost containment have largely failed or have shifted costs from acute to long-term care. Second, pressure from politicians and planners to provide for the medically indigent (those persons without insurance or private funds or access to health care through government assistance) grows. Some propose a national health plan, along the lines of European or Canadian practice. Others advocate employer-based, and if necessary state-supported, universal access via health insurance. Third, Americans are quite limited in their potential to say "No" in specific situations. The temptation to use advanced technology (at a high cost) to cure disease and disorders seems built into our social assumptions. Physicians and patients alike demand the best and want it immediately.

It is difficult to find anyone enamored of the present method of providing health care in the U.S. Such earlier strategies as increasing competition or inviting corporate intervention into health planning have yielded mixed results. Doctors (except the many physicians providing primary care) do well monetarily. Efforts at controlling costs have made many practitioners unhappy, in part because of the loss of authority over patient-care decisions. When the insurance company mandates a second opinion and tells the original doctor that "this surgery will cost $30,000 and the data do not support your hoped-for outcome. We refuse to pay!" both the clinician and the patient lose the chance to choose. Scrutiny of what were once routine physician-patient decisions is now based on both medical and economic necessity.

Managed care plans or Medicaid restrictions are designed to limit access by enrollees. Ten visits to the psychiatrist per year may be all that are allowed. A monthly doctor visit to the nursing home for a Medicaid patient (who may have qualified for government support by spending down to her last $2000 of savings) may be the mandatory limit. Money is the major scarce resource in contemporary health planning. Few doubt that reducing payments for health care affects the quality of patient care. Decisions about "who shall live" may depend on "who is paying"!

Allocating resources means making difficult choices. The demands seem infinite and advocates are loud and insistent. Strong voices state that utilizing dollars for prevention is both cost-effective and fair. Spending more money on prenatal care, immunization, environmental protection, nutrition, patient education, and community wellness programs could result in diminished demand for hospitalization and more effective use of emergency facilities and outpatient clinical services. Meanwhile, demands for health care accelerate as budgets tighten. At some inner city clinics, the average wait to see a nurse or doctor is 7 hours. A well baby appointment must be scheduled 5 months in advance.

Decisions at the level of macroallocation (the large-scale determination of societal interests) influence concrete judgments at the micro (or patient-care) level. The Medicare End Stage Renal Disease Program vastly increased the number of renal transplantation operations. Demands for other kinds of intervention are heightened. For example, the federal Medicare program has decided to support the funding of annual mammograms for older patients. Now the woman who could not afford such a screening prior to funding can see a radiologist for little or no payment. Discovering a lump in her breast may or may not extend her life. Certainly more breast surgeries and more chemotherapy and radiation treatments for a wider population will result. As many patients gain funded access to a resource formerly limited in availability, expenditures rise. Afficionados of cost containment will look back and ask, "Did we do the right thing in making mammograms so widely available?"

When we allocate scarce health care resources, the principle of justice haunts our deliberations, at both the micro and the macro level. Should a patient who is perhaps at fault for his present medical condition (e.g., the alcoholic who needs a new liver) be included in the pool of candidates or be excluded, and if so, on what grounds? If we want to be more inclusive, yet admit that resources will always be limited, what fair and equitable categorical grounds should we use to aid in making decisions? Should access be for everyone or should it be limited to those who will surely benefit. Should age be a criterion? What weight, if any, should be given to capacity to pay the bill? Does social worth count for anything? (Should convicted felons under life sentence for violent crimes be candidates for heart transplantation?)

Is it fair to offer high cost interventions such as bypass graft surgeries to more than a quarter million people per year while access to care for pregnant drug addicts is limited due to a lack of facilities? Should we base our priorities in health care on need, on effectiveness, or on concern for present or future generations? Answers to the policy dilemmas about allocating medical care will tell us not only what might be a just and fair health care system, it will also instruct us about the social values we truly prize.

■ FIVE ESSENTIAL CASES ■

Case 10-1

Physicians work in an economic, political, and social climate. The capacity to perform a procedure does *not* mandate that it take place. Factors such as cost, age, and quality of life often influence such choices. Are such factors extraneous or indispensable to responsible patient care?

Mr. B. is a 77-year-old man, a former engineer with a major corporation, with adult onset diabetes and mild cataracts that do not obstruct his mobility or his automobile driving. He gave up his pack-per-day smoking habit about 3 years ago. Since his retirement Mr. B.'s health care costs have been paid mainly by Medicare. For about 8 months he has experienced chest pain suggestive of angina that has recently worsened. Last week he had a severe spell and, after a long absence, went in to see his primary care physician, Dr. S. The doctor immediately prescribed nitroglycerine and scheduled a cardiac catheterization (angiogram).

The heart studies show multiple vessel coronary obstructions with a 75 to 90 percent narrowing. There is also some evidence of damage to the heart (decreasing left ventricular function). Otherwise, Mr. B. is mentally alert, intact, and has no debilitating problems. The patient has been married for 50 years and has two grown children. There are positive indications for coronary artery bypass graft (CABG) surgery (i.e., aside from the diabetes, present health status and major organ function, except for his heart, are unimpaired). Risks such as stroke resulting in mental impairment are statistically greater for Mr. B. than for a 50-year-old patient.

The cost of this surgery is estimated to be about $35,000, specifically $28,000 for 7 to 10 days of hospitalization, $2000 for anesthesia services, and $5000 for surgical services. In most nations with a national health service, patients over age 65 are not deemed candidates for such surgery.

Who has the "burden of proof" (a legal term with potential application in many other areas) in this case? Does this patient have to demonstrate a right, or a strong claim, to this expensive procedure? Does the paying party (in this case, Medicare) have to show that Mr. B. is not an appropriate candidate for CABG surgery? Where do the patient's doctors stand? Their dual roles as advocates for the health of Mr. B. and as professionals in a medical system that is trying desperately to limit rising health care costs are potentially in conflict.

Mr. B.'s situation is a common one: Chances of MI rise with age. Diabetes is an important complication. But what about the patient's age? All our data about outcomes is statistical. Mr. B.'s surgery is somewhat less likely to be successful than an operation on a person 30 years younger without diabetes. The risk of stroke rises with age. His recovery will likely be longer and slower. We can predict with confidence that the return of blood flow to Mr. B.'s heart, while surely giving him increased mobility and freedom from pain, will not add decades to his life. But in dollar costs, comparisons are indispensable. While the cost of surgery may seem very high, what would be the total expenses if Mr. B. has a severe heart attack, winds up in the ICU for several weeks, and requires extensive rehabilitative therapy? Cost-benefit analyses are rarely complete, but attempting to project relative costs is a useful exercise.

In countries such as England, only a handful of physicians would even offer the surgery to such a patient. Even less invasive procedures such as kidney dialysis are rarely provided for persons over 60, though this seems to be changing in response to the development of lower-cost peritoneal dialysis. But in the U.S., where there is a traditional presumption that the patient must be fully informed about benefits and risks of health care options, Mr. B.'s doctors will be pressed into service as gatekeepers. Not only will Dr. S. guide the patient through the maze of health care choices, he will also want to be attentive to matters of cost effectiveness.

The clinical options for Mr. B. are limited. Nonsurgical treatment entails the use of medications that can place less burden on the heart, lower the blood pressure, and reduce the risk of heart attack. Mr. B. will probably have to limit his exercise somewhat and "be careful." Is this a satisfactory quality of life? Only Mr. B. can say for certain. But to make a decision means to entertain choices. Dr. S. will have to be open and honest about the differences between a medical and a surgical course for Mr. B. The financial differences are enormous. Medication and monitoring cost less than one-tenth of surgery and follow-up. But if Mr. B., after discussion and reflection, chooses CABG surgery, the principle of autonomy suggests that his wishes should be carried out.

In discussing the allocation of scarce health care resources, we need to regard every case as a microcosm of larger policy issues. What sort of precedent would this decision to operate represent? The percentage of the population over 75 years of age is growing rapidly; health care expenditures for this group are disproportionate, as would be expected. Medicare and Medicaid claim an ever larger percentage of the federal budget. As life expenctancy rises, demands on the system from patients like Mr. B. also accelerate. There really is no such thing as an exception. If we affirm Mr. B.'s determination to have this expensive surgery, given his age and condition, we can hardly deny it to others in similar situations.

Mr. B.'s case forces physicians and administrators to face fiscal limits. It also evokes a debate about social values. Is longevity always preferable? What do the young owe the old and vice versa? Is the autonomously expressed patient wish—particularly one in which Mr. B. could rationally claim that the lifestyle projected by drug therapy was unsatisfactory to him—the end of the story? Or does a nation that pays for the health care of older persons have the right to say when costly interventions must cease?

Case 10-2

Institutions with limited budgets still want to do what is best for patients in need. Advanced technology often promises benefits, both diagnostically and therapeutically. If a hospital fails to use state-of-the-art machinery, it could be legally or ethically vulnerable.

The medical staff of H. Hospital (a community-supported hospital quite distant from the nearest tertiary care medical center) met recently and by a vote of 31–2 decided to request from the administration and board of trustees of the instituion an on-site magnetic resonance imaging (MRI) device. The staff's reasoning was quite explicit: (1) patient care depends on careful diagnosis, and the new imaging device is more advanced than their present machines; (2) although an MRI would probably not pay for itself in such a small town, it would be possible to come near to breaking even if it were utilized according to projections; (3) the local doctors want the hospital to own the device because they view a physician-invested MRI center as a conflict of interest and will not pursue it; (4) advice from the hospital's risk management department, which sought outside legal counsel, suggested that without the MRI, the prompt and accurate diagnosis of many diseases, disorders, and injuries might be postponed, with potentially disastrous results.

The legal counsel told the medical staff about a case in Washington, D.C., in which a female patient, complaining of a severe headache, was brought into the ER by her husband. That hospital lacked a CT scanner; the patient died the following morning. Her family sued and a jury awarded her survivors $240,000. The results of the lawsuit, the attorney told the assembled doctors, have heightened awareness of the need to stay up to date and even to try to stay a step ahead of the evolving standard of medical care.

The cost of an MRI device is likely to exceed $1 million. H. Hospital does have CT scanning facilities. At present, patients are sent to a distant, larger hospital for MRIs. It often takes 3 to 4 days to schedule an appointment, though results can quickly be faxed to the hometown doctor. Emergencies are handled via a medevac helicopter to the University Hospital 40 miles away. The radiologist at H. Hospital states that she feels qualified to interpret MRI results. There seems to be little doubt that a government certificate of need could be secured. But the hospital administrator is working with a very tight budget: This past quarter admissions are down 12 percent and some staff may have to be furloughed. The highest priority for future capital investment is a building addition that would provide more space for the pediatrics clinic serving a mostly Medicaid population.

(Based on Blake v. District of Columbia. Mp12623-80, D. C. Superior Court, June 30, 1981.)

The proportion of gross national product of health care expenditures has tripled since 1950. Estimates suggest that medical care will soon amount to 15 percent of all production, a higher percentage than in any other country. About one-quarter of this cost goes to doctors directly. Recent efforts at cutting down on unnecessary medical services are moderately encouraging. Health maintenance organizations (HMOs) have helped to limit hospitalizations. Regulatory plans such as changes in reimbursement processes based on a DRG system have slowed the growth of Medicare hospital costs.

A growing proportion of the health care budget is spent on advanced technology equipment and procedures, such as the MRI. The autonomatic implantable cardiac defribillator, which goes to work when a patient is experiencing a dangerous arrythmia, could help at least 25,000 patients each year. An estimated cost of more than $50,000 for each such patient would total more than $1 billion per year. An implantable artificial heart and a left-ventricular assist device could add $4 to 5 billion dollars a year to health care expenditures. There seems to be a rule when technologic possibilities emerge: If the machinery is there it must be used.

Many of the reasons the medical staff give for wanting to add an MRI device to the array of diagnostic tools at the hospital are solid and intelligent. Certainly the desire to find out what is wrong with patients flows from the principle of beneficence. One positive aspect of MRI devices is that they eliminate the need for surgical investigation of clinical problems; they are noninvasive, and they reduce patient apprehension and pain. If a local MRI device can keep patients at the community hospital, not only will local practitioners prosper, but sick people will avoid hospitalization in distant and larger institutions.

Financial costs can be very high, however. MRIs will not be the end of the story. Positron emission tomography and magnetic resonance spectroscopy are already on line. A commitment to state-of-the-art equipment opens the door to expenditures that could bankrupt a small local hospital. In an era in which rising health costs are matched by rising needs for primary care and preventive medicine and about 15 percent of the population lacks health insurance, it is very difficult for a community hospital with munificent ambitions to sort out this allocation problem. A pediatric clinic would serve a population manifestly in need, but would not likely reimburse the institution for the actual cost of services provided.

Added to the dilemma is another feature that influences most medical ethics scenarios: the fear of litigation. The legal counsel's noting of the Washington, D.C., case can only serve to heighten anxiety and to encourage purchase of the MRI. Is this realism, or is it a reflexive response to a single case in a very different jurisdiction? We need not abscribe scare tactic motives to the attorney. Some attention to actual legal vulnerability would seem to be necessary. Should possible damages from future lawsuits, if the MRI is not bought, be calculated into a cost-benefit analysis prior to a decision to buy? Some states and even counties have regional health planning commissions that provide guidance to institutions in the situation of H. Hospital. Is resource sharing an option? Could there be a downside to purchasing as well? Suppose utilization of the scanner was minimal and the local radiologist's experience was thus quite limited. Does this not increase the risk of error and of malpractice suits?

Finally, this case presses us to consider a much larger question. Who should determine whether or not such a device should be purchased? The state regulatory board may allow the MRI facility by granting its approval, but that does not mean that the community needs or wants it. Because H. Hospital is not a proprietary institution and relies on community fund-raising and other contributions for its operations, should local citizens and the political leadership of the town be involved in the purchasing decision? This would be an unusual occurrence. But in the absence of a public discussion or debate, the allocation issues will likely be settled by those with a narrower focus of interest.

<u>Case 10-3</u>

In a genuine emergency, ability of the patient to pay for immediate care is not a factor. But in situations in which it is possible to arrange transportation safely for a patient to another institution, the ethics of transfer (sometimes called dumping) can be troublesome.

Mr. W. walked into the ER of a large private institution, L. Hospital, late one evening. He had been in a fight while gambling with "some guys" he refused to identify and had rather deep cuts on his nose, shoulder, and forearm. The bleeding had been stopped, and Mr. W. was not in a life-threatening situation. Waiting to clean and sew up the wounds, at least for a short period, would not add significantly to Mr. W's risk of infection. The ER resident, Dr. D., told the patient that extensive suturing would be required. When asked about payment or insurance, Mr. W. stated, "I lost my job 7 weeks ago. I got no health insurance. I have about $8.00 in cash to my name. You can have it if you want!" L. Hospital does not have a formal policy about accepting indigent nonemergency patients; it conventionally avoids admitting patients without insurance. The state in which the hospital operates does not mandate care of those who cannot pay.

The resident is aware that the nearby (2 miles away) University hospital is supported by a tax levy that provides for the care of medically indigent patients. Dr. D. confers with the attending physician, Dr. F. Both doctors are satisfied that Mr. W. is stable and requires only preparation and suturing care. The senior physician points out that Mr. W. will require several hours of attention and that it is unlikely that anyone at L. Hospital will get paid for the work. Dr. D. points out that "at the moment we're not very busy." The attending physician, who has worked for many years in the ER, recommends that the patient be put in a cab and sent to the University Hospital, which has the resources and the staff to care for Mr. W. Dr. D. has reservations. "We'd certainly keep this guy here if he had the money," he tells the attending. "Is it fair to send him across town because he's lost his insurance?" Dr. F. replies, "If we take every nonemergency poor person who walks in the door, we'll have to close down the ER. Then who would we be serving?"

Hospitals receiving federal funds from Medicare, Medicaid, or government grants and loans are legally obliged to accept emergency patients without regard to ability to pay. A physician or other provider who refuses to give emergency treatment would also be vulnerable to legal sanction for failure to meet a duty to care, even if the patient were unknown to the doctor or hospital. Such general guidelines may not apply to Mr. W., for he does not seem to be in need of emergency care. No matter how we label an emergency—it is usually deemed to be an acute threat to life or well-being requiring immediate intervention—Mr. W. seems to be beyond the definitional border.

This case entails allocating resources in a concrete manner. If Mr. W. can be transferred swiftly and cooperatively to University Hospital, then L. Hospital will save monetary resources and be able to divert provider time to other, perhaps medically needier patients. University Hospital, on the other hand, will have its allocation decision made *for* it. Mandated to accept Mr. W., that institution, which treats the poor as a matter of course, will have yet one more nonpaying customer.

The debate between Dr. D. and Dr. F. seems to pit a youthful idealist against the voice of realism and experience (Dr. F. has "seen it all"). The final statements of both physicians are true: If Mr. W. had funds or were adequately insured he would never be turned away; if many others in Mr. W.'s status inundate the ER at L. Hospital, it could be financially overwhelmed. There are almost competing images of professional and institutional obligation here, too. A minimalist approach—sticking to legal requirements and going no further—would result in sending Mr. W. to the tax-supported institution. A more formally duty-based deontologic perspective would assert that Mr. W.'s claim for care is based on his injury, not on his capacity to pay.

This latter view is not unlimited. No emergency physician has to care for every patient who walks in the door, certainly not immediately. An adult with the sniffles would probably have to wait a very long time on a busy weekend evening while ER doctors took care of those with life-threatening injuries or illnesses. But Mr. W. has a real variety of injuries, and conditions of triage are not evident here. The resistance to providing care articulated by Dr. F. is primarily financial.

There may be other secondary reasons, tacit and not explicit, for rejecting Mr. W. as an L. Hospital patient. He is an "unattractive" patient who may have brought his injury upon himself. His self-reported behavior is not "middle class." He is also unemployed and could suffer the ignominy of that status. Mr. W. is not quite in the category of those notorious ER patients informally (and only among staff) called GOMERS (Get Out of My Emergency Room!). Such patients are often chronic alcoholics or mentally ill street people; prostitutes and drug addicts are also included under that rubric. But as Dr. D. has pointed out Mr. W. is also categorized: as a person without financial resources. Does he, as a result, belong at the University Hospital where such patients are routinely treated?

One utilitarian argument for retaining Mr. W., which may seem a bit cynical, is that the time and money expended on his care in the ER will not be very great. Were he in a nonemergency situation that required admission, with the possibility of extensive and expensive therapy, the motivation to "dump" him would be greater. Perhaps Mr. W. could squeeze by this time. But this is hardly a solution to the policy and process issue in this case. Is it the physician's task to govern a health care system's allocation plan? Suburban doctors read frequently about urban hospitals that are forced to shut down because of overserving medically indigent patients. Sending Mr. W. to the University Hospital may be wise, but does it contribute anything to solving the problem of a health care system that is based on a medically indigent population numbering in the tens of millions? What are the justice claims in the case of Mr. W and the ER debate? Should public hospitals be given even greater funds to help patients like Mr. W? Or should a *more-than-minimalist* ethic be imposed on all institutions, such as L. Hospital, which offer care via an ER?

Case 10-4

We rarely blame patients for their medical conditions, but some behaviors, quite clearly, lead to pathologies that require extensive and expensive interventions. Should scarce resources be withheld from those persons who seem at least partially responsible for their illnesses?

Malcolm B. is a 53-year-old chronic alcoholic. Married with two adult children, he has worked as a laborer since age 17. He avoided the health care system until last year. He presented in the hospital with spontaneous peritonitis. He spent 2 weeks in the hospital receiving IV treatment. At that time a diagnosis of alcoholic cirrhosis, advanced degree, was made.

Four months ago, Mr. B. had a recurrence of his peritonitis and again received IV treatment. He responded more slowly and was discharged on antibiotics. Last month he was again admitted, in an obvious state of deterioration with small liver, large varices on CT scan, and other symptoms.

Mr. B. is an apt candidate for liver transplantation. He does have a chronic illness: a swiftly degenerating liver as a result of cirrhosis. Aside from his liver disease, his organic status is quite good. (He does not suffer portal vein thrombosis, sepsis, or other complicating problems.) He has a family that will support him; they hope that he will give up drinking if given a second chance. Mr. B. agrees and states, "Believe me, I'll never touch the stuff again. I know it is a matter of life and death." He has told the hospital social worker to give him information about Alcoholics Anonymous as well as about other treatment programs. "If I get through this hospital stay," he says, "I'll be a new man."

The physicians believe Mr. B. to be sincere. He has never tried a rehabilitation program in the past, though the dangers of his heavy drinking were pointed out to him during both prior hospitalizations. The medical and nursing staff are divided: Some feel that the scarce organ should go to someone more deserving; others believe that Mr. B. should not be singled out and punished for his disease (alcoholism).

This case evokes a spectrum of provocative questions. What general criteria should be used in choosing patients as recipients of scarce organ resources? What weight should psycho-social and policy factors play in patient selection criteria? What do we mean in asserting that a patient is responsible for the behaviors that cause or exacerbate a medical condition? What is fair and just about either including or excluding patients with a history of risk-taking behavior?

A single standard, often strongly proclaimed, is frequently cited in decisions concerning the transplantation of a scarce bodily resource: It is wrong to waste a liver, heart, or kidney (i.e., a valuable organ hard to secure and difficult to transplant). Such an unofficial policy is, of course, future-oriented. We care about results. There are no voices asking anyone to place a new kidney into the body of a patient dying of cancer or of a person with only a minimal chance to survive the transplant surgery. To attempt either procedure would be nonsensical. But even if interested parties can agree that providing a valuable and rare organ to a terminal patient is irrational, few other agreements about patient status and social policy are secure in this area.

The case of Mr. B. seems to present this problem in crystalline fashion: Should this patient get a new liver if his physical condition is such that he will either reject the organ or need another were he to persist in his use of alcohol? One problem is that predicting future behaviors is notoriously difficult. If we deny Mr. B. a chance to get a new liver, we can be sure of only one thing: He will die soon. But if we transplant this patient we cannot know for certain what he will do on recovery from surgery. Is it fair to take this chance?

This leads to a related, and perhaps even more difficult, moral problem. Does Mr. B.'s past behavior—his knowing and untreated abuse of a dangerous substance—disqualify him for consideration for transplant? Is Mr. B. a worthy candidate? Reasonable physicians and ethicists have debated and disagreed about this subject. We are asking whether or not Mr. B. has placed himself outside the community of persons who can gain access to a scarce resource.

Patients are sometimes blamed for their ailments. Three pack-a-day smokers who develop lung cancer are said to be responsible for their disease. Obese patients who have made no effort to lose weight and who develop diabetes are sometimes castigated for such behavioral causes of their own problems. Persons who will not wear motorcycle helmets and who wind up in the ER with head trauma are often the subject of critical commentary. What does it mean to say that patients like this are at fault? Certainly it states that personal conduct that appears causative of medical problems is in need of scrutiny. But does it imply that the heavy drinker is to be denied a potentially life-saving therapy?

Who should decide this specific allocation determination regarding Mr. B.'s candidacy? Normally, the liver transplant team reviews the patient's record, tests, and evaluations and makes a recommendation or decision. But the questions raised by Mr. B.'s case, which include concerns about social morality, are not decided by medical expertise. Concepts and language play a large role. Is alcoholism a disease? If so, what shall we say about the physician who denies a patient with alcoholism the opportunity for both a new organ and a new lease on life? A "yes" decision for Mr. B. could be taken as a sign that, as a society, we regard heavy drinking as lamentable but as morally neutral.

Are physicians and other health professionals to become the functional equivalents of society's moral police? In the absence of a surgical team decision about Mr. B., who else would render a judgment? Should the voters, or their representatives, make such a policy? Tacitly, such decisions are made all the time. A state's decision to expend Medicaid funds on primary care rather than on heart transplantation means that some persons will die from advanced heart disease. But these persons usually remain anonymous. Mr. B. is alive, if not well; the consequences for him are obvious and could become public. (Begging, via the media, for scarce organs, or for funds to pay for their use, is not unknown.)

We do know that the availability of livers is limited and that there will perhaps always be a greater demand than supply of such organs. Should we, explicitly or implicitly, use social worth as a criteria? Should it be our rule that a patient who knows that a controllable risk can lead to a dangerously pathologic state, and yet still persists in this unadvisable behavior, is disqualified from the medical care that can cure disease or extend life?

Case 10-5

Health care resources are limited. If they are expended in a fashion that is not cost-effective, should patient or family demands for continuing care be affirmed or denied?

Mr. H.S. is a respirator-dependent patient in N. Rehabilitation Hospital. Eighty-six-years old and now completely unconscious, Mr. H.S. had suffered a cardiopulmonary arrest almost 2 years ago that left him without consciousness in a PVS. He is tube fed and receives antibiotics for infections, which are frequent. All efforts at weaning the patient from the ventilator have failed. The cost, paid for by Medicare and by supplemental insurance, for Mr. H.S.'s care is presently about $500 per day. In the nearly 2 years, this has amounted to more than one quarter million dollars.

Mr. H.S.'s only living family member is a son, D.S. His perspective on the case is clear, indeed adamant. "My father told me, many times, that God wanted him to stay alive for as long as possible. When I asked Dad if this included being hooked up to machines, he always said yes." The son then produced a letter from his father that stated, quite clearly, that resistance to death was his personal choice, even if the situation was hopeless. When D.S. was asked if he would agree to a limited treatment plan for his father, he refused. When he was told, quite bluntly, that the doctors believed that any further treatment, given that Mr. H.S. could no longer experience pain and had no chance of recovering any function, was futile, the son said that he didn't care. "Just take care of my Dad like he wanted!"

The physicians and nurses on the team conferred with hospital attorneys. There seemed to be no precedent for a court order that would discontinue treatment in the face of opposition of a family. The case was brought before the hospital's ethics committee, which made a good faith effort to mediate the dispute. D.S. refused to compromise and would not permit the transfer of his father to a long-term care facility. "Dad deserves the best treatment possible," he said, "and you folks know how to give it." The hospital administrator who mentioned to D.S. that costs of care were escalating dramatically got a similar rebuke.

Our analysis of this case focuses on its economic and policy dimensions. (See Chapter 6 for a discussion of ethical questions at the end-of-life.) First, the situation of a son or daughter having primary responsibility for the health care of a parent is not a rare occurrence. It is estimated that at least five million Americans undertake this task yearly. Americans are used to demanding health care and traditionally desire the best that they, or those who pay, can afford. When D.S. speaks for his father, he is not alone in pressing for a presumed right to continued treatment.

Respect for autonomy—either individually expressed or, as in the case of Mr. H.S., as stated by a surrogate—can be expensive. For example, physicians caring for a dying child in the NICU will often wait a long time before removing a ventilator—months, perhaps—until parents can accept the futility of the situation. Costs are not supposed to count. It is an unwritten rule: Doctors do not tell family members that they should stop treatment because of financial considerations.

Second, though estimates vary, a great deal of money is spent on patients like Mr. H.S. It is estimated that more than $150,000 per year per patient is spent on care of PVS patients. There may be more than 10,000 such patients in the United States each year. Such patients do not usually receive ventilatory support; they are tube fed. Estimated expenditures for Medicare clients during the last year of life range upward of $70,000; nearly 30 percent of Medicare's limited dollars are spent on such persons. A figure of one percent of the gross national product being expended for elderly patients in their last living year is also frequently heard.

Third, we must ask: To what extent is the age of the patient a factor in our assessment? A debate about how to limit health care expenditures often centers on patient age. For example, we do not give organ transplants to persons over 60 or so. (The argument is not a purely chronologic one; such persons have higher risk factors for disease and lower rates of recovery from complicated surgeries.) But should we seek a more general rule, especially with regard to patients like Mr. H.S. who will never recover bodily integrity or interactive functions? Should we say that all such patients should receive only pain medications and should be allowed to die peacefully and quietly? If we make this argument, it is easy to cloak it in such principles as beneficence. But we may be, at the same time, including economic factors that could be at once self-interested and socially significant.

A way of clarifying the conflation of economic and ethical dimensions of this case is to pursue a hypothetical variant. Suppose D.S. told the hospital that he would cease using Medicare and insurance funds for the cost of his father's treatment. Instead, he would sell the family house and use his own money for this care. Would our view of the merits of continuing treatment change? If so, how? The case of Mr. H.S. invites us to consider just what is public and what is private about health care. In an epoch of shrinking resources and growing expenses, the demand to limit care will accelerate. Following the rule of autonomy—listening to the many patients (or their surrogates) who do not want intensive care in terminal situations—will perhaps save some money. But if we affirm the principle, are we not forced to hear the voice of Mr. H.S. who, deeming cost irrelevant, *wants* to be sustained as long as it is medically possible?

■ PRACTICE MODEL CASE ■

Mr. B.L. is 82 years old and moderately demented as the result of a recent MI with complications. Prior to his heart attack, he lived at home alone (his wife died a decade ago). He is no longer capable of making medical decisions; he cannot understand the nature of his clinical situation and has a difficult time communicating his wishes, no matter what the subject. Mr. B.L. had never spoken in detail with anyone about arrangements for health care or long-term care, prior to his hospitalization. He has two adult sons with large families of their own. Mr. B.L. is a middle-class retiree, owns his own home (worth about $250,000), and his life insurance policies total $300,000; his two sons are his designated heirs.

After 5 weeks in the hospital, Mr. B.L. was discharged to a nursing home. Medicare covered only a small portion of his financial burden; the rest was paid for, temporarily, by his sons. The older son sought and got court-appointed guardianship of the patient. All parties agree that the quality of care at the long-term facility is quite good. Though Mr. B.L. is in bed for much of the day and night, he is often moved to a wheelchair and is placed outside in the sunshine on occasion. Efforts at physical rehabilitation continue, with only limited success. Mr. B.L. is quiet most of the time, eats by mouth with only limited assistance, and shows no signs of deterioration.

At a conference with the nursing home social worker, the sons (who have earlier discussed the matter privately) ask a simple question: "How much will it cost to keep Dad here, and who will pay for it?" The social worker reports that it is most likely that Medicare will reimburse very little of Mr. B.L.'s expenses and that either the family will have to pay or the patient will have to pay until his assets reach the Medicaid limit of $2000 (the spend-down requirement). At that time public assistance would provide financial support adequate to keep Mr. B.L. in the nursing home. The brothers realize that it is too late to redistribute their father's considerable assets in order to avoid this government mandate. Nursing home charges have approached an average $1000 per week.

"Suppose we just brought him home?" one of the brothers inquired. The social worker was concerned about who would provide the substantial custodial care that this patient requires. The brothers said that they and their families would take turns and could even stay over with Mr. B.L. on most evenings. They were willing to expend a small amount of money to bring a home health aide into the home, perhaps twice a week. The social worker noted that Medicare might support the visit of a home health aide two or three times a week. The brothers estimated that it would cost about $300 per week to supplement those arrangements. "We would rather spend our own money to help Dad at home and save everything he's accumulated during a lifetime," said the older brother.

The social worker has a very basic concern: Is Mr. B.L. well enough to live at home with limited assistance? The attending physician at the facility believes that he is, but points out that he could get very sick at any time. In addition, the social worker wonders about the motivation of the two brothers. He asks them, quite bluntly, about their reasons for advocating home care. They state, very candidly, that they see no reason why their father's assets should be completely depleted. "At his age," says the older brother, "he would want us to keep him at home and retain some of what he's saved for his grandchildren."

Patient

Unaware of the debate that is occurring around him, Mr. B.L. is the subject of a discussion about allocation of resources that could leave considerations for his well-being behind. Objectively we know that he is quite ill but stable. He will not recover much of his previous level of functioning, and he is at risk for all sorts of problems, including infection, stroke, deterioration of his heart, and pulmonary complications (including pneumonia) at any time. It is not a medical necessity, according to the physician, that he remain in the nursing home. But his wishes regarding where he ought to go are unknown.

Would Mr. B.L. be better off at home? He does retain minimal awareness of his surroundings—could that mean that the familiar terrain along with the proximity of close relatives will bring him pleasure? Shall we surmise that this is likely? Such guesswork is often avoidable in placement determinations. Mr. B.L. has long lived alone at home, but he is no longer capable of such independent existence. What is the trade-off here? Were the patient to remain in the nursing home (at much greater expense), he could be supervised around the clock. At home, his supervision is up to his sons and a function of the arrangements they have made for home care (at a much lower rate).

Though it is our natural inclination to focus on Mr. B.L. as the patient in this case, we are accustomed to seeing other, similarly situated persons as part of a larger and more complex definition of patient (see Chapters 3 and 5). We refer to pediatric dilemmas in which we speak of the child in the family. Attention to the needs of families is conventional in pediatrics ethics cases. Is Mr. B.L., a geriatrics patient, conceptually in the same situation? If so, concerns for the sons and their families might be in order. A more detailed investigation of family history and dynamics may be appropriate, no matter what our definition of patienthood.

Relationships

In a narrow, literal sense, Mr. B.L. is no longer capable of having relationships. His dementia makes content-based communication virtually impossible. But this case asks us to widen the scope of relationships quite broadly. Mr. B.L.'s sons certainly think of their father as present, hence their concern about having him live at home. The past web of connections among family members represents a historical foundation of plans, feelings, and memories that must be kept in mind.

The fact that the older son is a court-appointed guardian for Mr. B.L. creates opportunities and difficulties. Assuming that the nature of the guardianship appointment includes the obligation to make health care choices for Mr. B.L. on the grounds of his best interest (with court scrutiny, if necessary), at least we have a designated decision-maker. But who is to "guard the guardian" if determinations are made regarding this patient that are not overtly deleterious? Because guardians are usually pledged to economic responsibility, some might argue that a decision to save funds by bringing Mr. B.L. home is consistent with the conservatorship granted the older son.

Given the emphasis on cost of care in this case, we might examine a more global question about relationships. What are the moral obligations of the sons to their aging and very ill father? Are they entitled to the larger inheritance that will be theirs and their families' if health care and custodial costs for Mr. B.L. can be minimized? How can we balance cost-effectiveness with anxiety about patient well-being? What is the relationship between quantity and quality of life? What sense does it make to provide excellent and expensive nursing home care to a patient who will experience it only minimally and inevitably not at all? Does the fact that Mr. B.L. is 82 and quite ill mean that he should lose his claim on the common weal?

Advocacy

There is no reason to believe that Mr. B.L.'s sons wish to do harm to their father, but the level and intensity of their advocacy appears to be influenced by self-interest. Who, then, is to urge this silent patient's perspective? The social worker has taken on the role of advocate, but his capacity to act is weakened by the grant of guardianship to the older son. Of course, the social worker (or another interested party) could challenge the guardianship in probate court. Grounds for such a challenge, however, must be strong and convincing. Because the physician has already stated that Mr. B.L. could legitimately be brought home, a judge would not be likely to shift guardianship.

From the macro perspective, some healthcare economists and ethicists have argued that social values require advocacy too. In a society that cannot provide everything, the grounds for rationing should be rational and sensible. Does age-based or disability-based rationing meet these criteria? Should those who speak for Mr. B.L. recognize that the elderly owe it to generations that follow to provide only palliative care in the most cost-effective manner?

Conflicts

Placement is the surface issue: Should Mr. B.L. stay in the nursing home or should he receive family-based home health care? The clinical decision is influenced by medical, economic, interpersonal, and social factors. To deny Mr. B.L. nursing home care is not obviously unfair. But because money has been mentioned as a motivating element, we become morally suspicious. In fairness to the sons, home health care is *not* inferior care. Of the elderly population that is disabled and in need of assistance in daily living, three-quarters continue to live outside of long-term care facilities. Many choose to remain at home. The frail elderly and those who need active medical intervention often move from home to acute-care hospital to nursing home and back again. Care for chronic patients at home is routine and is now supported by public agencies, voluntary systems, and private, for-profit organizations.

Implicit in the case of Mr. B.L. is an argument about how much and in what mode government should be paying for the care of the debilitated elderly. The bulk of designated funds from Medicare goes to acute-care institutions and to physicians. Medicaid will eventually pay for nursing home care for those without means. Home care services receive very little payment from patients directly—Medicare, Medicaid, Social Security, and various grants are the principal sources of payment. Should there be a shift from expensive and interventionist acute-care spending to lower-tech, family-supported, home-based health care? This conflict is political and will not easily be settled in an epoch of scarce resources.

Oddly enough, cost containment measures have placed many patients in the situation of Mr. B.L. Incentives to move patients out of hospitals have meant that nursing homes, which sometimes lack the rehabilitation facilities and staffing necessary for the comprehensive care of ill patients, become swamped with problems. Finding economically sound ways of bringing Mr. B.L. home is challenging, for he will continue to need unskilled nursing care, transportation services to go to the doctor, laboratory services, medication and supplies, and special equipment. The shift of locale is a risk to more than the patient's well-being; it also brings to light the debate about the assessment of quality in health care.

Treatment or Nontreatment Options

Let us suppose that Mr. B.L. develops a high fever at home and one of his sons is providing family care at the time. Should the son call the ambulance service or rush his father to the hospital himself? Here, the crunch between quality and quantity of life becomes crucial. The fever — assume an infectious pneumonia as its cause — could be a life-threatening symptom. Should Mr. B.L. be placed on the roller coaster of ER admission, intensive care, hospitalization, and nursing home placement, until he again becomes the subject of whether or not to be brought home? A single treatment option is rooted in a concern for social values: Is it just to continue such expensive care for this patient?

Does Mr. B.L. have a right to health care that transcends the literal decision-making power granted to his son via guardianship? Is that right limited by the availability of resources? Is there a guaranteed minimum of basic care that should be available to all? Has Mr. B.L. exceeded that minimum? How will a trend to shift from extending life through new technologies to palliating pain and suffering determine the entitlement of this patient? As a society, we have not yet determined precise ways of limiting specific kinds of treatment. The sons' desire to save money could be sound and responsible. The extent to which they should influence treatment determinations is unexplored territory.

Interests

Mr. B.L. has given no prior statement about how he wishes his interests pursued. We can assume that he wishes to be comfortable and to experience whatever pleasures he can perceive. Though these interests are quite basic, they are still real. Judgments about placement must take into account prophecies about Mr. B.L.'s future and how he will experience it. For example, if avoiding the revolving door of acute illness and fervent intervention is a goal, then the patient might have an interest in being at home. Nursing homes are reluctant to put into effect limited-treatment plans: They almost inevitably call 911 when an acute episode occurs. Mr. B.L. could also have a more tangible interest in being at home because of the presence of familiar surroundings and close relatives. But such judgments are little more than guesses.

The sons have an interest that goes beyond the desire to inherit as much as possible. If they truly believe that Mr. B.L.'s own wishes to leave a patrimony to his children and grandchildren will be violated by spending down in the nursing home, they are speaking for their father and not only for themselves. The sons may also, perhaps unknowingly, be voicing the social policy perspective: Home health care is, in many cases, more supportive, efficient, and useful than institutional care. However, if taking the patient home results in neglect, we may legitimately say that *they* have abused Mr. B.L.'s best interests.

Do all parties have an interest in cost containment? The common wisdom in recent decades has asserted that the development of expensive technology along with heightened consumer demand, supplemented by institutional and professional greed, have combined to increase the cost of health care in this country beyond reason. The national medical care bill will reach $1 trillion annually very soon. Efforts at reversing retrospective payment plans have had some success, though the shift of costs to other parts of the system has also been observed. The growth of HMOs, with gatekeeper primary care physicians, has contributed to cost effectiveness. Managed care may well be the experience of most working Americans very soon. Yet costs have not stabilized.

Short of a fully-regulated national insurance scheme or a single-payer national health plan (both of which seem unlikely to develop), some form of system-wide rationing seems inevitable. (The present rationing system depends on a medically indigent population of more than 30 million people.) Should Mr. B.L.'s case be seen as an illustration of cost-effective limitation of care, an effort to meet the public's interest now?

Consequences

For the patient, the consequences are unpredictable. Remaining in the nursing home ought to guarantee a sound level of care, but how sick Mr. B.L. might become cannot be known. Oddly enough, nursing homes and hospitals are the natural sites of iatrogenic disease, especially through infection. Could this patient be safer at home? We know that Mr. B.L. will not get well and that he will die, if not sooner then later. He is not, however, terminal at the moment. Decisions about his final days will still have to be made; the likely surrogate will be his older son.

Life will change dramatically for the family should Mr. B.L. come home. Caring for a frail, elderly relative is a difficult and comprehensive task. The burdens are great and they do not lessen, day or night. Simply finding respite care or getting neighbors or friends to drop in is a difficult job. The relationships between formal and informal family caregivers is often frustrating. When a nursing aide gets stuck in traffic and the daughter-in-law must miss work, crisis time can draw near. The costs are also financial, for the estimates given the social worker of what the family is prepared to pay for Mr. B.L. are only suggestive. Who pays, and when, must also be worked out. Finally, the length of care could be weeks, months or years and cannot be predicted. The open-ended nature of the commitment must be taken into account in decision-making.

In the long term, for society as a whole, decisions about nursing home or home health care will depend on economic and political factors. A move toward long-term care insurance, possibly government subsidized, would change the equation completely. Recent changes in how hospice care is reimbursed and how patients might move from acute-care settings to hospice-based home terminal care will alter the system as a whole. Suffice it to say, Medicaid will probably never have to pay for Mr. B.L.'s care; if he stays in the nursing home it will take many years for the spend down to happen. If he goes home, his children or his own accumulated wealth will contribute to his management.

Ethical Principles

Autonomy is a memory for Mr. B.L. Beneficence obliges his sons to act in his best interest and his caregivers to protect those interests if they are impeded or harmed. Eventually, the principle of nonmaleficence might lead a substitute decision-maker to say "enough," and allow Mr. B.L. to die. In these regards, Mr. B.L.'s case resembles many other end-of-life scenarios (see Chapter 8). What distinguishes the case is a concern for the principle of justice.

Over and above our scrutiny of the moral and sometimes legal rights of the individual, justice as a concept moves us to look at the precedent value of our decisions, especially about the implications of how goods, services, and resources are distributed. At times the question is asked quite directly: If the ICU is filled and an emergency patient will die without access, who is well enough to be moved to a medical-surgical floor? Most of the time, however, inquiry is indirect, lacking a specific patient or client as a focus.

Should we treat like cases alike? Or are some patients (e.g., the altruist, the benefactor) more valuable than others? Does medical need trump individual desire for treatment? Should we provide access based on ability to pay or on other grounds? In triage situations, how do we define the probabilities of clinical success? Should we ration via considerations of social worth; first come, first served; or randomly as a testimonial to human equality? Are there situations in which we could advocate stopping a treatment program—say an experimental transplantation scheme involving only a few potential patients—in favor of expending funds on many people?

Justice for Mr. B.L. could perhaps be secured by guaranteeing government support of the elderly, no matter what their financial status. It could come through improved home health support. It could be a product of a national health policy that deemed medical care a definite, if limited, right, as in certain European nations and Canada. Or justice could remain a utopian ideal, a dream of fairness and equality that floats above everyday decision-making in a land of unlimited opportunity and medical scarcity.

■ CASES FOR DISCUSSION ■

Case A

Mr. F., a 65-year-old retired firefighter, was admitted to E. Hospital with a history of severe cardiac problems. Another heart attack seemed imminent, so extensive cardiac surgery was required. A few hours later it was apparent that one or more of the anastomoses was leaking. Mr. F. was operated on again and experienced a variety of technical problems resulting in massive bleeding, leading to shock, anoxia, and presumed irreversible brain damage.

The patient failed to show any sign of meaningful recovery and died 4 weeks after the second surgery. During the course of the hospitalization, Mr. F. had 280 blood gas determinations (expensive tests) and 36 blood transfusions, and his total hospital bill came to $111,000. Throughout the course of these events, Mrs. F., his wife of 30 years, was told by the treating physicians that they were doing all they could for her husband.

Questions

1. What arguments can be made for initially attempting the surgery on this patient?
2. After the complications of surgery during the second effort, should a review of costs and benefits to the patient have been offered to Mrs. F.?
3. Are there any limits—and if so, what are they—to the diagnostic and therapeutic regimes for a patient in Mr. F.'s condition?
4. What are the justifications for the expenditure of $111,000 in this case?

Case B

Dr. J. has been an obstetrician-gynecologist with a flourishing practice for 7 years. She has delivered more than 1000 babies (the figure includes her residency training). She enjoys the work, but economic frustrations and worries are growing. She has been sued twice for malpractice, after the birth of children with severe defects. Both times, after agonizing pretrial investigations, the lawsuits were dropped.

The annual premium Dr. J. must pay for malpractice insurance is $145,000. This is more than double the amount she paid 4 years ago. The reimbursement she receives from her patients via third-party payers, Medicaid, and out-of-pocket payments are insufficient to run an office, repay her educational loans, raise a family, and pay for the insurance premiums, which are particularly expensive in the state in which she practices. Given the current litigious climate she also feels pressure to order many tests that have only limited validity. Her OB/GYN colleagues tell her that such defensive medicine is unfortunate but can also be a source of income. Dr. J. feels uncomfortable with this admonition.

"I have been thinking of moving," she tells a colleague, "and shifting to a general, primary care practice. I could get licensed fairly swiftly in one of the unpopulated mountain states. I could be a family doctor and still deliver babies. My insurance coverage would cost around $25,000. I could simplify my concerns and still make twice as much as I do now." Dr. J. would have to give up her specialized practice if she makes such a move.

Questions

1. Are Dr. J.'s concerns about the legal and insurance issues reasonable ones? Or is the milieu in which such physicians practice one in which adjustment is the appropriate response?
2. Does the warning to practice defensive medicine via unnecessary testing mean that Dr. J. has no choice but to engage in the practice?
3. What do this physician's motives for shifting practice seem to be?
4. Given the rather large expenditure of time and government-supported funding that went into Dr. J.'s medical education, what implications for the allocation of scarce resources could be discovered in examining her proposed move from OB/GYN to general practice?

■ THINK PIECE: ALLOCATING RESOURCES ■

Medical ethics and medical economics necessarily overlap. The large questions are quite serious. How can we make the final days of life less painful and less costly? Should we shift from an interventive to a preventive model of health care? Should research funds be spent on terminal diseases such as cancer or on other ailments such as arthritis that are painful and chronic? If a national health plan would result in greater access for patients but also in diminished freedom for physicians, what would be the consequences for doctor-patient relationships? The public debate on large-scale issues has scarcely begun. It will be long and painful.

For every lofty, if speculative, issue in health care delivery and finance, we can find a closer-to-home illustration with real problems and real impacts. In a recent poll, respondents were given a lengthy list of social and community problems (e.g., toxic waste clean-up, crime prevention, bridge and road repair, and drug and alcohol treatment) and were asked to prioritize them. Seventy-six percent said that state government should spend tax dollars on long-term care for the elderly. The prospects of achieving federal or state support are minimal. It is not difficult to see why many persons advocate long-term care assistance by government. The cost of nursing home living forces most older persons to sell all of their assets to pay for long-term care. Having spent decades raising a family, pursuing a career, buying and paying off a house, and saving for retirement, older voters (and those with the capacity to imagine themselves older) are frightened by the prospects of using it all to pay for nursing home care. Can the public's desire for such a program be put into effect? What will it cost? Will all those other social problems simply fade into the background?

Another seemingly minor illustration: For years doctors have given patients free drug samples provided by the pharmaceutical industry. This practice is fundamentally unregulated (except for habit-forming drugs). There are beneficent reasons given: Poor patients cannot afford expensive prescriptions; starting the patient off immediately is medically useful to determine the therapeutic response and likely to result in compliant behavior; patients in general appreciate the special attention given them. There is another side to the story, however, one with fiscal implications. Samples of drugs are distributed to physicians by pharmaceutical companies via manufacturer's personnel who also provide physicians with information and who try to promote the use of the product. Leaving free samples with a doctor is a big business and the quantity of drugs so provided is immense, perhaps more than $500,000 worth every day of the work week. The promotional budget of a drug company is also enormous and costs are reflected in the price of drugs that are bought at the pharmacy. Many samples are disposed of not by being given to patients but by being consigned to the trash. Should a limitation be placed on the distribution of free drug samples? Who should decide?

A third, and final, micro example of a macro problem in health care finance and delivery: New remedies for infertility are being developed almost daily. Utilizing new diagnostic devices such as ultrasound and laparoscopy, specialists in reproductive medicine can devise specific plans to help infertile couples to achieve pregnancy and childbirth. The lengthy process of trying to get pregnant results in several million office visits per year. If a couple tries *in vitro* fertilization the cost for each attempt can exceed $7000. Some insurance companies will reimburse in whole or in part for such procedures; many will not. Is infertility a "disease" that deserves treatment? Who should pay for such care? If 35 million persons lack even basic access to the health care delivery system, should this fact have an impact on our policy regarding new reproductive technology?

Setting priorities in health care allocation is an unconscious, inchoate process in the United States. The chief executive officer of a large hospital has said, "The health care system in American is no system." Would broader, public participation in health care policy determination further or attenuate the state of present discontent? Can settling issues of fairness, justice, and cost at the societal level be translated into practical decisions at the micro level?

■ VOICES: HEALTH CARE PLANNER/ ■ ■ ADMINISTRATOR OF HMO ■

I think that there is a right to health care for all citizens, but that right is limited. An appropriate intervention to relieve pain and suffering is an absolute minimum need. But treatment of truly questionable merit should not be guaranteed. Let me give two examples. My father, at the age of 76 with a history of cardiovascular disease, was diagnosed as an emergency with 95 percent occlusion and was prepared for CABG surgery. Otherwise he was in pretty good health. Without the surgery he would probably die soon unless he stayed in bed and took a great deal of medication. He was operated on and lived 2 more years. Case number two: My best friend's father, a diabetic, with hypertension, chronic renal failure, and a candidate for dialysis went in for the identical problem. Against the better judgments of the doctors, the patient and family insisted on the surgery for the arterial blockage. This man never left the ICU and died in the hospital after 3 months of care. The bill was $350,000. *That* is a waste of resources.

My point is quite evident. Medical determinations—if rationally based on solid clinical data—about what will be effective for the given patient are usually economically sound. I don't want to limit that claim to just medical judgment. Humane concerns—that patients' lives not be dragged out forever—are usually cost-effective as well. If we are going to set limits on what patients can legitimately receive from the health care system, I don't believe that age is the most important factor. The value of a person's life is too subjective, too personal an experience, to set an arbitrary limit with a number. The physiology and the medical condition of the patient is the only logical factor in either giving or limiting treatment. It has to be based on degree of risk and survivability.

The economic cost of any given procedure probably does impact on a decision about whether to treat or not to treat. But in reality our society is never going to say no to an individual who truly wants an operation. Even insurance companies, with all of their efforts to limit cost, can't really say no. We are paying too much for things that shouldn't be done in the first place. We need to take the dollars we have and provide better care before people get sick. At the moment we are eliminating the very services (e.g., community health clinics) that save us money in the long term. We don't do much in the way of home health care, prenatal care, nutrition, sex education, immunizations, or birth control. But we pay billions to neonatal units and hospitals every year because of this failure to structure things logically.

Here's an example. The money we spent in ERs should be put into primary care. We did a survey recently and looked at our patients for a month as they went to the ER at a major hospital. Of the 134 patients who visited the ER, 68 percent were nonurgent care. They have a walk-in center at that hospital, just across the hall from the emergency area. But only one of those patients was triaged in that direction. This is crazy. We need a little bus that stops at the ER. Then we tell the patient, "Here at the ER we can see you in about 3 hours; if you want to take the bus outside, we will get you to a doctor 5 minutes away who can see you immediately." This is not just a homey example. It will really save money. We need to set up day surgery programs so that we can close beds in favor of a lower-cost unit. But there's not enough incentive to be creative.

I think that in the year 2010 we still will not have gone very far to make health care in the United States cost efficient. We will not be ready for centralized or regionalized decision-making. For example, there are too many doctors right now, but I don't think anyone will be willing to close medical schools. As for taking care of indigent patients, we already have enough money in the system to take care of them. There are too many empty beds and they are already being paid for by government or insurance companies. Can't we use these resources— and we should be using the money more wisely than just by putting patients into those beds—for those who lack coverage? We have so many specialized units in hospitals that are operating at 25 to 50 percent efficiency. All hospitals seem to think that they need every conceivable piece of equipment. How many MRI machines do we need? There is an incentive to have such stuff. You only get reimbursed for the services you provide. But in doing so we waste a lot of money. Still, we are not prepared as a society to give someone such as a regional health care authority the clout to close those wasteful units and to make wholesale system changes. State governments are too timid and insurance companies are not going to take the lead. Businesses may eventually demand a national health system, but I wouldn't bet on its being put into practice.

We are stuck with an iatrogenic model. We have created a system that is so dependent on the patient being acutely sick, and that is so driven by economics, that we can't undo it. We live in a disabling society. Everything becomes a health care problem. We shift around a little bit, keeping people in hospitals for a shorter time but then move them to long-term care facilities that are also expensive. There are some small improvements, but the system stays stuck. I am very skeptical about any real rational utilization of the delivery of health care. My hope is that we can improve slowly and prod the system into getting things straight. We could stop paying for psychiatric services when they are not needed: About 80 percent of what psychiatrists do can be done better by psychologists or others. This is only an example. But shaking up the system is required if anything substantial is to change.

RECOMMENDED READING

Callahan, D. *Setting Limits: Medical Goals in an Aging Society*. New York: Simon and Schuster, 1987.

Churchill, L. *Rationing Health Care in America: Perceptions and Principles of Justice*. Notre Dame, IN: University of Notre Dame Press, 1987.

Daniels, N. *Just Health Care*. New York: Cambridge University Press, 1985.

Fein, R. *Medical Care, Medical Costs*. Cambridge, MA: Harvard University Press, 1986.

Ginzburg, E. *The Medical Triangle*. Cambridge, MA: Harvard University Press, 1990.

Salmon, J. W., ed. *Issues and Directions: The Corporate Transformation of Health Care*. Amityville, NY: Baywood, 1990.

Glossary

Abandonment of patient. Termination of a doctor-patient relationship by the physician without reasonable notice or provision for continuity of health care.

Access. Degree to which the health care system aids or inhibits an individual or group in gaining entry and receiving needed services in light of constraints in financing and delivery of care.

Active euthanasia. Intentional or direct ending of a human life either in response to a competent request (voluntary active euthanasia) or without such a request (nonvoluntary active euthanasia).

Advance directives. Instructions (usually written) from a competent individual for future health care in the event of incompetency. Living wills and durable powers of attorney for health care documents are common examples. Legal provisions vary from state to state.

Assault. An intentional physical attack designed to make the victim fearful; produces reasonable apprehension of harm. Actionable under criminal and civil law.

Assent. Agreement to research or treatment given by a mature minor not legally old enough to give a valid informed consent.

Autonomy. Making decisions for oneself, in light of a personal system of values and beliefs.

Battery. The willful touching of one person by another without permission. Actionable under criminal and civil law.

Beneficence. The state or act of intentionally doing or producing good.

Best interest standard. A judgment based on an idea of what would be most beneficial to a patient, usually pursued in the absence of a patient's expressed wishes.

Bioethics committees. An interdisciplinary group that deals with conflicts of values in patient care in acute and long-term settings. Such committees discuss policy issues (e.g., regarding withholding and withdrawing of life-sustaining treatments).

Capitation. A method of payment for health services, often found in health maintenance organizations and preferred provider organizations. A provider is paid a fixed amount for each person served for a period of time, without regard to the number or nature of the services provided to each person.

Certificate of need (CON). Document provided by state regulators that limits capital expenditures by hospitals, nursing homes, and other institutional providers to prevent duplication of services and facilities.

Common law. Laws developed via precedents set in court decisions rather than those passed by legislatures.

Competent. A legal concept that describes people who are able to make decisions for themselves. Minors are presumed to be incompetent, except under certain specified conditions. The corollary medical-ethical term is *decisional capacity*.

Confidentiality. The professional-client promise not to reveal information without consent.

Consent. See Informed consent.

Contract. A legally enforceable promissory agreement between two or more people that creates, alters, or terminates a legal promise to undertake stated obligations.

Cost benefit analysis. An analytic procedure to aid in balancing a procedure's or program's fiscal cost with its benefits, frequently expressed in dollars. Sometimes referred to as risk-benefit analysis.

Cost containment. The effort to control the overall cost of the health care delivery system. Government and insurance regulations that endeavor to create a more cost-effective system.

Defendant. The person in a criminal case who is accused of committing a crime. The party in a civil action against whom suit is brought.

Deontologism. The ethical theory according to which actions are judged right or wrong based on their inherent characteristics or principles rather than on their consequences.

Deposition. A sworn statement made as part of the process of discovering the facts after a lawsuit has been filed.

Diagnosis related group (DRG). A patient classification system utilized in the Medicare prospective payment system that relates demographic, diagnostic, and therapeutic characteristics of patients to length of inpatient stay and amount of resources consumed.

Do not resuscitate (DNR). An order in a patient's record not to revive a patient who develops a cardiopulmonary arrest.

Double effect. A doctrine originating in Roman Catholic theology that holds that an evil effect is morally acceptable provided a proportional good effect will accrue, so long as the evil is not intended.

Durable power of attorney for health care. An advance directive that goes into effect in the event that a patient who has completed such a document loses decisional capacity. Allows an individual to name a person(s) who is empowered to make health care decisions when the individual becomes incapacitated.

Emancipated minor. A teenaged minor who is legally independent of parental control and who can thus give informed consent to medical treatments.

Emergency. A sudden unexpected occurrence or event causing serious threat to life and health.

Euthanasia. The act of either permitting a person to die or intentionally ending a person's life, generally rooted in motives of mercy, beneficence, or respect for patient dignity.

Felony. A serious criminal offense commonly punished by more than one year's imprisonment (e.g., murder or burglary).

Fidelity. Being faithful to a person or principle.

Gatekeeper. The role of a manager of a patient's care and treatment (by specialists and institutions) usually fulfilled by a primary care physician. Because the gatekeeper is charged with screening diseases and disorders and recommending or approving interventions as necessary, the role is designed to enhance cost effectiveness.

Good Samaritan law. A legal doctrine designed to provide immunity from liability for those who stop to render aid in an emergency.

Guardian ad litem. A court-appointed guardian who acts on behalf of a person involved in a lawsuit or court proceeding and who cannot act on her or his own behalf.

Health Care Financing Agency (HCFA). The federal agency within the Department of Health and Human Services that administers the Medicare and Medicaid programs at the federal level.

Health maintenance organization (HMO). A system for providing comprehensive prepaid health care in which providers deliver health services to a group of subscribers at a predetermined cost.

Iatrogenic. A clinical problem or disorder that results from factors found within the health care environment. An example is the development of an infectious disease contracted during hospitalization.

Indictment. A formal written accusation of a crime brought by a prosecuting attorney against a person charged with criminal conduct.

Informed consent. The legal and ethical requirement that no significant medical procedure can be performed until the competent patient has been informed of the nature of the procedure, risks and alternatives, as well as the prognosis if the procedure is not done. The patient must freely and voluntarily agree to have the procedure done.

Justice. The principle that states that fairness requires equals to be treated equally.

Living will. An advance directive document that allows a person in advance of a debilitating illness to state his or her preferences regarding the withholding or withdrawal of life-sustaining treatment or other significant medical interventions.

Macroallocation. The assessment and distribution of goods and services on a society-wide basis.

Malpractice. Negligent professional conduct or the improper discharge of professional duties that fails to meet the standard of care, resulting in harm to a person.

Managed care. An effort to contain health care costs by limiting inappropriate or excessive utilization of health care services.

Mature minor. A teenaged minor who may give consent because the physician judges that he or she understands the nature, purposes, and risks of the proposed treatment.

Medicaid. The federally aided, state operated and administered program that provides medical benefits for certain low-income persons in need of health and medical care. Typically people who are aged, blind, disabled, or members of families with dependent children with one parent absent are included; regulations vary from state to state.

Medicare. The federal health insurance program for people aged 65 and older who receive Social Security or Railroad Retirement benefits; it also incorporates persons who need kidney transplantation or dialysis, regardless of age or income.

Metaethics. The branch of ethics having to do with the meaning of moral terms and their justification.

Microallocation. The distribution of scarce resources on an individual or small-group scale.

Misdemeanor. An unlawful act of a less serious nature than a felony, usually punishable by fine or imprisonment for a period of less than 1 year.

Murder. The intentional and willful taking of a human life.

Negligence. An act or failure to act as an ordinary prudent person in the performance of duties.

Nonmaleficence. The state of not doing harm or evil; see also beneficence.

Passive euthanasia. Intentionally allowing a person to die by withholding or withdrawing treatment or by permitting the disease process to progress without further intervention.

Paternalism. Treating another person the way a parent treats a child in an attempt to promote the other's good either without acknowledgement or against the other's wishes.

Peer review. The evaluation by practicing physicians or others of the efficacy and efficiency of services ordered or performed by other practicing medical professionals.

Plaintiff. The party to a civil suit whose lawsuit seeks damages or other relief.

Preferred provider organization (PPO). A contractual arrangement in which providers negotiate with group purchasers, either directly or through the insurer or other third party, to provide health services for a given population.

Primary care. The first-line level of health care typically found in a person's entry into the health care system, usually involving preventive services as well as diagnosis and treatment of common illnesses.

Privileged communication. Information communicated to an attorney, physician, spouse, or counselor that may not be revealed, even in court, without the consent of the person who made the statement.

Proxy consent. Voluntary informed consent given on behalf of another who is for some reason incapable of giving it for himself or herself.

Rationality. The capacity to draw reasonable inferences from the known to the unknown.

Substituted judgment standard. Decisions based on an estimation of what an individual would have chosen.

Suicide. The intentional, uncoerced, and direct causation of one's own death.

Suit. Court proceeding in which a person who alleges injury seeks damages or other legal remedies from another. The term is not usually used in criminal cases.

Third-party payer. Any organization, public or private (e.g., an insurance company) that pays or insures health or medical expenses on behalf of beneficiaries or recipients; payments are usually based on premiums received from the insured, an employer, or a combination of the two.

Utilitarianism. The perspective that an action is morally justifiable because it produces the greatest balance of good over evil, taking into account all individuals affected.

Veracity. The principle that values telling the truth and establishes honesty in human relationships as a prime value.

Appendixes

A. THE HIPPOCRATIC OATH

I swear by Apollo Physician and Asclepius and Hygieia and Panaceia and all the gods and goddesses, making them my witnesses, that I will fulfil according to my ability and judgment this oath and this covenant:

To hold him who has taught me this art as equal to my parents and to live my life in partnership with him, and if he is in need of money to give him a share of mine, and to regard his offspring as equal to my brothers in male lineage and to teach them this art—if they desire to learn it—without fee and covenant; to give a share of precepts and oral instruction and all the other learning to my sons and to the sons of him who has instructed me and to pupils who have signed the covenant and have taken an oath according to the medical law, but to no one else.

I will apply dietetic measures for the benefit of the sick according to my ability and judgment; I will keep them from harm and injustice.

I will neither give a deadly drug to anybody if asked for it, nor will I make a suggestion to this effect. Similarly I will not give to a woman an abortive remedy. In purity and holiness I will guard my life and my art.

I will not use the knife, not even on sufferers from stone, but will withdraw in favor of such men as are engaged in this work.

Whatever houses I may visit, I will come for the benefit of the sick, remaining free of all intentional injustice, of all mischief and in particular of sexual relations with both female and male persons, be they free or slaves.

What I may see or hear in the course of the treatment or even outside of the treatment in regard to the life of men, which on no account one must spread abroad, I will keep to myself holding such things shameful to be spoken about.

If I fulfil this oath and do not violate it, may it be granted to me to enjoy life and art, being honored with fame among all men for all time to come; if I transgress it and swear falsely, may the opposite of all this be my lot.

B. AMERICAN MEDICAL ASSOCIATION'S PRINCIPLES OF MEDICAL ETHICS

The medical profession has long subscribed to a body of ethical statements developed primarily for the benefit of the patient. As a member of this profession, a physician must recognize responsibility not only to patients, but also to society, to other health professionals, and to self. The following Principles adopted by the American Medical Association are not laws, but standards of conduct which define the essentials of honorable behavior for the physician.

   I. A physician shall be dedicated to providing competent medical service with compassion and respect for human dignity.
  II. A physician shall deal honestly with patients and colleagues, and strive to expose those physicians deficient in character or competence, or who engage in fraud or deception.
 III. A physician shall respect the law and also recognize a responsibility to seek changes in those requirements which are contrary to the best interests of the patient.
  IV. A physician shall respect the rights of patients, of colleagues, and of other health professionals, and shall safeguard patient confidences within the constraints of the law.
   V. A physician shall continue to study, apply and advance scientific knowledge, make relevant information available to patients, colleagues, and the public, obtain consultation, and use the talents of other health professionals when indicated.
  VI. A physician shall, in the provision of appropriate patient care, except in emergencies, be free to choose whom to serve, with whom to associate, and the environment in which to provide medical services.
 VII. A physician shall recognize a responsibility to participate in activities contributing to an improved community.

(From American Medical Association, Principles of medical ethics. American Medical News August, 1980. p. 9.).

C. AMERICAN HOSPITAL ASSOCIATION'S PATIENT'S BILL OF RIGHTS

The American Hospital Association presents a Patient's Bill of Rights with the expectation that observance of these rights will contribute to more effective patient care and greater satisfaction for the patient, his physician and the hospital organization. Further, the Association presents these rights in the expectation that they will be supported by the hospital on behalf of its patients, as an integral part of the healing process. It is recognized that a personal relationship between the physician and the patient is essential for the provision of proper medical care. The traditional physician-patient relationship takes on a new dimension when care is rendered within an organizational structure. Legal precedent has established that the institution itself also has a responsibility to the patient. It is in recognition of these factors that these rights are affirmed.

1. The patient has the right to considerate and respectful care.
2. The patient has the right to obtain from his physician complete current information concerning his diagnosis, treatment, and prognosis in terms the patient can be reasonably expected to understand. When it is not medically advisable to give such information to the patient, the information should be made available to an appropriate person in his behalf. He has the right to know by name, the physician responsible for coordinating his care.
3. The patient has the right to receive from his physician information necessary to give informed consent prior to the start of any procedure and/or treatment. Except in emergencies, such information for informed consent should include but not necessarily be limited to the specific procedure and/or treatment, the medically significant risks involved, and the probable duration of incapacitation. Where medically significant alternatives for care or treatment exist, or when the patient requests information concerning medical alternatives, the patient has the right to such information. The patient also has the right to know the name of the person responsible for the procedures and/or treatment.
4. The patient has the right to refuse treatment to the extent permitted by law, and to be informed of the medical consequences of his action.

5. The patient has the right to every consideration of his privacy concerning his own medical care program. Case discussion, consultation, examination, and treatment are confidential and should be conducted discreetly. Those not directly involved in his care must have the permission of the patient to be present.

6. The patient has the right to expect that all communications and records pertaining to his care should be treated as confidential.

7. The patient has the right to expect that within its capacity a hospital must make reasonable response to the request of a patient for services. The hospital must provide evaluation, service, and/or referral as indicated by the urgency of the case. When medically permissible a patient may be transferred to another facility only after he has received complete information and explanation concerning the needs for and alternatives to such a transfer. The institution to which the patient is to be transferred must first have accepted the patient for transfer.

8. The patient has the right to obtain information as to any relationship of his hospital to other health care and educational institutions insofar as his care is concerned. The patient has the right to obtain information as to the existence of any professional relationships among individuals, by name, who are treating him.

9. The patient has the right to be advised if the hospital proposes to engage in or perform human experimentation affecting his care or treatment. The patient has the right to refuse to participate in such research projects.

10. The patient has the right to expect reasonable continuity of care. He has the right to know in advance what appointment times and physicians are available and where. The patient has the right to expect that the hospital will provide a mechanism whereby he is informed by his physician or a delegate of the physician of the patient's continuing health care requirements following discharge.

11. The patient has the right to examine and receive an explanation of his bill regardless of source of payment.

12. The patient has the right to know what hospital rules and regulations apply to his conduct as a patient.

No catalogue of rights can guarantee for the patient the kind of treatment he has a right to expect. A hospital has many functions to perform, including the prevention and treatment of disease, the education of both health professionals and patients, and the conduct of clinical research. All these activities must be conducted with an overriding concern for the patient, and, above all, the recognition of his dignity as a human being. Success in achieving this recognition assures success in the defense of the rights of the patient.

(Reprinted with the permission of the American Hospital Association, copyright 1972.)

D. AMERICAN MEDICAL ASSOCIATION'S POLICY ON WITHHOLDING OR WITHDRAWING LIFE-PROLONGING MEDICAL TREATMENT

The social commitment of the physician is to sustain life and relieve suffering. Where the performance of one duty conflicts with the other, the choice of the patient, or his family or legal representative if the patient is incompetent to act in his own behalf, should prevail. In the absence of the patient's choice or an authorized proxy, the physician must act in the best interest of the patient.

For humane reasons, with informed consent, a physician may do what is medically necessary to alleviate severe pain, or cease or omit treatment to permit a terminally ill patient whose death is imminent to die. However, he should not intentionally cause death. In deciding whether the administration of potentially life-prolonging medical treatment is in the best interest of the patient who is incompetent to act in his own behalf, the physician should determine what the possibility is for extending life under humane and comfortable conditions and what are the prior expressed wishes of the patient and attitudes of the family or those who have responsibility for the custody of the patient.

Even if death is not imminent but a patient's coma is beyond doubt irreversible and there are adequate safeguards to confirm the accuracy of the diagnosis and with the concurrence of those who have responsibility for the care of the patient, it is not unethical to discontinue all means of life-prolonging medical treatment.

Life-prolonging medical treatment includes medication and artificially or technologically supplied respiration, nutrition or hydration. In treating a terminally ill or irreversibly comatose patient, the physician should determine whether the benefits of treatment outweigh its burdens. At all times, the dignity of the patient should be maintained.

(From American Medical Association Withholding or Withdrawing Life-Prolonging Medical Treatment. Current Opinions of the Council on Ethical and Judicial Affairs of the AMA Chicago: AMA, 1986.)

E. ADVANCE DIRECTIVES: LIVING WILL AND HEALTH CARE PROXY

Death is a part of life. It is a reality like birth, growth and aging. I am using this advance directive to convey my wishes about medical care to my doctors and other people looking after me at the end of my life. It is called an advance directive because it gives instructions in advance about what I want to happen to me in the future. It expresses my wishes about medical treatment that might keep me alive. I want this to be legally binding.

If I cannot make or communicate decisions about my medical care, those around me should rely on this document for instructions about measures that could keep me alive.

I do not want medical treatment (including feeding and water by tube) that will keep me alive if:

- I am unconscious and there is no reasonable prospect that I will ever be conscious again (even if I am not going to die soon in my medical condition), *or*
- I am near death from an illness or injury with no reasonable prospect of recovery.

I do want medicine and other care to make me more comfortable and to take care of pain and suffering. I want this even if the pain medicine makes me die sooner.

I want to give some extra instructions: [*Here list any special instructions, e.g., some people fear being kept alive after a debilitating stroke. If you have wishes about this, or any other conditions, please write them here.*]

The legal language in the box that follows is a health care proxy. It gives another person the power to make medical decisions for me.

> I name ————————————, who lives at ———————— ————————————, phone number ————————— to make medical decisions for me if I cannot make them myself. This person is called a health care "surrogate," "agent," "proxy," or "attorney in fact." This power of attorney shall become effective when I become incapable of making or communicating decisions about my medical care. This means that this document stays legal when and if I lose the power to speak for myself, for instance, if I am in a coma or have Alzheimer's disease.
>
> My health care proxy has power to tell others what my advance directive means. This person also has power to make decisions for me, based either on what I would have wanted, or, if this is not known, on what he or she thinks is best for me.
>
> If my first choice health care proxy cannot or decides not to act for me, I name ————————————, address ———————————— phone number ————————, as my second choice.

(continued)

I have discussed my wishes with my health care proxy, and with my second choice if I have chosen to appoint a second person. My proxy(ies) has(have) agreed to act for me.

I have thought about this advance directive carefully. I know what it means and want to sign it. I have chosen two witnesses, neither of whom is a member of my family, nor will inherit from me when I die. My witnesses are not the same people as those I named as my health care proxies. I understand that this form should be notarized if I use the box to name (a) health care proxy(ies).

Signature _____

Date _____

Address _____

Witness' signature _____

Witness' printed name _____

Address _____

Witness' signature _____

Witness' printed name _____

Address _____

Notary [to be used if proxy is appointed] _____

Drafted and distributed by Choice In Dying, Inc. — the national council for the right to die. Choice In Dying is a national not-for-profit organization which works for the rights of patients at the end of life. In addition to this generic advance directive, Choice In Dying distributes advance directives that conform to each state's specific legal requirements and maintains a national Living Will Registry for completed documents.

(Reprinted with permission of
CHOICE IN DYING, INC.
the national council for the right to die)

F. CONSENT TO TREATMENT PROCESS

POLICY

The Hospital recognizes that any adult person with the requisite mental capacity has the right to permit or refuse treatment. It is the policy of the Hospital to render treatment to any person only after obtaining consent of the person seeking treatment or of the person authorized to consent on behalf of the person seeking treatment. The Hospital also recognizes that in certain circumstances consent is implied by law and in these circumstances the Hospital will render treatment based upon the implied consent.

PROCEDURE

I. General Consent

Signatures on the back of the head sheet by the person seeking treatment or the person authorized to consent on behalf of the person seeking treatment manifests a desire to receive routine diagnostic and therapeutic treatment. It is *not* satisfactory evidence of an informed consent for invasive procedures, including surgery, research or procedures for which risks are greater than those associated with routine diagnostic and therapeutic procedures.

II. Informed Consent

A. For invasive procedures, including surgery, research or procedures for which risks are greater than those associated with routine diagnostic and therapeutic procedures, the responsible faculty or resident physician on the treating service, before preparatory sedation, must conduct an informed consent discussion with the patient or other person authorized to consent. During that discussion, the condition to be treated, the proposed risks and consequences, reasonable alternative treatment, administration of anesthesia, and the identity of the physician(s)/surgeon(s) performing the procedure are to be reviewed.

F. CONSENT TO TREATMENT PROCESS (continued)

Note: Decisions to refuse treatment or leave the Hospital against medical advice require informed consent and can only be made by patients with decision-making capacity, see Section V. below.

B. Following the informed consent discussion, the physician conducting that discussion is to fill out the relevant consent form. Information is to be as specific as possible (e.g., "open repair of fracture, left femur" is preferable to "fix broken leg"). That physician then:

1. obtains the signature of the consenting individual on the form;

2. fills in the date and time; and

3. signs as witness.

It may be helpful to have a nurse present for this discussion in order to obtain information that will be helpful in responding to the patient's concerns. Such involvement is optional, however, and does not in any way remove from the physician complete responsibility for obtaining and documenting consent.

C. The completed, signed consent form suffices as documentation of consent. The preoperative/pre-procedural progress note should state that the form has been completed and signed. A nurse involved in the informed consent discussion with the patient may document appropriately in progress/nursing notes.

D. Multiple or additional procedures to be performed at the same time may be covered in a single consent form. A separate form must be obtained for later procedures.

E. Unless an emergency as defined in Section IV. exists, the patient will not be premedicated or transported if the

F. CONSENT TO TREATMENT PROCESS (continued)

consent form and supporting note are not completed. Nursing is to notify the responsible physician and the unit where the procedure will be performed of any deficiency preventing transport. In an emergency (Section IV.), that physician must document the emergent nature of the case in a progress note. The name of the faculty physician consulted, or his cosignature, must be included in the note.

F. If the patient is premedicated before consent has been obtained and before a consent form has been signed, the case should be delayed for 24 hours unless the responsible physician can document an emergency (Section IV.) that requires proceeding on schedule and the faculty physician concurs in writing. However, if an informed consent discussion was conducted with the patient, and the patient was in agreement with the planned procedure, the case may proceed after written documentation of that fact is placed in the progress notes by the physician who conducted the discussion. Questions should be directed to Risk Management or, if Risk Management's legal staff cannot be reached, to Patient Relations.

G. If a procedure on an inpatient must be rescheduled, the consent form is valid for up to seven (7) days after it is obtained. If the patient is discharged and readmitted for the rescheduled procedure, a new consent form must be obtained even if fewer than seven (7) days have elapsed. Consent forms for same day admission and same day surgery procedures are valid for thirty (30) days but may be revalidated for an additional seven (7) days.

H. Nursing staff in the operating room or other areas where the procedure is to be performed are to check for a completed consent form or a progress note documenting the reasons for performing the surgery on an emergency basis (II.E.) or on the basis of a consent discussion under II.F. Responsibility for obtaining valid consent for the

F. CONSENT TO TREATMENT PROCESS (continued)

procedure, however, remains with the physician supervising the procedure.

III. Minors

See "Consent to Treatment of Minors."

IV. Emergencies

An emergency exists when delay is likely to result in substantial risk to the patient's life, a significant probability of loss of limb or bodily function, a major disfigurement, or psychiatric damage with irreversible harm.

A. Under these circumstances, when treatment is required for an adult, who by virtue of his condition, is incapable of consenting, or for a child whose parent or guardian is unavailable, the law implies consent to administer emergency medical services. The circumstances necessitating such action must be clearly documented in the patient's medical record by the responsible physician. The name of the faculty physician consulted in determining the emergent nature of the case, or his co-signature, should be included in that physician's note. A consent form is not required. Indicated treatment is performed under authority of the emergency note.

B. Reasonable attempts should be made to contact the patient's family prior to initiation of emergency treatment. If that attempt fails or if time does not allow, the responsible physician is to initiate efforts to contact the family promptly after the completion of emergency treatment. These attempts are to be documented in the patient's medical record.

V. Mental Incompetence

A. Determination of Capacity to Consent

F. CONSENT TO TREATMENT PROCESS (continued)

Informed consent cannot be obtained when the patient is mentally incapable of giving an informed consent whether or not he has been adjudicated incompetent. However, without such adjudication (i.e., appointment of a legal guardian), capacity to consent is presumed and the patient must consent to all procedures unless that capacity is questioned. Capacity to consent means the ability to understand the condition to be treated, the proposed procedure and what it is expected to accomplish, the known significant risks, reasonable alternative treatment, administration of anesthesia and the identity of the physician(s)/surgeon(s) performing the procedure. It is the treating physician's responsibility to determine whether the patient has the capacity to give informed consent. Psychiatric or other appropriate consultation should be requested to aid in this determination if there is doubt about the patient's ability to understand the proffered information well enough to give informed consent. However, the determination of capacity to consent remains a decision of the responsible physician.

B. Emergency Treatment of the Incompetent Patient

See IV. above.

C. Non-Emergency Treatment of a Patient Lacking Capacity to Consent

1. When treatment of a patient lacking capacity to consent is medically indicated, but a medical emergency does not exist (see IV. above), consent must be obtained from a substitute source. If a legal guardian has not been appointed, the priority list of legal next of kin from whom consent can be accepted is: 1) spouse, if marriage intact, 2) adult child, 3) parent, 4) adult brother or sister. When legal next of kin are unavailable, unresponsive or unknown, consult policy on "Substituted Consent for Mentally Incapacitated Patients."

F. CONSENT TO TREATMENT PROCESS (continued)

2. Even before identifying a substitute source of consent, it is appropriate to initiate routine diagnostic and therapeutic measures reasonably necessary to determine the nature and scope of the patient's medical problem and/or to alleviate pain and suffering.

   However, *before* invasive procedures, including surgery, research, or procedures for which risks are greater than those associated with routine diagnostic or therapeutic procedures are initiated, an informed consent must be obtained from the person authorized to consent. In the event it becomes medically advisable to perform a non-emergency procedure falling into one of these categories and no guardian or legal next of kin can be located, contact Patient Relations.

VI. The Psychiatric Patient

A. General Medical Treatment with Elective Surgery

   Patients hospitalized on the psychiatric service or admitted from a State hospital have the same right as any other patient to permit or refuse treatment as long as they are capable of consenting. If the patient is incapable of consenting (IV.A.), a substitute consent may be obtained as previously described (IV.C.) only for the cases falling under VI.B. below.

B. Emergency procedures (IV.) may be performed, when the patient is incapable of consenting, on the authorization of the patient's guardian, spouse, or next of kin. Should such a person be unable or unwilling to consent, court approval is necessary unless the delay involved in obtaining it would endanger the patient. If so, the procedure may be authorized by the Director of Inpatient Psychiatry. He and the responsible physician must execute an affidavit describing the circumstances necessitating their action. The affidavit must then be filed with the Probate Court within five days

F. CONSENT TO TREATMENT PROCESS (continued)

after the procedure, and a copy placed in the patient's medical record. Due to the need for legal action, Risk Management must be notified before the procedure is initiated. If Risk Management legal staff cannot be reached, Patient Relations is to be contacted.

C. Major aversion intervention may not be used with voluntary patients without the "informed, knowing, and intelligent written consent of the patient or his guardian." With involuntary patients, consent to major aversive interventions requires compliance with a very complicated procedure mandated by State law. Contact Risk Management for details.

D. Sterilization, psychosurgery, or any unusually hazardous treatment procedures may only be undertaken with the patient's informed consent *and* court approval. There is no provision for substituted consent.

E. Electro-Convulsive Therapy must be administered under the conditions set forth under appropriate state law.

G. EXAMPLE OF DO NOT RESUSCITATE AND TREATMENT OF CRITICALLY ILL PATIENT PROCESS

POLICY

I. To render care and treatment appropriate to the patient's condition.

The appropriateness of treatment plans, in critically ill patients including those in whom death would not be unexpected, depends on:

A. The medical evaluation of the responsible physician (taking into account the patient's particular situation as well as the assessments of other staff), *and*

B. The desire of the patient (either in written or oral statements) or whomever may speak for him.

II. *To affirm* that no person has the right to speak for a conscious adult who has decision-making capacity; and *to respect* the right of those adults to refuse treatment.

In the event a patient lacks decision-making capacity, the Hospital will allow an appropriate legal representative (See "Substituted Consent for Mentally Incapacitated Patients" policy) to speak for him—*unless* the patient has previously (when he had decision-making capacity) spoken for himself.

III. To make the patient the primary focus of decisions concerning appropriate care and treatment. The decision to initiate or withhold or withdraw treatment shall be based upon the patient's desires implemented in a manner consistent with this policy. When a patient lacks decision making capacity, the patient shall still be the primary focus of decisions made by the person speaking for the patient concerning appropriate care and treatment. Any decision to initiate, withhold or withdraw in this latter circumstance shall include an effort to determine the patient's desire through consideration of prior

G. DO NOT RESUSCITATE AND TREATMENT OF CRITICALLY ILL PATIENT PROCESS (continued)

statements by the patient, the patient's ethical, religious and moral beliefs and patient's values.

IV. To share with the patient's family (unless the patient objects), as well as with the principal members of the treatment team, the reasoning behind significant treatment decisions.

PROCEDURE

I. General Responsibilities of Physician and Nursing Staff

A. When difficult treatment decisions are anticipated, it is the responsibility of both physicians and nurses to communicate fully with each other, with the patient, and also (given patient consent) with the patient's family/guardian. The basic policy to be followed is outlined in the following statement.

It is especially important in managing critically ill patients that the patients themselves, patients' families, and all the members of the health care staff be appraised of the goals of management of these patients who are critically ill and in whom death is not entirely unexpected. Even though mechanical resuscitative efforts and other therapeutic measures might not be appropriate, total care effort from the point of view of family, physician, nurses, and other members of the staff needs to be continued and accelerated where appropriate in order that the feeling of abandonment in patients and their families be avoided.

Conservative management of critically ill patients will include special attention to patient's needs for relief of pain, relief of anxiety, and any other relief of bodily discomforts that may arise. Supportive care from all members of the health care team including the physicians, students, nurses, and others attending to the patient is critically

G. DO NOT RESUSCITATE AND TREATMENT OF CRITICALLY ILL PATIENT PROCESS (continued)

important. Detailed communications with members of the patient's family regarding expectation of relief of discomfort, and duration of life are part of the supportive process. Enteral or parenteral nutrition and/or fluids and the use of antibiotics where there is fever or obvious infection are not necessarily part of every patient's program of management. (EXCEPTION: State and federal laws must be followed with respect to any withholding or withdrawal of treatment from infants. State law requires nutrition, hydration and medication to be continued in most circumtances.) Oral pharyngeal suction in an effort to improve the patient's comfort and nasogastric suction to decrease abdominal distention and distress may be used as deemed necessary. Cardiopulmonary resuscitative efforts in these cases will not be used. Under special sets of circumstances on prior agreement with the patient and/or members of the family, vasopressors, cardiac arrhythmic drugs and external ventilatory support may be considered.

B. If it becomes apparent that certain relevant therapeutic measures might better be withheld or withdrawn, the patient and/or the patient's family/guardian are to be consulted in such a way as to gain their understanding and agreement with a reasonable treatment plan. The physician's documentation of that discussion (along with other recent records) must support the proposed course of action. Persistent disagreement over the course of treatment should be handled by initiation of the procedures outlined elsewhere in this policy.

Note: An order to withhold or to withdraw particular treatment measures *is not* to be taken as an order to diminish other medical and nursing care appropriate to the patient. The responsible physician and the head nurse are to ensure that the physical and emotional needs of the patient continue to be addressed effectively, and that the patient's family/guardian is aware of that ongoing commitment.

G. DO NOT RESUSCITATE AND TREATMENT OF CRITICALLY ILL PATIENT PROCESS (continued)

C. If agreement is reached to withhold or withdraw cardio-pulmonary life support, appropriate orders must be written. *Full cardiopulmonary resuscitation will always be initiated unless there are written orders* by the responsible resident or attending physician specifically describing desired treatment as well as treatment limitations. *Verbal (oral) orders to withhold or withdraw cardiopulmonary life support will NOT be honored* (unless given at the patient's bedside at the time of an arrest).

Operational Policy Statement

If conservative management is to be utilized, a specific statement in the orders should be placed stating: "Conservative management of the critically ill will be utilized in this patient."

A check list of what procedures and/or support measures are to be and not to be utilized will be placed in the chart and cleared by the appropriate attending physician.

D. When an order to initiate conservative management is written, the corresponding Progress Note must contain documentation of the discussion with, and agreement of, the patient and/or the patient's family/guardian.

If that order is written by a resident physician, it must also document the attending physician's knowledge about, and agreement with, the decision.

E. To remain in effect, all orders to withhold or withdraw cardiopulmonary life support must be reviewed daily. If still appropriate, they must be reaffirmed with a progress note supporting that conclusion.

F. Existing orders to withhold full cardiopulmonary resuscitation from a patient must be carefully reviewed with any

G. DO NOT RESUSCITATE AND TREATMENT OF CRITICALLY ILL PATIENT PROCESS (continued)

physicians who are requested to perform or assist with procedures on that patient. Agreement must be reached among all responsible physicians on appropriate action should the patient arrest during the procedure.

II. Patients with Decision-Making Capacity

A. An adult patient with the mental and emotional capacity to make decisions concerning his treatment may always request that medically recommended care and treatment, *including measures believed necessary to preserve life*, be withheld or withdrawn. When that occurs, the responsible physician, along with other appropriate pesonnel, must thoroughly explore that request with the patient. The exploration should include a careful assessment of the patient's mental status (utilizing psychiatric consultation as necessary) and the consistency of his request with the values expressed in other decisions in his life. It must also include a clear description of the possible consequences of making this particular choice.

B. If the patient appears to be making a choice that is *not* substantially influenced by mental illness, temporary stress or anxiety, and if the patient remains firm in his decision, the physician is legally required to respect it. If, however, the exploration raises significant questions about the stability of the patient's expressed motivations and desires, and the decision poses a serious threat to the patient's well-being (or fetal/dependent minor well-being), Patient Relations or Risk Management must be consulted before a course of action is chosen.

C. In all cases where the patient's decision poses a serious threat to his well-being, before writing any necessary orders, the responsible physician will document:

1. The patient's desires.

G. DO NOT RESUSCITATE AND TREATMENT OF CRITICALLY ILL PATIENT PROCESS (continued)

2. Disclosure of the risks, benefits and possible alternatives.

3. Evidence concerning the patient's comprehension.

4. Factors supporting the patient's decision-making capacity.

III. Patients Without Decision-Making Capacity

A. Adult patients without decision-making capacity have the same rights to refuse treatment as other adult patients. If the patient, before losing decision-making capacity, has clearly (and verifiably) expressed his desires regarding specific treatment measures, the patient's desires will be honored—*unless* his course has changed significantly from that foreseen at the time he expressed those desires.

1. Evidence of a patient's desires can consist of written or oral communications to his physician, immediate family or others close to him. Oral expressions must be substantiated by another source, and principal family members must agree that the evidence does represent the will of the patient.

2. If it can be documented that the patient's life or the course of his illness has changed significantly from that foreseen at the time the patient expressed his desires, or if there is suspicion/disagreement about the reliability of the presented evidence, the person speaking for the patient while he lacks decision-making capacity will make the decision.

H. IN THE MATTER OF KAREN QUINLAN, AN ALLEGED INCOMPETENT [THE SUPREME COURT OF NEW JERSEY, 1976]

CONSTITUTIONAL AND LEGAL ISSUES

I. The Free Exercise of Religion

Simply stated, the right to religious beliefs is absolute but conduct in pursuance thereof is not wholly immune from governmental restraint. So it is that, for the sake of life, courts sometimes (but not always) order blood transfusions for Jehovah's Witnesses (whose religious beliefs abhor such procedure), forbid exposure to death from handling virulent snakes or ingesting poison (interfering with deeply held religious sentiments in such regard), and protect the public health as in the case of compulsory vaccination (over the strongest of religious objections).... The Public interest is thus considered paramount, without essential dissolution of respect for religious beliefs.

We think, without further examples, that, ranged against the State's interest in the preservation of life, the impingement of religious belief, much less religious "neutrality" as here, does not reflect a constitutional question, in the circumstances at least of the case presently before the Court. Moreover, like the trial court, we do not recognize an independent parental right of religious freedom to support the relief requested.

II. Cruel and Unusual Punishment

Similarly inapplicable to the case before us is the Constitution's Eighth Amendment protection against cruel and unusual punishment which, as held by the trial court, is not relevant to situations other than the imposition of penal sanctions. Historic in nature, it stemmed from punitive excesses in the infliction of criminal penalties. We find no precedent in law which would justify its extension to the correction of social injustice or hardship, such as, for instance, in the case of poverty. The latter often condemns the poor and deprived to horrendous living conditions which could certainly be described in the abstract as "cruel and unusual punishment." Yet the constitutional base of protection from "cruel and unusual punishment" is plainly irrelevant to such societal ills which must be remedied, if at all, under other concepts of constitutional and civil right.

So it is in the case of the unfortunate Karen Quinlan. Neither the State, nor the law, but the accident of fate and nature, has inflicted upon her conditions which though in essence cruel and most unusual, yet do not amount to "punishment" in any constitutional sense.

Neither the judgment of the court below, nor the medical decision which confronted it, nor the law and equity perceptions which impelled its action, nor the whole factual base upon which it was predicated, inflicted "cruel and unusual punishment" in the constitutional sense.

III. The Right of Privacy

It is the issue of the constitutional right of privacy that has given us most concern, in the exceptional circumstances of this case. Here a loving parent, *qua* parent and raising the rights of his incompetent and profoundly damaged daughter, probably irreversibly doomed to no more than a biologically vegetative remnant of life, is before the court. He seeks authorization to abandon specialized technological procedures which can only maintain for a time a body having no potential for resumption or continuance of other than a "vegetative" existence.

We have no doubt, in these unhappy circumstances, that if Karen were herself miraculously lucid for an interval (not altering the existing prognosis of the condition to which she would soon return) and perceptive of her irreversible condition, she could effectively decide upon discontinuance of the life-support apparatus, even if it meant the prospect of natural death. To this extent we may distinguish [a case] which concerned a severely injured young woman (Delores Heston), whose life depended on surgery and blood transfusion; and who was in such extreme shock that she was unable to express an informed choice (although the Court apparently considered the case as if the patient's own religious decision to resist transfusion were at stake), but most importantly a patient apparently salvable to long life and vibrant health;—a situation not at all like the present case.

We have no hesitancy in deciding, in the instant diametrically opposite case, that no external compelling interest of the State could compel Karen to endure the unendurable, only to vegetate a few measurable months with no realistic possibility of returning to any semblance of cognitive or sapient life. We perceive no thread of logic distinguishing between such a choice on Karen's part and a similar choice which, under the evidence in this case, could be made by a competent patient terminally ill, riddled by cancer and suffering great pain; such a patient would not be resuscitated or put on a respirator in the example described by Dr. Korein, and *a fortiori* would not be kept *against his will* on a respirator.

Although the Constitution does not explicitly mention a right of privacy, Supreme Court decisions have recognized that a right of personal privacy exists and that certain areas of privacy are guaranteed under the Constitution. The Court has interdicted judicial intrusion into many aspects of personal decision, sometimes basing this restraint upon the conception of a limitation of judicial interest and responsibility, such as with regard to contraception and its relationship to family life and decision.

The Court in *Griswold* found the unwritten constitutional right of privacy to exist in the penumbra of specific guarantees of the Bill of Rights "formed by emanations from those guarantees that help give them life and substance." Presumably this right is broad enough to encompass a patient's decision to decline medical treatment under certain circumstances, in much the same way as it is broad enough to encompass a woman's decision to terminate pregnancy under certain conditions.

The claimed interests of the State in this case are essentially the preservation and sanctity of human life and defense to the right of the physician to administer medical treatment according to his best judgment. In this case the doctors say that removing Karen from the respirator will conflict with their professional judgment. The plaintiff answers that Karen's present treatment serves only a maintenance function; that the respirator cannot cure or improve her condition but at best can only prolong her inevitable slow deterioration and death; and that the interests of the patient, as seen by her surrogate, the guardian, must be evaluated by the court as predominant, even in the face of an option *contra* by the present attending physicians. Plaintiff's distinction is significant. The nature of Karen's care and the realistic chances of her recovery are quite unlike those of the patients discussed in many of the cases where treatments were ordered. In many of those cases the medical procedure required (usually a transfusion) constituted a minimal bodily invasion and the chances of recovery and return to functioning life were very good. We think that the State's interest *contra* weakens and the individual's right to privacy grows as the degree of bodily invasion increases and the prognosis dims. Ultimately there comes a point at which the individual's rights overcome the State interest. It is for that reason that we believe Karen's choice, if she were competent to make it, would be vindicated by the law. Her prognosis is extremely poor, — she will never resume cognitive life. And the bodily invasion is very great, — she requires 24-hour intensive nursing care, antibiotics, and the assistance of a respirator, a catheter and feeding tube.

Our affirmance of Karen's independent right of choice, however, would ordinarily be based upon her competency to assert it. The sad truth, however, is that she is grossly incompetent and we cannot discern her supposed choice based on the testimony of her previous conversation with friends, where such testimony is without sufficient probative weight. Nevertheless we have concluded that Karen's right of privacy may be asserted on her behalf by her guardian under the peculiar circumstances here present.

If a putative decision by Karen to permit this non-cognitive, vegetative existence to terminate by natural forces is regarded as a valuable incident of her right of privacy, as we believe it to be, then it should not be discarded solely on the basis that her condition prevents her conscious exercise of the choice. The only practical way to prevent destruction of the right is to permit the guardian and family of Karen to render their best judgment, subject to the qualifications hereinafter stated, as to whether she would exercise it in these circumstances. If their conclusion is in the affirmative this decision should be accepted by a society the overwhelming majority of whose members would, we think, in similar circumstances, exercise such a choice in the same way for themselves or for those closest to them. It is for this reason that we determine that Karen's right of privacy may be asserted in her behalf, in this respect, by her guardian and family under the particular circumstances presented by this record . . .

DECLARATORY RELIEF

We thus arrive at the formulation of the declaratory relief which we have concluded is appropriate to this case. Some time has passed since Karen's physical and mental condition was described to the Court. At that time her continuing deterioration was plainly projected. Since the record has not been expanded we assume that she is now even more fragile and nearer to death than she was then. Since her present treating physicians may give reconsideration to her present posture in the light of this opinion, and since we are transferring to the plaintiff as guardian the choice of the attending physician and therefore other physicians may be in charge of the case who may take a different view from that of the present attending physicians, we herewith declare the following affirmative relief on behalf of the plaintiff. Upon the concurrence of the guardian and family of Karen, should the responsible attending physicians conclude that there is no reasonable possibility of Karen's ever emerging from her present comatose condition to a cognitive, sapient state and that the life-support apparatus now being administered to Karen should be discontinued, they shall consult with the hospital "Ethics Committee" or like body of the institution in which Karen is then hospitalized. If that consultative body agrees that there is no reasonable possibility of Karen's ever emerging from her present comatose condition to a cognitive, sapient state, the present life-support system may be withdrawn and said action shall be without any civil or criminal liability therefor on the part of any participant, whether guardian, physician, hospital or others. We herewith specifically so hold.

I. CRUZAN V. DIRECTOR, MISSOURI DEPARTMENT OF HEALTH [U.S. Supreme Court, 1990]

Petitioner Nancy Cruzan is incompetent, having sustained severe injuries in an automobile accident, and now lies in a Missouri state hospital in what is referred to as a persistent vegetative state: generally, a condition in which a person exhibits motor reflexes but evinces no indications of significant cognitive function. The State is bearing the cost of her care. Hospital employees refused, without court approval, to honor the request of Cruzan's parents, co-petitioners here, to terminate her artificial nutrition and hydration, since that would result in death. A state trial court authorized the termination, finding that a person in Cruzan's condition has a fundamental right under the State and Federal Constitutions to direct or refuse the withdrawl of death-prolonging procedures, and that Cruzan's expression to a former housemate that she would not wish to continue her life if sick or injured unless she could live at least halfway normally suggested that she would not wish to continue on with her nutrition and hydration. The State Supreme Court reversed. While recognizing a right to refuse treatment embodied in the common-law doctrine of informed consent, the court questioned its applicability in this case. It also declined to read into the State Constitution a broad right to privacy that would support an unrestricted right to refuse treatment and expressed doubt that the Federal Constitution embodied such a right. The court then decided that the State Living Will statute embodied a state policy strongly favoring the preservation of life, and that Cruzan's statements to her housemate were unreliable for the purpose of determining her intent. It rejected the argument that her parents were entitled to order the termination of her medical treatment, concluding that no person can assume that choice for an incompetent in the absence of the formalities required by the Living Will statute or clear and convincing evidence of the patient's wishes.

Held:

1. The United States Constitution does not forbid Missouri to require that evidence of an incompetent's wishes as to the withdrawal of life-sustaining treatment be proved by clear and convincing evidence.

(a) Most state courts have based a right to refuse treatment on the common-law right to informed consent, see, *e.g., In re Storar*, 52

N.Y.2d 363, 438 N.Y.S.2d 266, 420 N.E.2d 64, or on both that right and a constitutional privacy right, see, *e.g., Superintendent of Belchertown State School v. Saikewicz*, 373 Mass. 728, 370 N.E.2d 417. In addition to relying on state constitutions and the common law, state courts have also turned to state statutes for guidance, see, *e.g., Conservatorship of Drabick*, 200 Cal.App.3d 185, 245 Cal.Rptr. 810. However, these sources are not available to this Court, where the question is simply whether the Federal Constitution prohibits Missouri from choosing the rule of law which it did.

(b) A competent person has a liberty interest under the Due Process Clause in refusing unwanted medical treatment. Cf., *e.g., Jacobson v. Massachusetts*, 197 U.S. 11, 24–30, 25 S.Ct. 358, 360–363, 49 L.Ed. 643. However, the question whether that constitutional right has been violated must be determined by balancing the liberty interest against relevant state interests. For purposes of this case, it is assumed that a competent person would have a constitutionally protected right to refuse lifesaving hydration and nutrition. This does not mean that an incompetent person should possess the same right, since such a person is unable to make an informed and voluntary choice to exercise that hypothetical right or any other right. While Missouri has in effect recognized that under certain circumstances a surrogate may act for the patient in electing to withdraw hydration and nutrition and thus cause death, it has established a procedural safeguard to assure that the surrogate's action conforms as best it may to the wishes expressed by the patient while competent.

(c) It is permissible for Missouri, in its proceedings, to apply a clear and convincing evidence standard, which is an appropriate standard when the individual interests at stake are both particularly important and more substantial than mere loss of money, *Santosky v. Kramer*, 455 U.S. 745, 756, 102 S.Ct. 1388, 1396, 71 L.Ed.2d 599. Here, Missouri has a general interest in the protection and preservation of human life, as well as other, more particular interests, at stake. It may legitimately seek to safeguard the personal element of an individual's choice between life and death. The State is also entitled to guard against potential abuses by surrogates who may not act to protect the patient. Similarly, it is entitled to consider that a judicial proceeding regarding an incompetent's wishes may not be adversarial, with the added guarantee of accurate factfinding that the adversary process brings with it. The State may also properly decline to make judgments about the "quality" of a particular individual's life and simply assert an unqualified interest in the preservation of human life to be weighed against the constitutionally protected interests of the individual. It is self-evident that these interests are more substantial, both on an individual and societal level, than those involved in a common civil dispute. The clear and convincing evidence standard also serves as a societal judgment about how the risk of error should be distributed between the litigants. Missouri may permissibly place the increased risk of an erroneous decision on those seeking to terminate life-sustaining treatment. An erroneous decision not to terminate results in a maintenance of the status quo, with at least the potential that a wrong decision will eventually be corrected or its impact mitigated by an event such as an advancement in medical science or the patient's unexpected death. However, an erroenous decision to withdraw such treatment is not susceptible of correction. Although Missouri's proof requirement may have frustrated the effectuation of Cruzan's not-fully-expressed desires, the Constitution does not require general rules to work flawlessly.

2. The State Supreme Court did not commit constitutional error in concluding that the evidence adduced at trial did not amount to clear and convincing proof of Cruzan's desire to have hydration and nutrition withdrawn. The trial court had not adopted a clear and convincing evidence standard, and Cruzan's observations that she did not want to live life as a "vegetable" did not deal in terms with withdrawal of medical treatment or of hydration and nutrition.

3. The Due Process Clause does not require a State to accept the "substituted judgment" of close family members in the absence of substantial proof that their views reflect the patient's. This Court's decision upholding a State's favored treatment of traditional family relationships, *Michael H. v. Gerald D.*, 491 U.S.——, 110. S.Ct. 22, 106 L.Ed.2d 634, may not be turned into a constitutional requirement that a State must recognize the primacy of these relationships in a situation like this. Nor may a decision upholding a State's right to permit family decisionmaking, *Parham v. J.R.*, 442 U.S. 584, 99 S.Ct. 2493, 61 L.Ed.2d 101, be turned into a constitutional requirement that the State recognize such decisionmaking. Nancy Cruzan's parents would surely be qualified to exercise such a right of "substituted judgment" were it required by the Constitution. However, for the same reasons that Missouri may require clear and convincing evidence of a patient's wishes, it may also choose to defer only to those wishes rather than confide the decision to close family members.

760 S.W.2d 408, affirmed.

REHNQUIST, C.J., delivered the opinion of the Court, in which WHITE, O'CONNOR, SCALIA, and KENNEDY, JJ., joined. O'CONNOR, J., and SCALIA, J., filed concurring opinions. BRENNAN, J., filed a dissenting opinion, in which MARSHALL and BLACKMUN, JJ., joined. STEVENS, J., filed a dissenting opinion.

Index